The Pathophysiology of Human Immunologic Disorders

The Pathophysiology of Human Immunologic Disorders

Edited by

Jeremiah John Twomey
M.B. (NUI), F.A.C.P.

Professor of Medicine
Baylor College of Medicine
and
Director, Immunohematology Research
Veterans Administration Medical Center
Houston, Texas

Urban & Schwarzenberg
Baltimore-Munich 1982

Urban & Schwarzenberg, Inc.
7 E. Redwood Street
Baltimore, Maryland 21202
USA

Urban & Schwarzenberg
Pettenkoferstrasse 18
D–8000 München 2
West Germany

Printed in the United States of America

NOTICES

The Editors (or Author(s)) and the Publisher of this work have made every effort to ensure that the drug dosage schedules herein are accurate and in accord with the standards accepted at the time of publication. The reader is strongly advised, however, to check the product information sheet included in the package of each drug he or she plans to administer to be certain that changes have not been made in the recommended dose or in the contraindications for administration.

The Publishers have made an extensive effort to trace original copyright holders for permission to use borrowed material. If any have been overlooked, it will be corrected at the first reprint.

Library of Congress Cataloging in Publication Data

The Pathophysiology of human immunologic disorders.

Includes index.
Contents: Human T cell differentiation/Leonard Chess and Yolene Thomas—Disorders of B lymphocytes/Alexander R. Lawton—Disorders of macrophages/Jeremiah J. Twomey—[etc.]
1. Immunopathology. I. Twomey, Jeremiah John, 1934- [DNLM: 1. Immunologic diseases—Physiopathology. WD 200 P297]
RC582.15.P37 1982 616.07'9 82-8672
ISBN 0-8067-1921-4 AACR2

Cover design: Roger MacLellan
Compositor: Brushwood Graphics
Printer: Port City Press
Manuscript editor: Susan Lohmeyer
Indexer: Robert Rosenberg
Production and design: John Cronin

ISBN 0-8067-1921-4 Baltimore

ISBN 3-541-71921-4 Munich

Dedicated to my father
Daniel J. Twomey, M.B. (NUI)
(1898-1971)

Contents

Contributors

Leonard Chess, M.D.
Associate Professor of Medicine
Director, Division of Rheumatology
College of Physicians and Surgeons
Columbia University
New York, New York 10032

Edgar G. Engleman, M.D.
Assistant Professor of Pathology
and Medicine
Stanford University School of Medicine
Stanford, California 94305

Richard J. Ford, M.D., Ph.D.
Department of Anatomic Pathology
M.D. Anderson Hospital
and Tumor Institute
Houston, Texas 77030

H. Hugh Fudenberg, M.D.
Professor and Chairman
Department of Basic and Clinical
Immunology and Microbiology
Medical University of South Carolina
Charleston, South Carolina 29425

Ronald B. Herberman, M.D.
Laboratory of Immunodiagnosis
National Cancer Institute
Bethesda, Maryland 20205

Richard Hong, M.D.
Department of Pediatrics
Department of Medical Microbiology
University of Wisconsin
Center for Health Sciences
Madison, Wisconsin 53792

Alexander R. Lawton, M.D.
Professor of Pediatrics
Vanderbilt University
School of Medicine
Nashville, Tennesee 37232

Abby L. Maizel, M.D., Ph.D.
Department of Anatomic Pathology
M.D. Anderson Hospital
and Tumor Institute
Houston, Texas 77030

James T. Rosenbaum, M.D.
Fellow, The Arthritis Foundation
Division of Immunology
Stanford University School of Medicine
Stanford, California 94305
Visiting Associate Scientist
Kuzell Institute for Arthritis Research
Institutes of Medical Science
San Francisco, California 94115

R.D. Rossen, M.D.
Professor
Microbiology and Immunology
Internal Medicine
Baylor College of Medicine
Chief, Clinical Immunology
Veterans Administration Medical Center
Houston, Texas 77211

Gregory W. Siskind, M.D.
Department of Medicine
Cornell University Medical College
New York, New York 10021

Josef S. Smolen, M.D.
The Arthritis and Rheumatism Branch
National Institutes
of Arthritis, Metabolism,
and Digestive Diseases
Bethesda, Maryland 20205

Alfred D. Steinberg, M.D., F.A.C.P.
The Arthritis and Rheumatism Branch
National Institutes
of Arthritis, Metabolism,
and Digestive Diseases
Bethesda, Maryland 20205

Yolene Thomas, Ph.D.
Research Associate
College of Physicians and Surgeons
Columbia, University
New York, New York 10032

Jeremiah J. Twomey, M.B., F.A.C.P.
Professor of Medicine
Baylor College of Medicine
Director, Immunohematology Research
Veterans Administration Medical Center
Houston, Texas 77211

Gabriel Virella, M.D., Ph.D.
Professor
Department of Basic and Clinical
Immunology and Microbiology
Medical University of South Carolina
Charleston, South Carolina 29425

Marc E. Weksler, M.D.
Wright Professor
Department of Medicine
Cornell University Medical College
New York, New York 10021

Preface

I personally find most introductions extremely dull. Yet there they are, invariably thrust into the forefront of every textbook. They are intended to encourage you to buy the book. That seems contradictory, since something that turns you off is not likely to encourage you to read on. In your typical introduction, a few paragraphs are devoted to each chapter; they first briefly summarize the content and then tell you why you should read it. The effect is like a collection of good shirts just back in a semilyophylized state from a bad laundry. The concluding section tells of the nice things people did to help get the book out. Rather than introducing the book in such a pedantic fashion, let me tell you why I undertook this one.

In immunology, research with experimental animals has held center stage for many years. The sophistication of experimental immunology lured many young investigators and garnered prominence at scientific meetings and in the literature. This trend was also cause for concern. Would intellectual gratification take precedence over clinical urgency? Would this burgeoning mass of experimental data ever prove applicable to human systems? Would taxpayers tire of funding research that seemed preoccupied with mice, guinea pigs and chickens, rather than mankind?

While experimental immunobiology was experiencing rapid growth, clinical immunology was in a decline. Students found even the most obscure of immunologic syndromes detailed in many texts but had to turn to animal models to learn how the immune system worked. The absence of inbred human models and the red tape needed to keep human experimentation within ethical boundaries discouraged students from careers in clinical investigation. Perhaps we fell short at the bedside by not generating enough enthusiasm about important questions raised by disease.

Clinical investigation has recently picked up considerable momentum. This surge is largely due to technical developments such as the hybridoma technique for producing monoclonal antibodies and cell sorting. This new information can be readily applied to clinical settings. The similarities that are emerging between human and animal systems have clearly vindicated the basic scientist. Experience with basic immunology is suggesting new approaches to clinical problems. The leap from cage to bedside has been taken.

This recent union of basic and clinical immunology is permitting incisive research on clinical problems. Old concepts are being remolded. Ideas for new research are appearing at a remarkable rate and undoubtedly exceed the funding available to undertake many projects that would benefit humanity. It is time to pause and take stock. In effect, this book examines where we stand regarding human immunobiology and immunopathology in 1981. It is compiled in editorial style, in the hope that it will evoke ideas for further investigation while you read. That is why I undertook this book.

For those of you who do not know, compiling a textbook is a lot of work. It will not make you rich. It will not justify additional funds for your own research. Your peers will not think any more of you as an investigator after reading it. The fact is that it is a work of personal gratification. My gratification will be enhanced if you enjoy reading our book.

Nobody has the time to author a complete textbook anymore. Indeed, our interests have become so focused that there are few scientists with the range of information that would justify complete authorship. Nowadays you edit a book and call upon colleagues to "contribute" chapters. This is where the trouble begins. Initial enthusiasm is replaced by exasperation with the encroachment this makes upon the contributor's time, already overcommitted. Those that are punctual remind you that their chapters are not like Bordeaux and do not improve with age while awaiting others that are tardy. Most chapters are delivered to the editor with pride. You must be careful not to hurt this pride when making suggestions as to how the manuscript could be improved or made to conform with the overall style of the text.

The caliber of scientists who joined in this venture is gratifying. The literary style of conventional reviews was vetoed because compulsive overcrowding of data destroys literary composition. Yet another description of clinical syndromes was redundant. Basic experimental immunobiology could only serve as background for human systems which receive unashamed priority herein. Bibliographies were to identify sources of information and not to serve as a substitute for a literature search when preparing future manuscripts. Instead, contributors to this book were asked to present their views on specific topics. That should not be cause for concern. Divergent opinion has often served as a catalyst for important research. This interest in the future is the spirit of this book.

A few comments are indicated about the spirit to whom this book is dedicated. Daniel Twomey grew up in rural Ireland during the convulsions that preceded the birth of the Republic. He practiced medicine in this countryside for 30 years. There is no record of the many textbooks and medical journals he read by candlelight during those years. He would not take vacations in case ''somebody might get sick'' while he was away. He was humble enough to attend the funerals of deceased patients, but too proud to attend if the family had called in another general practitioner on the case! He serves as a constant reminder to me that the raison d'etre for medical research is to improve the lot of my fellow man.

JEREMIAH JOHN TWOMEY

Chapter 1

Human T Cell Differentiation

Leonard Chess and Yolene Thomas

Introduction

The induction and physiologic regulation of B cell differentiation is governed in large part by T cells and, perhaps more importantly, by interactions among T cells (Armerding and Katz, 1974; Cantor et al., 1976; Cantor and Boyse, 1977a). One of the major paradigms to emerge during the last decade is that the various homeostatic immunoregulatory functions of T cells are effected by distinct subsets of T cells that can be distinguished by cell surface differentiation antigens. Antibodies to these surface differentiation antigens are extremely useful tools in identifying and isolating these subsets. For example, the evidence for functional subsets of murine T cells came from the elegant studies by Cantor and Boyse (1977a and b) which demonstrated that genetically defined cell surface alloantigens (lyt) can be used to identify and isolate functionally distinct T cells at different stages of differentiation.

Recently, using the technique of Köhler and Milstein (1975) for the production of myeloma-lymphocyte hybrid cell lines, monoclonal antibodies reactive with human T cell surface antigens have produced. To date, the most extensive series of monoclonal antibodies which have been developed are the OKT and Leu series (Engleman et al., 1981; Evans et al., 1981; Kung et al., 1979; Ledbetter et al., 1981). For ease in discussion and data evaluation, we will largely restrict our discussion of these reagents to the OKT series of monoclonal antibodies since these have been the best characterized to date from a functional point of view. These antibodies were functionally assessed in earlier studies by Reinherz et al., (1979a and b, 1980a and b), and more recently by our laboratory and others (Biddison et al., 1981; Friedman et al., 1981; Janossy et al., 1980; Thomas et al., 1980, 1981a, b and d). The OKT3 antibody defines an antigen present on most human peripheral T cells (90 to 95%), the OKT4 antibody identifies 50 to 60% of human T cells and the OKT8 antibody identifies 30 to 40% of human peripheral T cells. Interestingly, initial studies demonstrated that the T cell marker, OKT4, is directed at T cell sets containing helper cells, while OKT8 reacts with the suppressor and cytotoxic T cell effectors. More detailed analysis of these subsets, however, has demonstrated that this preliminary subdivision represents an oversimplification of the spectrum of T cell functional diversity.

In this review, we will concentrate upon some recent developments in our understanding of the functional properties of isolated T cell subsets, with emphasis on human T cell subset interactions in the induction and homeostatic control of B cell differentiation and T cell effector function. For example, it has been shown that the generation of suppressor-effector activity in human peripheral T cells requires cooperation between two subsets of cells: one within the

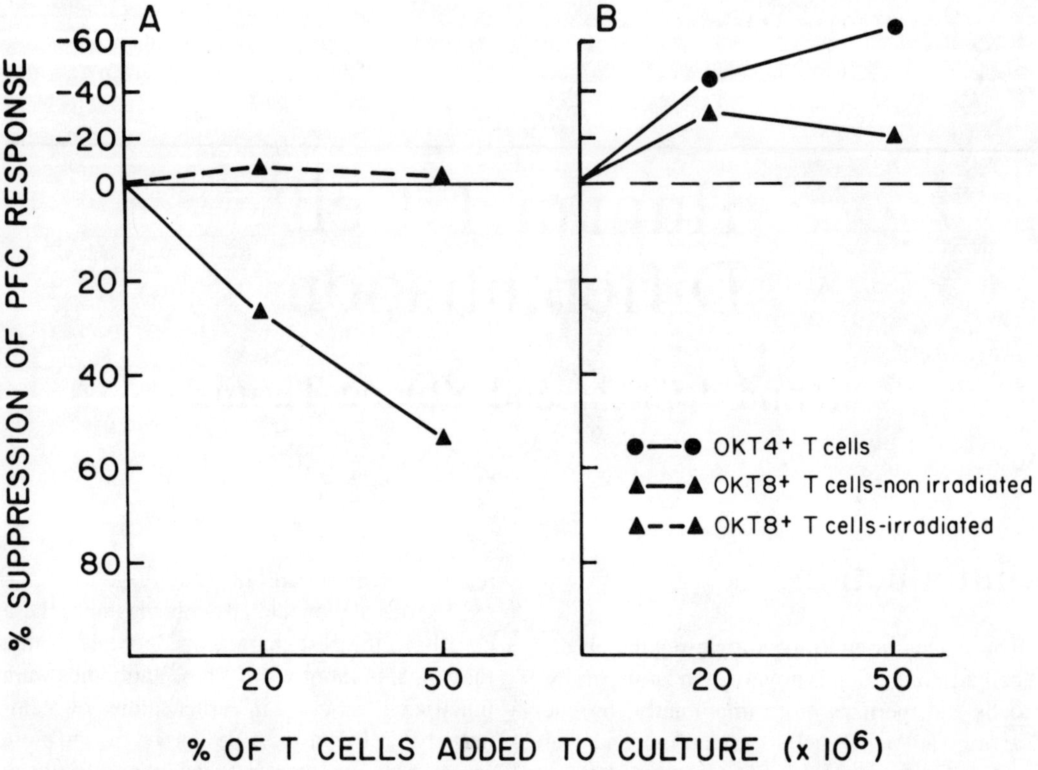

Fig. 1.1 Cooperative interaction between $OKT4^+$ and $OKT8^+$ is involved in the generation of suppressor activity. A) The standard cultures contained 0.1×10^6 $OKT4^+$ T cells and 2.0×10^6 B cells in addition to 10 μg PWM. To this system was added graded numbers of either untreated $OKT8^+$ T cells (▲——▲) or irradiated $OKT8^+$ cells (▲---▲). B) The standard cultures contained 1×10^6 irradiated $OKT4^+$ T cells and 2.0×10^6 B cells in addition to 10 μg PWM. To this system were added graded numbers of either $OKT4^+$ T cells (●——●) or $OKT8^+$ T cells (▲——▲). After 5 days, cultures were harvested and assayed for PFC activity. Suppression was calculated as follows:

$$\% \text{ Suppression} = 1 - \frac{\text{PFC (experimental culture)}}{\text{PFC (standard culture)}} \times 100$$

$OKT4^+$ population and the other within the $OKT8^+$ population. Moreover, evidence is emerging that there exists important functional heterogeneity within the $OKT4^+$ and $OKT8^+$ populations. The evidence for this heterogeneity arises from studies which have depended in part on the relative radiosensitivity of distinct immunoregulatory functions of cells contained within these sets and the use of additional monoclonal probes reactive with fractions of $OKT4^+$ and/or $OKT8^+$ cells. For instance, recent studies have revealed that the $OKT4^+$ T cell subset contains at least four distinct types of cells: radiosensitive helper cells; radioresistant helper cells; radiosensitive inducer of suppressor cells; and, after activation, radiosensitive suppressor cells. Furthermore, the radioresistant $OKT4^+$ helper cells and radiosensitive $OKT4^+$ helper cells can be identified and isolated by virtue of an additional cell surface antigen, OKT17. Since the Leu 3 monoclonal antibody identifies essentially the same subset as the OKT4 antibody, it is obvious that heterogeneity will also exist within the Leu 3^+ population. In other studies, functional microheterogeneity has been found within the $OKT8^+$ population (essentially identical in the Leu 2 population) and it has been possible to distinguish suppressor from cytotoxic cells after activation using newer monoclonal probes.

Functional Properties of Isolated Human Lymphocyte Subsets and Their Interactions

OKT8⁺ Cells Require the Cooperation of Radiosensitive OKT4⁺ Cells to Mediate Suppressor Activity

There is compelling evidence that distinct T cell subsets are involved in the regulation of B cell differentiation (Cantor et al., 1976; Gershon, 1974; Jandinski et al., 1976). However, with respect to the development of human suppressor and effector cells, the question arose whether or not obligatory interactions between different T cell subsets were required before suppressor activity could be expressed. One of the first indications that T-T interactions are essential for the development of mature suppressor T cells was reported in 1978 by Broder et al. They observed that in patients with T cell leukemias whose blast cells induced suppression of B cell differentiation the leukemic cells required radiosensitive normal T cells to induce suppression.

To formally address the possibility in normal individuals, we investigated whether OKT4⁺ cells collaborated with OKT8⁺ cells in mediating suppression in pokeweed mitogen (PWM) induced B cell differentiation. Thus, graded numbers of OKT8⁺ cells were added to cultures containing purified B cells and either nonirradiated OKT4⁺ (Figure 1.1a) or irradiated OKT4⁺ cells (Figure 1.1b). As can be seen in Figure 1.1a, only the addition of nonirradiated OKT8⁺ cells resulted in suppression of plaque-forming cell activity. In contrast (Figure 1.1b), when nonirradiated OKT8⁺ cells were added to a mixture of B cells plus irradiated OKT4⁺ cells, the suppression of immunoglobulin production did not occur. However, a complete suppressor effect was restored when small numbers of nonirradiated OKT4⁺ cells were reintroduced into the cultures (Thomas et al., 1980). It is clear, therefore, that the absence of suppression observed in the presence of irradiated OKT4⁺ cells is not due to unfavorable OKT4⁺/OKT8⁺ cell ratios. Taken together, these results demonstrate that cooperative interactions between two distinct populations of radiosensitive cells, one within the OKT4⁺ population and the other within the OKT8⁺ group, must occur before suppressor activity can be expressed. These data suggest also that OKT8⁺ do not deliver negative signals to B cells alone, independent of OKT4⁺ cells. Further evidence that OKT8⁺ cells require OKT4⁺ cells to suppress has come from experiments in which B cells triggered by helper factors in the absence of OKT4⁺ cells could not be suppressed by OKT8⁺ cells (Thomas et al., 1981d).

T Cell Subsets Involved in the Regulation of the Production (and/or Release) of MLC-Derived Helper Factor(s)

The mechanisms by which T cell subsets exert their regulatory influences on other T cell sets and B cells is only partially understood. Among these regulatory mechanisms, the release of soluble mediators which are known to play a role in T-T and T-B cooperation is of particular interest (Armerding and Katz, 1974; Geha et al., 1974; Marrack and Kappler, 1975; Pickel et al., 1976; Schimpl and Wecker, 1977). Therefore, experiments were undertaken to characterize the T cell subsets responsible for the production of helper function in response to alloantigens. Cell-free supernatants were obtained after 48 hours of culture of either unselected T cells, OKT4⁺ or OKT8⁺ cells cocultured with irradiated (2000 R) allogeneic stimulator cells. Varying dilutions of these supernatants were added to purified B cells and the induction of antibody synthesis was measured after 6 days of cell culture. The results depicted in Figure 1.2 clearly show that OKT4⁺ responder cells, but not OKT8⁺ cells, appear to be the predominant T cell subset involved in the production of allogeneic helper factor(s) that can trigger B cell differentiation.

Since, in several experiments, purified OKT4⁺ cells produced a more potent supernatant than did unselected T cells, further experiments were conducted to explore a possible negative

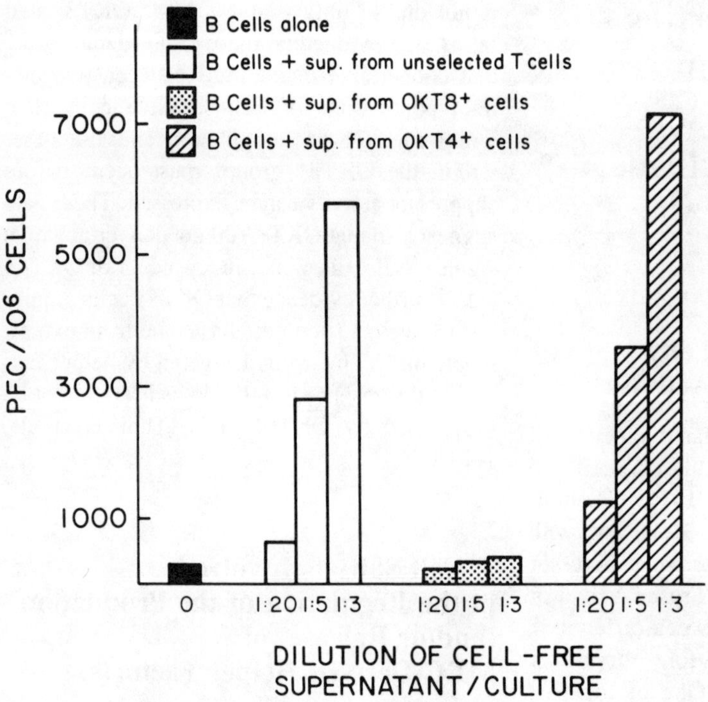

Fig. 1.2 OKT4⁺ T cells produce MLC helper factor(s) which trigger B cell differentiation. Peripheral T cells were treated with anti-OKT8 + C. Residual viable cells (2×10^6) were then cultured with 4×10^6 T cell depleted, irradiated E negative cells. In control culture, unselected T cells were treated with complement alone. After 48 hours, various concentrations of cell-free supernatants were harvested and assayed for B cell helper activity after 6 days of culture. As control for B cell purity, additional B cell cultures were supplemented with PWM.

regulatory influence of $OKT8^+$ cells in the production of helper factors. Thus, increasing numbers of $OKT4^+$ cells, $OKT8^+$ cells or irradiated $OKT8^+$ cells were added to a constant number of $OKT4^+$ cells prior to activation; subsequently, the 48-hour cell-free supernatants were assayed for B cell helper activity. As shown in Figure 1.3, addition of graded numbers of unirradiated $OKT8^+$ cells progressively decreased helper factor activity. Conversely, further addition of $OKT4^+$ cells or irradiated $OKT8^+$ cells did not decrease this activity. Thus, the modulation by $OKT8^+$ cells in the production of helper factors is not simply the result of cell crowding but, rather, is due to an active suppression of $OKT4^+$ cells by radiosensitive $OKT8^+$ cells.

Functional Heterogeneity Within the $OKT4^+$ Population

The first evidence of functional heterogeneity of the $OKT4^+$ population was shown in studies of the regulation of B cell immunoglobulin production by the $OKT4^+$ subset (Thomas et al., 1980). For example, addition of graded numbers of radiosensitive $OKT4^+$ cells to B cells did not result in a linear increase of plaque-forming cells (which would be predicted if the $OKT4^+$ were exclusively inducer cells). Instead, decrease of the net helper activity was observed. Because of this observation, it was proposed that suppressor cells may be generated from precursors within the $OKT4^+$ population alone.

To address this possibility, we investigated whether $OKT4^+$ cells were able to suppress B cell differentiation independent of $OKT8^+$ cells after in vitro pokeweed mitogen activation. Thus, graded numbers of activated $OKT4^+$ cells were added to secondary cultures containing B cells and either nonirradiated fresh $OKT4^+$ cells (Table 1.1, part A) or irradiated fresh $OKT4^+$ cells (Table 1.1, part B). As shown in Table 1.1, part A, addition of activated $OKT4^+$ cells to cultures containing nonirradiated fresh $OKT4^+$ cells resulted in a reduction of the plaque-forming cell response. By contrast, addition of identical populations of activated $OKT4^+$ cells to cultures containing irradiated fresh $OKT4^+$ cells failed to decrease the plaque-forming cell response (Table 1.1, part B). However, addition of a small percentage of nonirradiated fresh

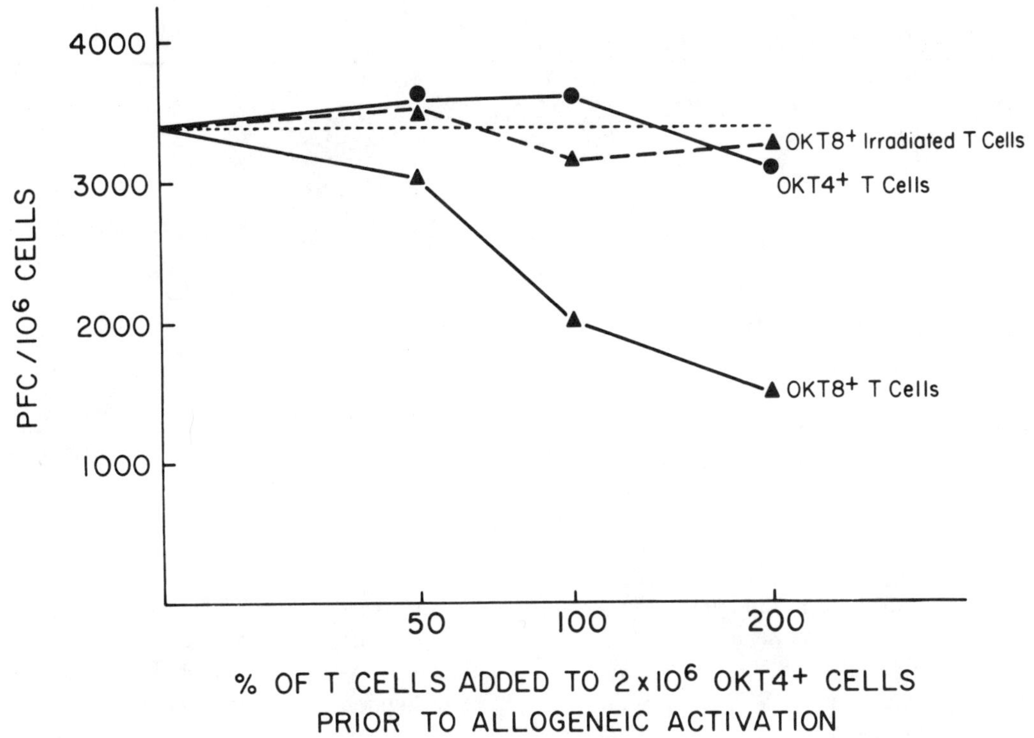

Fig. 1.3 Radiosensitive OKT8⁺ cells regulate the production of MLC-derived helper factor(s); 2×10^6 OKT4⁺ cells were cultured in the presence of graded numbers of either OKT4⁺ cells (●——●), OKT8⁺ cells (▲——▲) or irradiated (1250 R) OTK8⁺ cells (▲---▲) prior to allogeneic activation. After 48 hours of culture, cell-free supernatants were harvested and then added at a final concentration of 33% to cultures of highly purified B cells. Each culture was assayed for PFC activity after 6 days of culture.

OKT4⁺ cells (0.1×10^6) allowed for re-expression of suppression (Table 1.1, part C). These data strongly support the idea that suppression can be generated by polyclonal activation of the OKT4⁺ subset. It should be noted that suppression induced by activated OKT4⁺ cells is not secondary to the emergence of OKT8⁺ cells in culture because: each population after activation maintained the original OKT3⁺, OKT4⁺, OKT8⁻ surface phenotype when reanalyzed by immunoflourescence on the Cytoflurograf; and when activated OKT4⁺ cells were treated with OKT4 or OKT8 in the presence of C′, only OKT8-treated (but not OKT4-treated) cells maintained their capacity to suppress B cells plus fresh OKT4⁺ cells. We emphasize, however, that although activated OKT4⁺ can exert potent feedback suppression, they can also function as helper cells in inducing B cell differentiation.

Further Dissection of the Functional Heterogeneity Within the OKT4⁺ and OKT8⁺ Populations by Additional Monoclonal Antibodies

Additional insight into the heterogeneity of OKT4⁺ T cell function has been developed from studies using an additional monoclonal antibody, OKT17, reactive with a fraction of activated OKT4⁺ cells (Thomas et al., 1981b). This antibody recognizes a cell surface antigen present on the majority of thymocytes and resting normal peripheral T cells. In contrast, OKT17 is unreactive with normal B cells, B cell lines, T cell lines or SIg⁺CLL. Moreover, this monoclonal antibody is unreactive with null cells or macrophages. These observations demonstrate that OKT17 identifies a cell surface differentiation antigen unique to T cells. Interestingly,

Table 1.1 Suppression Mediated by Activated OKT4$^+$ Cells Requires the Presence of Radiosensitive Cells Within the Resting OKT4$^+$ Population

Numbers of Fresh OKT4$^+$ Cells Present in the Secondary Culture[a]	Activated OKT4$^+$ Cells (First Culture) Added	PFC/10^6 Cells	Suppression (%)[b]
A. 0.1 × 10^6 non-irradiated	0	13.890 ± 1800	0
	0.2 × 10^6	8.100 ± 420	42
	0.4 × 10^6	7.500 ± 750	47
	1.0 × 10^6	5.190 ± 900	63
B. 1 × 10^6 irradiated	0	8.640 ± 608	0
	0.2 × 10^6	18.450 ± 2404	0
	0.4 × 10^6	12.600 ± 180	0
	1.0 × 10^6	8.310 ± 180	4
C. 1 × 10^6 irradiated + 0.1 × 10^6 non-irradiated	0	19.880 ± 300	0
	0.2 × 10^6	15.240 ± 1780	24
	0.4 × 10^6	9.440 ± 1321	53
	1.0 × 10^6	6.960 ± 600	65

[a] For 5 days, 2.0 × 10^6 fresh B cells were cultured in the presence of 10 μ_g of PWM. To these cultures various numbers of fresh OKT4$^+$ and activated OKT4$^+$ cells (first culture) were added.

[b] Suppression percentage was calculated as before (Fig. 1.1).

following activation, the antigen recognized by OKT17 is lost from a subset of OKT4$^+$ cells, but not from activated OKT8$^+$ cells. Thus, we investigated whether the OKT17 could serve as a marker to further dissect the functional heterogeneity within the OKT4$^+$ population. Graded numbers of activated unselected OKT4$^+$ cells as well as activated OKT4$^+$17$^+$ cells or OKT4$^+$17$^-$ were added to secondary autologous cultures containing B cells plus fresh OKT4$^+$ cells in the presence of PWM (Figure 1.4). Consistent with previous studies, activated unselected OKT4$^+$ cells suppressed B cell differentiation. The addition of small numbers of activated OKT4$^+$17$^+$ cells also suppressed B cell immunoglobulin production. In marked contrast, OKT4$^+$17$^-$ cells had minimal inhibitory activity. Thus, these data suggest that the suppressor cells within the activated OKT4$^+$ cells are restricted to a distinct subset of OKT4$^+$ cells bearing the OKT17 marker.

Although activated OKT4$^+$ cells can exert potent feedback suppression, activated OKT4$^+$ cells also contain helper cells. In particular, the helper function induced by activated OKT4$^+$ cells is relatively radioresistant. In contrast, the helper function mediated by fresh OKT4$^+$ cells is exquisitely radiosensitive over a wide range of T cell concentrations. Irradiated, unactivated OKT4$^+$ cells only induce B cell differentiation at high ratios of T cells to B cells. Because of these observations, we proposed the possibility that radiosensitive and radioresistant helper activities represent functions of distinct T cell subsets within the OKT4$^+$ population. Recent studies provide support for the presence of both a relatively radiosensitive, as well as a radioresistant, helper OKT4$^+$ population; these differ in terms of their reactivity with OKT17 antibody. For example, activated OKT4$^+$17$^-$ helper cells are radiosensitive, whereas activated OKT4$^+$17$^+$ helper cells are radioresistant (Figure 1.5 and Thomas et al., 1981b).

As mentioned previously, the reciprocal T cell population, OKT8$^+$, does not provide helper activity but contains cytotoxic effector cells and radiosensitive cells important in the suppression of B cell differentiation. Recently, Irigoyen et al., (1981) described a monoclonal antibody, PVR 11, which reacts with CTL effector cells within the OKT8$^+$ population but is unreactive with suppressor-effector cells. This dissociation of effector-suppressor and cytotoxic effect has been confirmed by other studies (Thomas et al., 1981c) using another monoclonal antibody, OKT20. This surface antigen is present on a small percentage of resting lymphocytes but is expressed in varying proportions on activated T cells. Functional analysis of normal resting human T lymphocytes demonstrated that the OKT20-depleted T cell subset was able to generate cytotoxic cells and to suppress antibody production to the same extent that OKT8$^+$ cells did. On the other hand, when unselected T

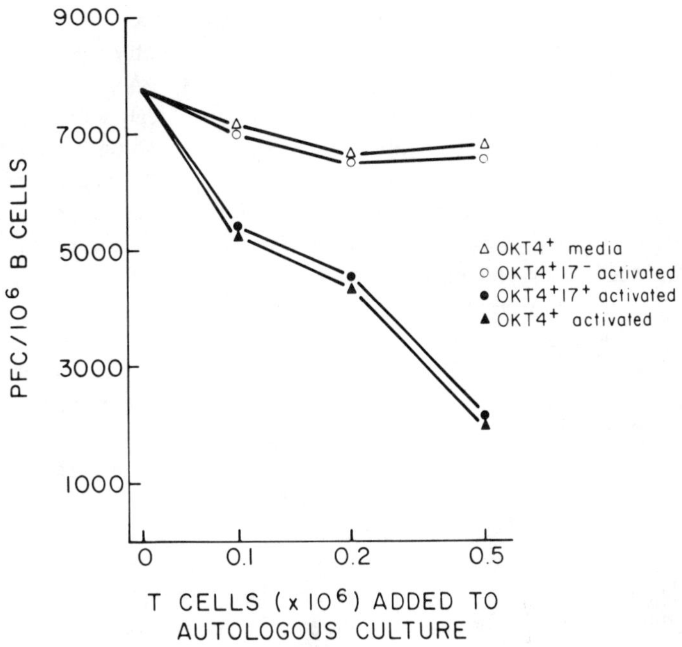

Fig. 1.4 Activated OKT4⁺17⁺ cells, but not activated OKT4⁺17⁻ cells, will suppress B cell differentiation induced by fresh OKT4⁺ cells. The standard culture contained 0.05×10^6 fresh OKT4⁺ cells and 1×10^6 B cells in addition to 10 μg of PWM. To this system were added graded numbers of either OKT4⁺ cells cultured with medium alone (Δ——Δ), OKT4⁺ cells, (▲——▲), OKT4⁺17⁻ cells (○——○) or OKT4⁺17⁺ cells (●——●) cultured with PWM during 60 to 70 hours of previous culture. After 5 days, cultures were harvested and assayed for PFC activity.

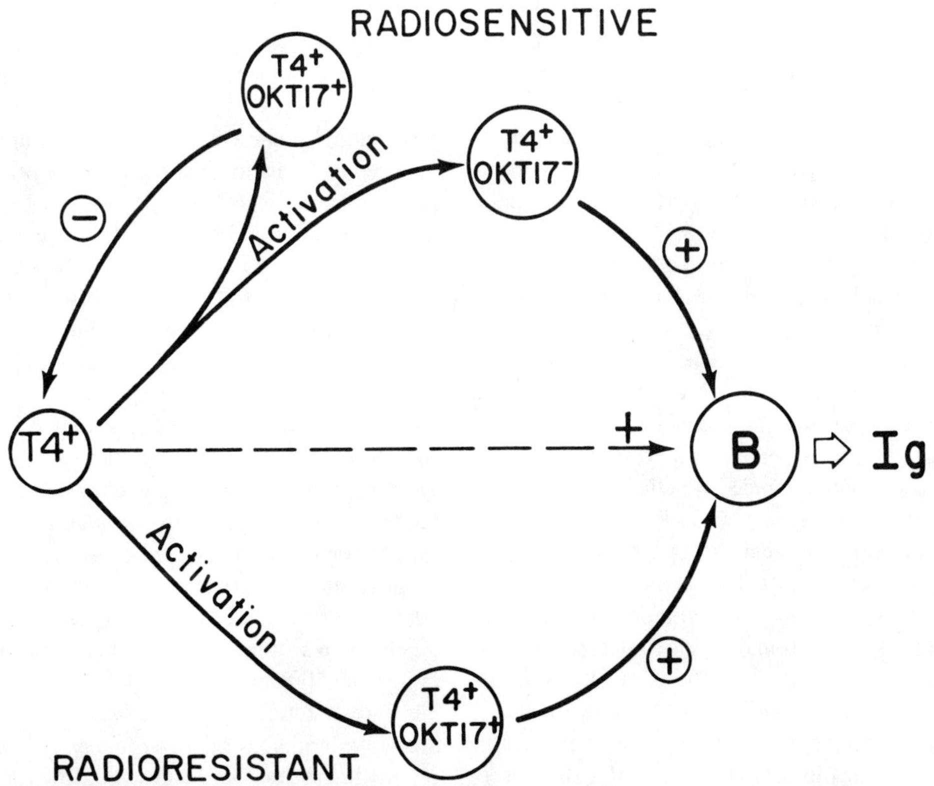

Fig. 1.5 Heterogeneity within the OKT4⁺ population.

lymphocytes were cultured for 6 days in mixed lymphocyte reaction and then depleted of OKT20 reactive cells, the cytotoxic effector T cells were eliminated. In contrast, OKT20-depleted T cells after identical activation were still able to suppress antibody production. Taken together, these data suggest that, following activation of $OKT8^+$ cells, the OKT20 differentiation antigen becomes selectively expressed on cytotoxic effectors but not on suppressor cells.

Summary

In this review we have focused on studies of the interactions of T cell subsets important in regulating human immune responses in normal individuals. These studies took advantage of the fact that, during the ontogeny of human T cells, functionally discrete subsets emerge that can be identified and isolated by virtue of distinct cell membrane differentiation antigens. These antigens, in turn, have been identified by monoclonal antibodies specifically reacting with the particular membrane differentiation antigens. Although we have presented evidence predominantly using the OKT series of antibodies, it is clear that other monoclonal antibodies identifying essentially identical populations will reveal similar functional properties. More importantly, the present data suggest that the currently available monoclonal antibody probes do not address the full range of functional subsets that exist within the human T cell peripheral pool.

In this regard, the evidence that the cell population identified by the OKT4 antibody contains at least four separable functional subsets including both helper and suppressor cells is of paramount importance. Whether these subsets contained within the OKT4 population arise from a common precursor or whether functionally distinct $OKT4^+T8^-$ cells emerge during thymic dependent differentiation is currently unknown. Additional monoclonal probes directed exclusively at fractions of $OKT4^+$ cells may allow for resolution of this problem. Until this question is resolved, the precise evolutionary relationship between human T cell subsets and murine T cell subsets will remain unclear. It is possible, for example, that contained within the $OKT4^+$ cells there exists a major precursor population analogous to the murine Lyt 1^+, 2^+, 3^+ subset which can be driven to differentiate along either helper or suppressor pathways. If such a cell exists, the current probes (OKT, Leu series, etc.) do not distinguish this population from the majority of differentiated helper cells. Thus, both helper cells and putative precursors are $OKT3^+$, $OKT4^+$, $OKT8^-$, Leu 3^+ and Leu

Despite the need for resolution of these ambiguities, the currently available monoclonal probes have been extremely useful with respect to the analysis of T-T and T-B interactions in man. The essential points to emerge so far are that suppressor cells contained within the $OKT8^+$ population require the presence of radiosensitive $OKT4^+$ cells in order for suppressor-effector function to be effected and the suppressor effects operate predominantly on $OKT4^+$ helper cells and not on B cells. In addition, it is important to emphasize that all inductive (helper) functions of human T cells are contained within the $OKT4^+$ population, although even here the evidence for microheterogeneity of $OKT4^+$ inducer cells is compelling. This evidence stems largely from dissection of the $OKT4^+$ population with the newer monoclonal probe OKT17. This latter antibody also seems to distinguish the radiosensitive and radioresistant helper cells.

The clinical significance of the current analysis of human T cell subsets is clearly worthy of comment. The bottom line probably will be that for straightforward clinical problems there will be straightforward results. Conversely, for complex problems the current probes may yield ambiguous results. An example of a relatively straightforward problem is that of acquired agammaglobulinemia, where at least one defect seems to be an excess of circulating $OKT8^+$ suppressor cells. On the other hand, complex diseases such as diffuse autoimmune states may not be readily assessed by phenotypic analysis of T cell subsets without detailed functional studies of T-T and T-B interactions. It is our optimistic view that future progress with monoclonal probes will address the heterogeneity of human T cells in greater detail and will allow for more precise analysis of human diseases.

References

Armerding, D., and Katz, D.H. 1974. Activation of T and B lymphocytes in vitro. II. Biological and biochemical properties of an allogeneic effect factor (AEF) active in triggering specific B lymphocytes. J Exp Med 140:19.

Biddison, W.E., Sharrow, S.O., and Shearer, G.M. 1981. T cell subpopulations required for the human cytotoxic T lymphocyte response to influenza virus: Evidence for T cell help. J Immunol 127(2):448.

Broder, S., Poplack, D., Whang-Peng, J., Durm, M., Goldman, C., Muul, L., and Waldmann, T.A. 1978. Characterization of a suppressor-cell leukemia. Evidence for the requirement of an interaction of two T cells in the development of human suppressor effector cells. N Engl J Med 298(2):66.

Cantor, H., and Boyse, E. 1977a. Regulation of the immune response by T cell subclasses. Contemp Top Immunobiol 7:47.

Cantor, H., and Boyse, E. 1977b. Regulation of cellular and humoral immune responses by T cell subclasses. Cold Spring Harbor Symp Quant Biol 41 Pt 1:23-32.

Cantor, H., Shen, F.W., and Boyse, E.A. 1976. Separation of helper T cells from suppressor T cells expressing different Ly components. II. Activation by antigen: After immunization, antigen-specific suppressor and helper activities are mediated by distinct T cell subclasses. J Exp Med 143(6):1391.

Engleman, E.G., Benike, C.J., Glickman, E., and Evans, R.L. 1981. Antibodies to membrane structures that distinguish suppressor/cytotoxic and the helper T lymphocyte subpopulations block the mixed leukocyte reaction in man. J Exp Med 154(1):193.

Evans, R.L., Wall, D.W., Platsouscas, C.D., Siegal, F.P., Fikrig, S.M., Testa, C.M., and Good, R.A. 1981. Thymus-dependent membrane antigens in man: Inhibition of cell-mediated lympholysis by monoclonal antibodies to TH2 antigen. Proc Natl Acad Sci USA 78(1):544.

Friedman, S.M., Hunter, S.B., Irigoyen, O., Kung, P.C., Goldstein, G., and Chess, L. 1981. Functional analysis of human T cell subsets defined by monoclonal antibodies: II. Collaborative T-T interactions in the generation of TNP-altered-self-reactive cytotoxic T lymphocytes.

Irigoyen, O.H., Rizzolo, P., Thomas, Y., Hemler, M.E., Shen, H.H., Friedman, S.M., Strominger, J.L., and Chess, L. 1981. Dissection of distinct human immunoregulatory T cell subsets by a monoclonal antibody. Recognizing a cell surface antigen with wide tissue distribution. Proc Natl Acad Sci USA 785:3160.

Geha, R.S., Schneeberger, R., Rosen, F.S., et al. 1974. Interaction of human thymus-derived and non-thymus-derived lymphocytes in vitro. Induction of proliferation and antibody synthesis in B lymphocytes by a soluble factor released from antigen-stimulated T lymphocytes. J Exp Med 138:1230.

Gershon, R.K. 1974. T cell control of antibody production. Contemp Top Immunobiol 3:1.

Jandinski, J., Cantor, H., Tadakuma, T., Peavy, D.L., and Pierce, C.W. 1976. Separation of helper T cells from suppressor T cells expressing different Ly components. I. Polyclonal activation: Suppressor and helper activities are inherent properties of distinct T cell subclasses. J Exp Med 1436:1382.

Janossy, G., Tidman, N., Selby, W.S., Thomas, J.A., Granger, S., Kung, P.C., and Goldstein, G. 1980. Human T lymphocytes of inducer and suppressor type occupy different microenvironments. Nature 288:81.

Köhler, G., and Milstein, C. 1975. Continuous cultures of fused cells secreting antibody of predefined specificity. Nature 256(5517):495.

Kung, P.C., Goldstein, G., Reinherz, E.L., and Schlossman, S.F. 1979. Monoclonal antibodies defining distinctive human T cell surface antigens. Science 206:347.

Ledbetter, J.A., Evans, R.L., Lipinski, M., Cunningham-Rundles, C., Good, R.A., and Herzenberg, L.A. 1981. Evolutionary conservation of surface molecules that distinguish T lymphocyte helper/inducer and cytotoxic/suppressor subpopulations in mouse and man. J Exp Med 153:310.

Marrack, P.C., and Kappler, J.W. 1975. Antigen-specific and nonspecific mediators of T cell/B cell cooperation. I. Evidence for their production by different T cells. J Immunol 114(3):1116.

Pickel, K., Hammerling, U., and Hoffmann, R. 1976. Ly phenotype of T cells releasing T cell replacing factor. Nature 264:72.

Reinherz, E.L., Kung, P.C., Breard, J., Goldstein, G., and Schlossman, S.F. 1980a. T cell requirements for generation of helper factor(s) in man: Analysis of the subjects involved. J Immunol 124:1883.

Reinherz, E.L., Kung, P.C., Goldstein, G., and Schlossman, S.F. 1979a. Further characterization of the human inducer T cell subset defined by monoclonal antibody. J Immunol 123(6):2894.

Reinherz, E.L., Kung, P.C., Goldstein, G., and Schlossman, S.F. 1979b. Separation of functional subsets of human T cells by a monoclonal antibody. Proc Natl Acad Sci USA 76(8):4061.

Reinherz, E.L., Kung, P.C., Goldstein, G., and Schlossman, S.F. 1980b. A monoclonal antibody reactive with the human cytotoxic/suppressor T cell subset previously defined by a heteroantiserum termed TH2. J Immunol 124:1301.

Reinherz, E.L., Kung, P.C., Pesando, J.M., Ritz, J., Goldstein, G., and Schlossman, S.F. 1979c. Ia determinants on human T cell subsets defined by monoclonal antibody. Activation stimuli required for expression. J Exp Med 150(6):1472.

Schimpl, A., and Wecker, E. 1977. Replacement of T cell function by a T cell product. Nature (New Biology) 237:15.

Thomas, Y., Rogozinski, L., Irigoyen, O., Friedman, S.M., Kung, P.C., Goldstein, G., and Chess, L. 1981a. Functional analysis of human T cell subsets derived by monoclonal antibodies. IV. Induction of suppressor cells within the OKT4⁺ population. J Exp Med 154(2):459.

Thomas, Y., Rogozinski, L., Irigoyen, O., Shen, H., Talle, M.A., Goldstein, G., and Chess, L. 1982. Functional analysis of human T cells subsets derived by monoclonal antibodies V. Suppressors cells within the activated OKT4⁺ population belong to a distinct subset. J Immulol 128(3):1386.

Thomas, Y., Rogozinski, L., Rothman, P., Goldstein, G., and Chess, L. Further dissection of the functional heterogeneity within the OKT4⁺ and OKT8⁺ human T cell subsets. J Clin Immunol. 1982 (in press).

Thomas, Y., Sosman, J., Irigoyen, O., Friedman, S.M., Kung, P.C., Goldstein, G., and Chess, L. 1980. Functional analysis of human T cell subsets defined by monoclonal antibodies. I. Collaborative T-T interactions in the immunoregulation of B cell differentiation. J Immunol 125(6):2402.

Thomas, Y., Sosman, J., Rogozinski, L., Irigoyen, O., Kung, P.C., Goldstein, G., and Chess, L. 1981d. Functional analysis of human T cell subsets defined by monoclonal antibodies. III. Regulation of helper factor production by T cell subsets. J Immunol 126:1948.

Van Wauwe, J.P., DeMey, J.R., and Goossens, J.G. 1980. OKT3: A monoclonal anti-human T lymphocyte antibody with potent mitogenetic properties. J Immunol 124(6):2708.

Chapter 2

Disorders of B Lymphocytes

Alexander R. Lawton

Introduction

Current concepts of the development and function of B lymphocytes have largely been developed, and can best be discussed, within the theoretical framework of MacFarlane Burnet's clonal selection theory (1959). Clonal selection represents a synthesis of two earlier theories concerning the genesis of antibody responses. Paul Erlich's "side-chain" theory (1900) postulated the existence of cells bearing antitoxic side chains on their surface membranes. Toxins interacting with these side chains were viewed as provoking enhanced synthesis and release of these antitoxins into the serum. In 1955, Nils Jerne proposed a revolutionary theory of antibody formation based upon principles of natural selection. In contrast to the then prevailing view that antigens somehow served as templates for directing synthesis of complementary antibodies (instructionist theories), Jerne viewed antigens as selecting, from a preformed pool of "natural" antibodies, molecules having complementary binding sites. He suggested that the immune complexes thus formed would be ingested by cells of the reticuloendothelial system and induce formation of antibodies of identical specificity. Burnet's fundamental contribution was to meld Jerne's idea of selection with Erlich's concept of cell-bound receptors by proposing that the locus of selection was a lymphocyte bearing on its membrane an antibody receptor of a unique and predetermined specificity. The entire repertoire of antibody molecules was viewed as being genetically determined and distributed among families of lymphocytes called clones. Each clone was distinguished by the identical specificity of its receptor antibodies. Antigens combined with the receptors of specific clonal precursors, triggering expansion by cell division and differentiation to plasma cells secreting antibodies identical in specificity to the cell-bound receptor. The major elements of the clonal selection theory have been amply verified for B cells, for which immunoglobulin molecules serve as the cell-bound receptors for antigen.

Current understanding of the pathogenesis of immunodeficiencies originated with the discovery in chickens (Warner et al., 1962; Cooper et al., 1966) and mice (Claman et al., 1966; Mitchell and Miller, 1968) that immunologic functions were mediated by two developmentally independent but functionally interacting cell types. These are T cells originating in the thymus and B cells developing within the avian bursa of Fabricius or the mammalian bone marrow. Cooper, Good and their colleagues (Cooper et al., 1967) were the first to recognize the pathogenetic significance of these observations in human immunodeficiencies and lymphoid malignancies. The application of these concepts in subsequent years has largely depended upon the development of the means to identify, enumerate and study the functions of lymphocytes from man and experimental animals in vitro. As it is difficult to find a better example of fruitful interplay between basic and clinical research than has occurred in the field of cellular and clinical immunology during the last decade, it seems appropriate to discuss disorders of human B cells within the broader context of knowledge of B cell development and function derived from experimental animals as well as man.

Normal B Cell Differentiation

The fundamental requirement of clonal selection is the generation of a population of lymphocytes each of which expresses a unique receptor specificity. The logic of a selective theory argues that this primary differentiation event should occur independently of environmental antigens and that the totality of clones (each defined by its receptor specificity) expresses most of the potential inherited repertoire of receptor specificities. By this argument, B cell differentiation occurs in two distinct stages. These are an antigen-independent process of clonal development and the series of proliferation and differentiation events which follow interaction of selected clones with antigens to which they have complementary receptors. The latter process of clonal selection is synonymous with an immune response. The significance of this conceptual division of B cell differentiation into discrete phases depends upon the extent of inherited (germ line) antibody diversity and on the mechanisms for creating diversity. If the germ line repertoire is small, then only a few "primary" clones need be generated. If it is large and involves complex mechanisms, the process of clonal development assumes great significance. Due to some extraordinary revelations on the structure and organization of immunoglobulin genes during the past 3 years (see Early and Hood, 1981), it is now possible to appreciate the magnitude of the differentiation problem and to sketch the outlines of how the process occurs.

Immunoglobulin Genes

Immunoglobulin molecules are encoded in three unlinked families of tandemly arranged genes. Two families specify kappa and lamda light chain genes, respectively, while the third codes for the heavy chains (μ, δ, γ, α, ξ) that determine immunoglobulin class. Three or more separate genes within a family contribute to the formation of a light or heavy polypeptide chain. The specificity-determining variable regions of light chains are encoded by genes designated by V (variable) and J (joining). For heavy chains there is an additional coding sequence: D (diversity). Genes designated C (constant) encode the carboxy-terminal end of the molecule which determines isotype (light chain type or heavy chain class) (Fig. 2.1).

The specificity of an immunoglobulin molecule for antigen depends upon the association and folding of V regions of light and heavy chains to form a cavity. The amino acid residues which form the walls of this cleft are called complementarity-determining regions. Each V gene encodes two complementarity-determining regions, while J and D genes contribute to a third. These observations clearly indicate that combinational association plays an important role in generation of antibody diversity. Since combination of one V gene with different J or D genes may produce different combining sites, the number of potential germ line specificities is the product of the numbers of each gene. Current estimates (based on studies in mice) suggest that each light chain family in humans will contain more than 100 V genes and several J genes; the heavy chain family is expected to contain similar numbers of V and J genes, respectively, and an unknown number of D genes. Since combination of different light and heavy chains may also contribute to diversity, the potential repertoire of specificities generated by all combinations of these genes should easily exceed 10^6.

The formation of functional immunoglobulin genes is accomplished by a series of translocations within each tandemly linked family. A particular light chain V gene moves from its original germ line location and is spliced to one of the several J genes. The DNA separating the two genes in the germ line is deleted by this

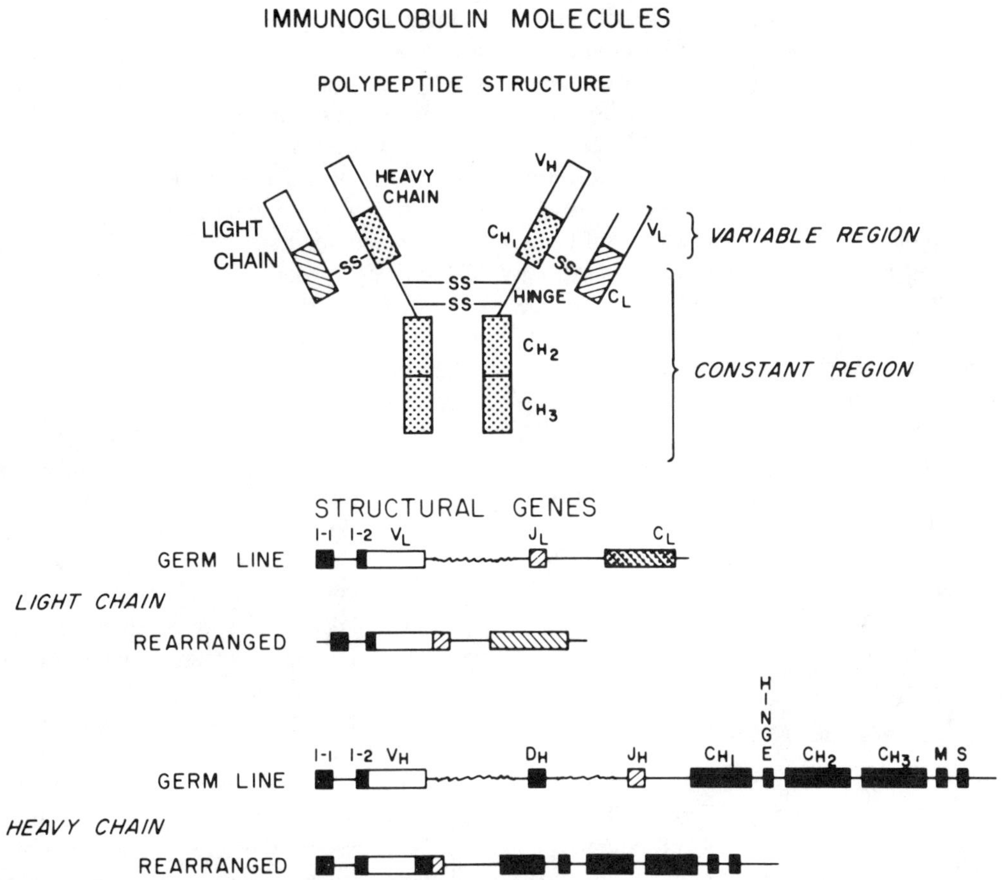

Fig. 2.1 Immunoglobulins are bilaterally symmetrical molecules made up of paired light and heavy chains joined by disulfide bonds. The amino terminal ends of each pair (V_H + V_L)form an antibody-combining site. Each polypeptide is divided into structural domains of ~110 amino acids in length, containing an internal disulfide bond. Heavy chains have a flexible hinge region separating the CH1 and CH2 domains.

The organization of the structural genes encoding each chain is shown in the bottom of the diagram. Light chain V regions are encoded by three genes. Genes designated 1-1 and 1-2 code for a hydrophobic leader sequence which initiates transport of the nascent chain across the membrane of the endoplasmic reticulum and is subsequently cleaved off. V_L codes for the first 97 amino acids and J_L codes for the remainder of the V region (98-110). During differentiation, a V_L gene is translocated and spliced to one of the J_L genes; the intervening DNA indicated by the way lines is excised.

An additional minigene, called D_H, codes a part of the sequence of the heavy chain V region. The C_H region is coded by a split gene in that each domain, including the hinge, is encoded by a separate exon. The intervening DNA separating the exons (introns, designated by solid lines) are transcribed but subsequently spliced out of the mature messenger RNA. Most, if not all, heavy chains have alternative C terminal amino acid sequences which determine whether they will be secreted or become attached to the B cell membrane. These are coded by exons designated m and s; the alternatives are selected by RNA processing. V_H, D_H and J_H genes, all at separate locations in germ line DNA, are rearranged during differentiation to form a contiguous coding sequence for the V_H region.

process. At this point messenger RNA may be transcribed which encompasses VJ, the intervening DNA sequence separating J and C and the C gene. This large mRNA is processed to remove the noncoding intron between J and C before translation into the light polypeptide chain. Formation of transcriptionally actively heavy chain genes is similar but involves more extensive rearrangements (Fig. 2.2). V and D genes are apparently spliced before translocation to one of the J genes which are located on the 5′ side of the μ gene. An additional series of translocations occurring at a later stage of B cell differentiation accounts for expression of immunoglobulin class diversity, as will be discussed in a subsequent section. "Errors" in splicing may provide additional amplification of diversity by addition or deletion of codons or by changing the reading frame.

One additional phenomenon must be introduced before attempting to integrate this genetic information with the biological aspects of B cell development. Individual B lymphocytes express only one of the two types of light chains (isotype exclusion) and only one of the homologous chromosomal segments encoding the selected light chain and heavy chain family (allelic exclusion). Repression of genetic information such that each lymphocyte expresses only a single receptor specificity is as important an element in clonal selection as the expression of most or all of the potential diversity by the entire population of clones.

Pre-B Cells and Development of Clonal Diversity

The earliest morphologically identifiable cells in the B lineage are termed pre-B cells. They were first observed in studies of B cell ontogeny in mice as medium to large lymphoid cells containing cytoplasmic μ chains but no cell surface immunoglobulin (Raff et al., 1976). Pre-B cells appeared in fetal liver several days prior to the development of the first lymphocytes bearing surface IgM receptors. In adult animals, cells with pre-B morphology are found exclusively in the bone marrow.

The biologic characteristics of pre-B cells defined by studies in mice and man suggested that these cells might function as the primary generators of clonal diversity (Cooper et al., 1977). Large pre-B cells divide very rapidly, having a mean generation time which is probably on the order of 8–12 hours. These cells express μ heavy chains but no light chains. Their progeny are smaller cells which divide at a much slower rate; some of these have begun to express light chains but still lack surface immunoglobulin. Small pre-B cells then express surface IgM receptors, probably without further cell division, and thus become functional B lymphocytes (Fig. 2.3).

Initial evidence that the gene rearrangements involved in generation of diversity occurred in pre-B cells came from immunoflourescence studies demonstrating expression of V region markers in these cells. In patients wth multiple myeloma, a large fraction of bone marrow pre-B cells were shown to express the myeloma idiotype (Kubagawa et al., 1979). Pre-B cells from rabbits heterozygous for heavy chain V allotypes expressed these markers and demonstrated allelic exclusion (Gathings et al., 1981).

Burrows et al. (1979) produced stable hybridoma cell lines of mouse pre-B cells by fusing fetal liver cells with a nonproducer plasmacytoma cell line. These hybridomas synthesized μ chains but not light chains, confirming their pre-B cell origins. These investigators pointed out the potential importance of asynchronous onset of heavy and light chain synthesis for generation of diversity; a pre-B cell expressing a particular V_H gene may generate a large progeny in which a variety of different V_L genes are expressed. This mechanism greatly increases the likelihood of expression of each V_H gene with all available V_L genes. Riley et al. (1981) extended the hybridoma approach to verify this hypothesis. They fused an Abelson virus-induced pre-B cell line to a myeloma variant which produced no light chains. Several of the resulting hybridomas were light chain producers and different κ light chains, all derived from genes donated by the pre-B cell parent, were expressed by different hybridomas.

Recent studies on immunoglobulin gene rearrangements in human B cell lines indicated that the same general strategy of sequential activation regulates expression of kappa and lambda gene families (Hieter et al., 1981). Cell lines expressing κ light chains contain λ light chain genes in the embryonic configuration. In contrast, lines expressing λ light chains have either deleted κ genes or have them in a rearranged form. These observations suggest that activation of kappa genes precedes that of lambda genes.

A reasonably coherent picture of the generation of diversity within a population of rapidly dividing pre-B cells is now emerging. The initial event is the formation of a functional Cμ gene (Maki et al., 1980). This requires two distinct gene rearrangements; these are translocation of

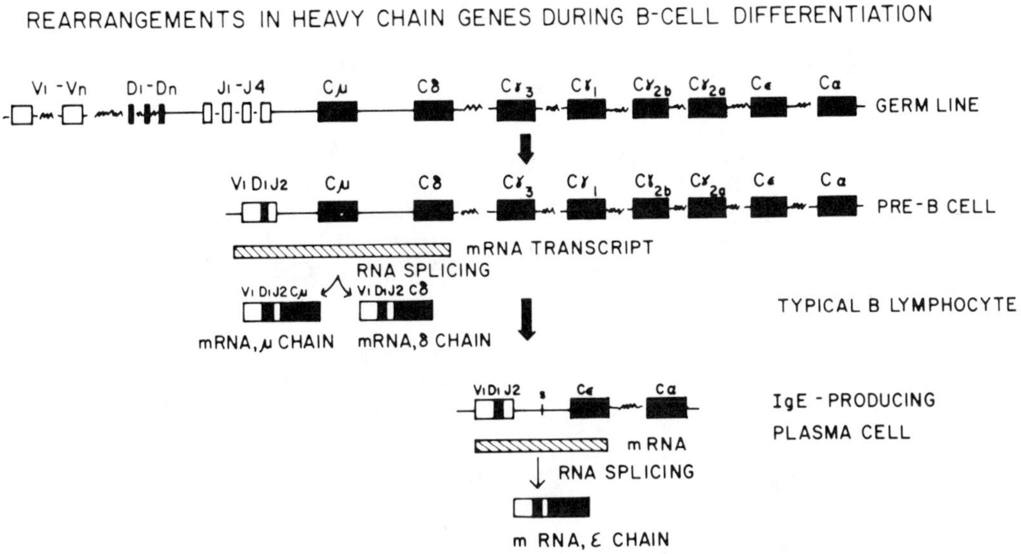

Fig. 2.2 Sequential alterations in the content and context of immunoglobulin genes occur during B cell differentiation. The heavy chain gene family of the mouse, shown here, consists of four sets of genes arranged in tandem. V, D and J genes determine the specificity of the heavy chain, while C genes code for immunoglobulin class. The first rearrangement of the germ line configuration results in approximation of one member each of the V, D and J gene sets; DNA separating the selected genes is deleted. This rearrangement results in a transcriptionally active gene extending from V to Cδ. A large nuclear mRNA transcript may then be processed to yield cytoplasmic mRNA for μ chains (in pre-B cells) or both μ and δ chains (in B lymphocytes).

A second rearrangement occurs in mature plasma cells. In the IgE-producing cell illustrated, the VDJ genes and part of the intervening sequence separating J and Cμ have been translocated to a switch site(s) located to the left of the Cξ gene. Intervening Cμ, Cδ and Cγ genes have been deleted.

A rearrangement of the first type occurs in a similar fashion for the κ and λ light chain families.

V_H to one of several D_H genes and translocation of the V_H–D_H hybrid to one of four J_H genes. These gene splicing events appear to be rather imprecise, being subject to two sorts of error. Errors which serve to insert or delete codons without shifting the reading frame or introducing stop codons serve to increase diversity (see Early and Hood, 1981). Errors of the opposite sort result in abortive rearrangements (Coleclough et al., 1981). A successful rearrangement occurring on one chromosome may serve to suppress attempts at rearrangements involving the homologous chromosome. Similar events then occur for the kappa light chain family, leading either to productive or non-productive rearrangements of Vκ and Jκ genes. Failure to produce a valid rearrangement of kappa genes is followed by activation of the lambda gene family.

This process is highly efficient as a generator of diversity in two respects. The asynchrony in onset of H and L chain expression maximizes the chances that all possible combinations of germ line V_H and V_L genes will be expressed. The imprecision of splicing of V_H–D_H, D_H–J_H, and V_L–J_L genes serves to create somatic diversity, although at some cost in terms of cell wastage. The pre-B cell has two critically important biologic attributes which facilitate this process. First, it divides at an extraordinarily high rate, allowing expression of successful gene rearrangements and permitting the necessary wastage. Second, proliferation of pre-B cells is not dependent on stimulation by antigens, since these cells lack cell surface antigen receptors. The existence of this cell type confirms a prediction of the clonal selection hypothesis by clearly separating the process of clonal development from the selective events which drive an immune response.

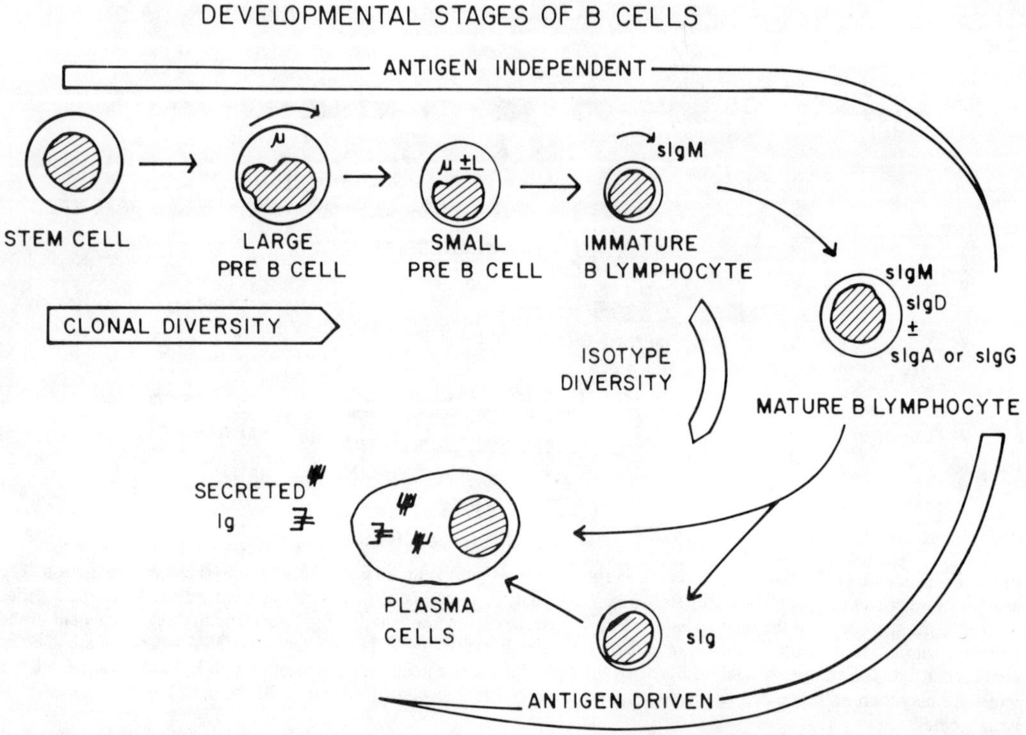

Fig. 2.3 Isotype diversity is generated within each clone of developing B cells and ultimately by the translocation of VDJ genes from Cμ to other C_H genes, as illustrated in Figure 2.1. Since light chain expression is unaltered, the process assures that each clone contains members which may secrete any of the immunoglobulin classes with their different biologic activities.

This simplified diagram shows the predominant phenotypes of B lymphocytes observed in the fetus, neonate and adult, with the solid lines indicating the sequence of switching suggested by this ontogenetic data. The broken lines indicate alternative pathways for switching suggested by studies showing that single B lymphocytes may generate clones expressing various combinations of immunoglobulin classes.

Immature B Lymphocytes

The most primitive B lymphocytes, distinguished from pre-B cells by the expression of cell surface immunoglobulin, differ from their more mature counterparts in several respects (see Fig. 2.3). From a functional standpoint, immature B cells are easily rendered tolerant by contact with specific antigens or inactivated by exposure to anti-immunoglobulin antibodies. Neonatal murine B cells exposed to hapten-carrier conjugates in the presence of T lymphocytes which have been primed to the carrier generate an immune response; if the same cells are challenged in the absence of T cells primed to the carrier, they become refractory to subsequent antigenic stimulation (Metcalf and Klinman, 1976). Tolerance susceptibility among splenic B cells is gradually lost during the first week of postnatal life, but approximately one-third of bone marrow B cell precursors remain susceptible in adult animals (Metcalf and Klinman, 1977). The kinetics of specific tolerance induction is paralleled by sensitivity of newborn B cells to suppression by anti-μ antibodies. Newborn mice injected wth anti-μ fail to develop B lymphocytes. If anti-μ treatment is not begun until 1 week of age, B cell development is not suppressed (Lawton and Cooper, 1974). In vitro experiments have suggested that tolerance induction and anti-μ suppression are related to the phenomenon of receptor modulation. Adult B cells exposed to anti-μ antibodies are stripped of their IgM receptors by the process of cap formation and endocytosis; on removal of the antibody, surface IgM receptors are rapidly reexpressed. The surface immunoglobulin of neonatal cells is modulated at much lower concentrations of anti-μ and neither re-expression of sIgM nor of the capacity to undergo further differentiation occurs during subsequent culture (Raff et al., 1975). It seems very likely that this phenomenon, termed clonal abortion by Nossal and Pike (1975), plays an important role in the acquisition of B cell tolerance to self antigens.

Development of Isotype Diversity

Isotype diversity, or the capacity to produce antibodies of different classes and subclasses, is generated within each developing clone of B lymphocytes by a series of rearrangements of heavy chain gene segments. As indicated in Figure 2.2, expression of IgM by pre-B cells follows the translocation of particular V and D genes to one of several J genes located on the 5′ side of the gene for the constant region of IgM (Cμ). Other heavy chain constant region genes are arranged on the 3′ side of Cμ, in the order: Cδ, $C\gamma_3$, $C\gamma_1$, $C\gamma_{2b}$, $C\gamma_{2a}$, Cξ, Cα. Each gene is separated from its neighbors by an untranslated sequence of DNA containing one or more splice sites. Cμ and Cδ are relatively close together, being separated by ~2.5 kilobases; the intervening sequences between the remaining genes are believed to be approximately ten times as large. Analysis of cloned DNA from plasmacytomas producing IgA or IgG immunoglobulin has revealed that at least one copy of each of the C genes located to the left (5′ side) of the expressed C gene has been deleted and that the intervening sequence (IS) between the J gene and the expressed C gene is derived partially from the IS flanking germ line Cμ and partially from the IS flanking the expressed C gene in its germ line location (see Early and Hood, 1981). Thus, switching is ultimately accomplished by translocation of genes coding for the immunoglobulin variable region (V, D, and J) from a position adjacent to Cμ to a new location next to one of the other C genes. By this process each clonal precursor generates a family of B cells having the same antibody specificity and light chain classes.

Although the terminal mechanisms of switching seem clear, the intermediate steps and regulation of this process remain controversial. Observations of the ontogeny of B cell expression isotype diversity in mouse and man have suggested the model shown in Figure 2.4 (Gathings et al., 1977; Abney et al., 1978; Gandini et al., 1981). Expression of sIgG, or sIgA, occurs initially on separate populations of B lymphocytes which also express sIgM. At a slightly later stage of development, B lymphocytes expressing sIgG or sIgA also bear *both* sIgM and sIgD. Probably as a consequence of antigen-driven proliferation and maturation, expression of sIgD and sIgM is lost as differentiation to memory cells and plasma cells proceeds.

Coexpression of sIgM and sIgD by single cells is apparently accomplished by post-transcriptional modification of a single large messenger RNA transcript containing information for VJD, Cμ and Cδ sequences (Early and Hood, 1981). This RNA is spliced to yield separate mRNA molecules encoding the μ and δ heavy chains. However, it is unlikely that RNA splicing can account for coexpression of IgM and IgG or IgA molecules by single cells, as the intervening DNA sequences separating these constant genes are very large. It is possible that cells expressing IgM and IgA, for example, have already excised the Cμ gene and are utilizing a long-lived mRNA for the μ heavy chain. However, this explanation does not easily account for the sequence in which the Cα gene is expressed prior to the Cδ gene.

The mechanisms regulating both the expression and sequence of switching are equally controversial. During ontogeny, expression of isotype diversity occurs at a rather precise time and without obvious antigenic stimulation. On the other hand, single precursor cells stimulated by antigens may generate progeny which produce various combinations of several different isotypes (Gearhart et al., 1975). It seems most logical to assume that the switching process is linked to proliferation of B cells, such that each round of cell division, whether driven by antigen or not, has a certain frequency of generating a progeny expressing a different isotype.

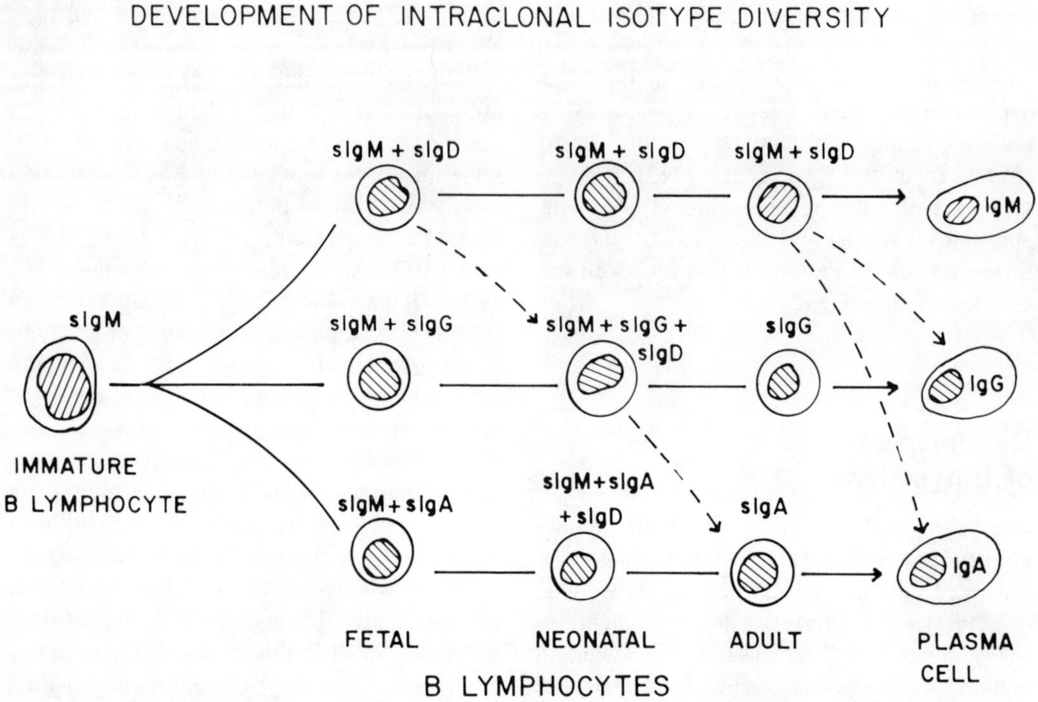

Fig. 2.4 B cell differentiation occurs in two discontinuous stages. The first is antigen-independent and comprises the selection and rearrangements of immunoglobulin genes which create a diverse clonal repertoire. This process occurs primarily in large rapidly dividing pre-B cells which express cytoplasmic μ chains and in their immediate progeny which begin to express light chains. Immature B lymphocytes are the first antigen-sensitive B cells, because they express cell surface IgM receptors and are distinguished functionally by a high degree of tolerance susceptibility.

Expression of isotype diversity marks the transition from immature to mature B lymphocyte; this process occurs in an antigen-sheltered environment but may also be antigen-driven.

The steps in the lower half of the diagram follow selection by specific antigen and are regulated by T cells and macrophages. The generation of expanded clones of memory cells and antibody-secreting plasma cells are synonymous with the humoral immune response.

Differentiation Markers of B Lymphocytes

B lymphocytes as a population bear a variety of cell surface antigens in addition to the surface immunoglobulin which is their primary distinguishing feature. Certain of these are acquired subsequent to the initial expression of sIgM and thus may serve to mark more mature cells. However, there are as yet no markers or combinations of markers on human B lymphocytes which are clearly associated with discrete functions.

Receptors for Epstein-Barr (E-B) virus are expressed by pre-B cells and B lymphocytes and probably by cells committed to the B lineage which have not yet expressed any immunoglobulin. Human DR antigens, glycoproteins encoded by the D locus of the major histocompatibility complex, are expressed on all B cells, including pre-B cells (Cooper et al., 1978; Pearl et al., 1979). It is interesting that this is not the case in the mouse. Ia antigens in this species are expressed on only a small proportion of $sIgM^+$ lymphocytes at birth, but on virtually all B cells by 2 weeks of age (Kearney et al., 1977). Most human B lymphocytes bear receptors for the Fc fragment of IgG and for C_3, the third component of the complement. Of these markers, only the EB virus receptor is uniquely associated with cells of the B lineage.

Approximately one-half of the human peripheral blood B lymphocytes bear a receptor for mouse erythrocytes (Gupta et al., 1976). The population of cells bearing this receptor is highly enriched for expression of sIgM, sIgD and the complement receptor, but relatively depleted in Fc receptor-positive cells. Interestingly, most of the B cell precursors capable of being triggered to plasma cell differentiation by the pokeweed mitogen (PWM) do not form rosettes with mouse erythrocytes (Lucivero et al., 1981).

Monoclonal antibodies reactive with unique subpopulations of human B cells have already been described (Brooks et al., 1981). It seems certain that this approach will produce new information on differentiation pathways and functional distinctions among B cells, as it already has for T cells.

Antigen-driven B Cell Differentiation

Up to this point the discussion has dealt with the primary differentiation events through which clonal and isotype diversity of B cells is generated. In man, this process begins by about the eighth week of gestation; by the time of birth there is extensive development of both sorts of diversity (Gathings et al., 1977). Clonal generation does not depend upon exposure to external antigens; rather, it is probably regulated by the same sorts of genetically programmed signals that direct differentiation of other cell lines, such as erythrocytes or granulocytes. This process normally proceeds in the bone marrow throughout most or all of adult life, continually seeding peripheral tissues with newly formed clones of virgin B cells.

An immune response is initiated when an antigenic determinant (epitope) binds to complementary receptors expressed by one or more B cell clones. Under the proper circumstances, this binding event triggers the cell to proliferate and to generate a differentiated progeny of plasma cells secreting antibodies having the same specificity as the original cell-bound receptor molecule. A particular epitope is likely to encounter many clones whose receptors are capable of binding with varying affinities. Those clones having receptors of highest affinities will continue to be stimulated as concentrations of the epitope diminish. This continuous selection results in an increase of the average affinity of the antibody molecules produced as the immune response proceeds. Most antigens have many different epitopes, each capable of stimulating a large number of different clones. Consequently, the population of antibodies produced to natural antigens is usually extremely heterogeneous.

Not all B lymphocytes triggered by an encounter with antigen differentiate into plasma cells; some remain as rather long-lived memory B lymphocytes. Several factors contribute to the formation of immunoglogic memory at the B cell level. One is clonal expansion; antigen-induced proliferation of selected clones results in a larger fraction of cells having complementary receptors among the total B cell population. Also, clones having higher binding affinity are expanded to a greater degree than those with lower affinity, resulting in a memory population of relatively high affinity cells. A third factor concerns physiologic differences between virgin and memory B cells.

Memory cell populations have different and generally less stringent requirements for stimulation than do unprimed B cells (Klinman, 1972). This phenomenon may be related to changes in the expression of cell surface immunoglobulin which occurs consequent to antigenic stimulation. Virgin precursors for IgG and IgA responses bear receptors of the IgM class and either already express or are rapidly induced to express IgD and IgA receptors as well. Memory B lymphocyte precursors which produce high affinity IgG antibodies have IgG receptors only, while those which will produce lower affinity antibodies may retain expression of IgM and/or IgD (Herzenberg et al., 1980). This pattern of alterations in expression of isotype is consistent with the ontogeny of isotype expression. In neonatal humans and mice, virtually all cells bearing sIgA or sIgG also express both sIgM and sIgD, while in adults the majority of sIgA or sIgG positive cells bear only that isotype (Abney et al., 1978; Gandini et al., 1981). Athymic mice retain the neonatal pattern, presumably because in the absence of helper T cells and their B cells are not stimulated to proliferate (Gathings, W.E.; Cooper, M.D., and Mond, J., unpublished data).

As is discussed in Chapters 1 and 3, antigen-induced triggering of B lymphocytes is highly regulated by direct interaction with antigen-presenting and T cells macrophages and/or factors produced by these cell types. The detailed mechanisms of T cell regulation are just beginning to be elucidated. The general pattern of organization appears to be a complex series of autoregulatory circuits, in which helper T cells induce suppressor T cells which serve to limit helper function.

B cells and their products contribute to these regulatory interactions in at least two ways. Antibodies with specificity for the immunizing antigen serve a role by reducing the antigen concentration and thereby limiting further stimulation. In addition, immunization triggers an autoregulatory response based on idiotype. Idiotypes are antigenic determinants associated wth the combining sites of antibody molecules. Jerne (1974) envisioned the immune system as a network of idiotypes and anti-idiotypes. Introduction of an antigenic determinant (epitope) stimulated a response and thus raised the concentration of idiotype associated with that particular antibody specificity. This response in turn provoked an auto-anti-idiotypic response. Anti-idiotypic antibodies may either amplify or suppress the original response and also serve to induce production of antibodies to their own idiotypes. This idea has received firm experimental support [for example, see Bona et al. (1981)] and clearly offers infinite possibilities for regulating the intensity and duration of an immune response.

Abnormal B Cell Differentiation

Abnormal B cell differentiation in man encompasses several conditions, including the malignancies involving B cells, autoimmune disorders and immunodeficiency states. Each of these is discussed in other chapters of this volume. The goal in this section is to outline some general relationships, actual or potential, between the normal processes of B cell differentiation and developmental or functional arrests which result in failure to produce appropriate antibody responses.

Stem Cell Defects

Defective development of precursors for B lineage cells occurs in a subgroup of infants with severe combined immunodeficiency. These lymphopenic patients lack both T and B cells in their circulation; bone marrow from some has had no detectable pre-B cells (Pearl et al., 1979).

Patients who acquire hypogammaglobulinemia in association with epithelial thymoma also appear to have a defect in differentiation of an early progenitor B cell. Two patients lacked both circulating B lymphocytes and pre-B cells in bone marrow (Pearl et al., 1979). These patients may develop other disorders consistent with defective function of hemopoietic stem cells, including eosinopenia, erythroid aplasia or aplastic anemia (Jeunet and Good, 1968). There is evidence that excess activity of suppressor T cells occurs in these patients; this might play a role in the pathogenesis of the stem cell dysfunction (Litwin & Zanjani, 1977; Moretta et al., 1977). The relationship of these acquired stem cell defects to thymoma is not understood.

Defective Differentiation of Pre-B Cells

With few exceptions, males with congenital x-linked agammaglobulinemia (X-LA) have had a normal frequency of pre-B cells in their bone marrow despite the virtual absence of B lymphocytes or plasma cells in the circulation or lymphoid tissues (Pearl et al., 1978). The failure of these patients to generate B lymphocytes has been confirmed using several B cell markers; they lack lymphocytes bearing DR antigens or EB virus receptors, as well as surface immunoglobulin. The fundamental defect in this disease thus appears to be a defect in the capacity of pre-B cells to generate a progeny of B lymphocytes. In one patient, large marrow pre-B cells failed to incorporate thymidine at the same high rate as do normal pre-B cells (Pearl et al., 1978).

Fu et al. (1981) have recently developed a series of cell lines using EB virus to transform bone marrow from X-LA patients. Some of these lines have the typical pre-B cell phenotype, containing cells which are positive for cytoplasmic μ chains but lack sIg. Others have morphologic and growth characteristics distinct from the usual B cell lines. This group has recently reported that both types of lines produce messenger RNA for J chain, a polypeptide associated with polymeric immunoglobulins (McCune et al., 1981). This suggests that the "round cell" lines also belong to the B lineage and could be the precursors of pre-B cells. The existence of these lines should be of great value in searching for the x-linked defect responsible for the arrest in pre-B cell maturation.

Partial arrests in the generation or function of pre-B cells may occur in other hypogammaglobulinemic states. Approximately one-third of the patients with common variable immunodeficiency (CVI) have very low or undetectable numbers of circulating B lymphocytes (Preud'homme et al., 1973). In some patients, the number of B cells fluctuates from time to time and may increase dramatically with infection. Some patients with CVI and B lymphocyte deficiency have a corresponding lack of pre-B cells; in one patient, an increase in circulating B lymphocytes was associated with the appearance of pre-B cells in marrow (Pearl et al., 1979).

Defects in Generation of Clonal or Isotype Diversity

The immense complexity of the genetic rearrangements which contribute to the generation of immunoglobulin chains suggests that mistakes should occur frequently; in fact, abortive rearrangements of the various genes involved presumably leading to non-functional B cells seem to occur frequently in normal B cell development (Coleclough et al., 1981). This rather sloppy process appears to be acceptable in an evolutionary sense because it also has the potential of increasing diversity and because of the size of the antibody specificity repertoire is so large.

In chickens one can limit clonal diversity by removal of the bursa of Fabricius at or slightly before the time of hatching. Such birds have a life-long deficiency of circulating B lymphocytes but may eventually develop normal concentrations of circulating IgM and IgG (Kincade et al., 1973). Primary antibody responses are absent or meager, but repeated stimulation leads eventually to antibody production. Huang and Dreyer (1978) have shown that antibodies produced by these birds have limited charge heterogeneity, suggesting that they are derived from many fewer clones than antibodies of normal birds.

Patients with defects in generation of diversity might be expected to have low numbers of B lymphocytes. Because the available clones of lymphocytes could function normally, immunoglobulin levels might be relatively high, but specific antibody responses should be low or might vary depending upon the antigen used. In the extreme case, immunoglobulins might have restricted electrophoretic heterogeneity. A few patients with these clinical features have been described (Lawton et al., 1975; Cooper et al., 1979). However, it is exceedingly difficult to distinguish between underproduction of B cells with normal diversity and production of too few clones of normal size.

Deficiency in production of kappa light chains has been observed. One patient lacked B lymphocytes bearing kappa chains as well (Zegers et al., 1976). Such a deficiency should be associated with a gap in antibody diversity, since the V and J genes associated with the kappa family would not be expressed. This defect could be caused either by deletion of structural defects of the Cκ gene or in the Jκ complex of genes to which Vκ genes must be joined. Imbalances in expression of κ and λ light chains among serum immunoglobulins of immunodeficient patients are frequent. In some instances this appears to be a regulatory defect, since κ/λ ratios among B lymphocytes are normal (Preud'homme and Seligmann, unpublished; see Cooper et al., 1979).

Abnormal Development or Expression of Isotype Diversity

A number of patients have had associated deficiencies in expression of sIgG and sIgA on B lymphocytes and of the corresponding immunoglobulin classes in serum (Cooper et al., 1973; Preud'homme et al., 1973, 1977). Among these are patients with severe combined immunodeficiency and others with common variable immunodeficiency. It must be the case that several different genetic defects, some of which must be regulatory, may contribute to the failure to accomplish intraclonal isotype switching. Study of the context of immunoglobulin C_H genes in such patients may have much to teach us about normal pathways of switching.

Defects in Terminal Differentiation of B Cells

Many patients with panhypogammaglobulinemia or with selective deficiencies of one or more immunoglobulin classes in serum have normal numbers and isotype diversity of circulating B lymphocytes. Reduced to the simplest possible terms, failure of B lymphocyte differentiation might result from abnormalities in development of function of immunoregulatory T cells or intrinsic B cell abnormalities.

The central role of T cells in regulating function of B cells in humans has been shown in many ways, but is perhaps most dramatically demonstrated in a subgroup of patients with severe combined immunodeficiency. These patients have a normal population of B lymphocytes in blood and bone marrow but lack T cells and fail to produce antibodies. Incubation of bone marrow cells from these patients on monolayer cultures of thymic epithelium may result in induction of E rosette-forming cells and, in parallel, of the capacity to generate an antigen-specific plaque-forming cell response (Gelfand et al., 1980). In similar patients, transplantation of cultured thymic epithelium has resulted in partial correction of both T and B cell function (Hong et al., 1976, 1978). Patients with Di George's syndrome (a birth defect in which tissues derived from the third and fourth pharyngeal pouch areas, including thymus and parathyroids, fail to develop normally) have variable, but sometimes relatively normal, B cell function. This may be explained by observations that such patients frequently have a histologically normal, though tiny, thymus (Lischner and Huff, 1975).

The largest group of patients with defects in terminal B cell differentiation is included in the subset of common varied immunodeficiency in which normal numbers of B cells are present. Most studies of pathogenetic mechanisms in these patients have employed an in vitro culture system in which pokeweed mitogen is used to stimulate B lymphocytes to differentiate to immunoglobulin secreting plasma cells (Wu et al., 1973). This system has been particularly useful because the B cell response is entirely T cell-dependent, being regulated by the balance between irradiation-sensitive suppressor T cells and irradiation-resistant helper T cells (Waldmann et al., 1974; Janossy and Greaves, 1975; Keightley et al., 1976; Fauci et al., 1976; Siegal and Siegal, 1977). Moreover, both helper and suppressor activities are relatively uninfluenced by histocompatability differences between T and B cells. Thus it has been possible to use cocultures of normal and hypogammaglobulinemic lymphocytes to independently assess T and B cell function of lymphocytes from hypogammaglobulinemic patients.

Initial studies using this sytem indicated that the in vivo defect in immunoglobulin synthesis in some patients could be overcome in vitro, while lyphocytes from others failed to respond (Wu et al., 1973). Waldmann and coworkers (1974) were the first to assess the role of T cells in these patients; they found that lymphocytes from most of their patients suppressed B cell differentiation by normal lymphocyte populations and identified the suppressors as T cells.

Subsequent studies from several laboratories have emphasized the heterogeneity of defects which may be encountered in these patients (Geha et al., 1974; Broom et al., 1976; Siegal et al., 1976; De La Concha et al., 1977; Waldmann et al., 1976b, 1980). Excess T suppressor activity is common, but is frequently associated with what appears to be an intrinsic abnormality of B cells. Several further cautions concerning the role of suppressor T cells have emerged. Siegel et al. (1976) found that suppressor activity in some patient's cells varied depending upon the source of normal cells used in the assay.

Several laboratories have reported that some patients with x-linked agammaglobulinemia or thymoma have excessive T suppressor activity (Waldmann et al., 1980). Both of the latter groups of patients have defects in primary B cell development. Although it is possible that suppressor T cells could inhibit primary B cell development, there is no evidence in experimental animals to support such a notion.

Blaese et al. (1974, 1977) developed a model of "infectious agammaglobulinemia" in chickens which is highly relevant to this point. Birds rendered agammaglobulinemic by neonatal bursectomy lack circulating B lymphocytes. T cells from these agammaglobulinemic birds transferred into normal chickens rendered the latter agammaglobulinemic, but the recipient chickens maintained normal numbers of B lymphocytes. By limiting dilution assays it was determined that the original donors developed suppressor T cells specific for different immunoglobulin isotypes. In this experimental system, suppressor T cells appear to develop as a consequence of agammaglobulinemia in donor birds and act on terminal phases of B cell differentiation in recipients. An additional mechanism which may contribute to secondary development of suppressor activity was suggested by studies on a patient with thymoma and hypogammablobulinemia (Moretta et al., 1977). This patient had increased proportions of T cells bearing receptors for IgG (T_γ cells); this subset of T cells had the capacity to suppress B cell differentiation. Studies using normal patients revealed that T_γ cells were suppressive, but only after they had bound IgG immune complexes. These observations suggest that treatment of some hypogammaglobulinemic patients with gammaglobulin injections may contribute to generation of active suppressor cells.

These considerations raise doubts about a primary pathogenetic role for suppressor T cells in hypogammaglobulinemia, but by no means negate the importance of this mechanism in contributing to the maintenance of the hypogammaglobulinemic state.

Defects in development or function of helper T cells have been described in a few patients. Heterologous or monoclonal antibodies were used to define deficiencies of the inducer T cell subset in two patients (Reinherz et al., 1979; Reinherz and Schlossman, 1980). Another patient had normal numbers of $T4^+$ inducer cells which could not be activated by antigens to proliferate or to release helper factors for B cell differentiation. T cells of the patient failed to provide help for B cell differentiation by lymphocytes from an HLA-matched sibling, while B cells and suppressor T cells were functionally normal (Reinherz et al., 1981).

Isolated deficiency of IgA may be another example of a B cell defect resulting from T cell dysfunction (reviewed by Cooper et al., 1981). Most patients with IgA deficiency have circulating B lymphocytes bearing IgA (Lawton et al., 1972; Preud'homme et al., 1973), although recent reports suggest that the frequency of these cells is somewhat lower than normal (Conley and Cooper, 1981). Studies have indicated that lymphocytes from some of these patients may be stimulated by PWM to generate IgA-containing plasma cells, although such responses are usually less than normal (Wu et al., 1973; Waldmann et al., 1976a; Delespesse et al., 1976; Cassidy et al., 1979). An interesting parallel situation occurs in the normal newborn. IgA-bearing B lymphocytes are present in frequencies similar to those in adult blood, but most infants lack detectable IgA in serum. PWM-stimulated cultures of cord blood lymphocytes rarely contain IgA plasma cells (Wu et al., 1976). Cocultures of cord B cells with adult T cells do stimulate an IgA response, although of lesser magnitude than is obtained with adult B cells. Conversely, cord T cells do not support as vigorous a response from adult B cells as is obtained using adult T cells (Hayward and Lawton, 1977). It has recently been shown that the IgA-bearing lymphocytes from most IgA-deficient patients are phenotypically similar to neonatal IgA^+ cells; that is, the $sIgA^+$ cells bear both sIgM and sIgD (Conley and Cooper, 1981). IgA-bearing cells from athymic mice also retain this neonatal phenotype. These observations suggest that T cells may be involved in the differentiation step from "immature" to "mature" B cells and that such a step may precede acquisition of the capacity to undergo terminal differentiation. The selective nature of IgA deficiency would require that the T cell dysfunction be specific for this isotype. Precedence for this exists with regard to T suppressor cells (Waldmann et al., 1976a; Atwater and Tomasi, 1978).

Intrinsic Abnormalities of B Cells

Geha et al. (1974) described a group of hypogammaglobulinemic patients whose lymphocytes were stimulated in the presence of a T cell-derived factor to differentiate into IgG-containing cells. No release of IgG could be demonstrated. The failure of IgG secretion was correlated with a defect in glycosylation of the intracellular IgG (Ciccimara et al., 1976). An apparent block in secretion of IgA has also been described in IgA-deficiencies (Waldmann et al., 1976a). The significance of these in vitro observations is not entirely clear. Patients with panhypogammaglobulinemia or isolated IgA deficiency have a corresponding lack of plasma cells containing immunoglobulin in their lymphoid tissues, suggesting that synthesis as well as secretion must be defective in vivo.

At the present time, the majority of patients with defects of terminal B cell differentiation appear to have intrinsic abnormalities of their B cells, the nature of which are undefined. It is interesting that these defects seem to operate primarily on differentiation rather than proliferation, since affected patients often have generalized lymphadenopathy, prominent germinal centers on lymph node biopsy and nodular lymphoid hyperplasia of the intestine.

Summary

Only 10 years have elapsed since the techniques of cellular immunology were first applied to study the disorders of immunity in man. A great deal has been learned about the cellular defects which contribute to immune dysfunction. Each newly discovered step in B cell differentiation soon has been followed by descriptions of patients in whom differentiation is blocked around that step. Almost every aspect of regulatory T cell function defined in experimental animals has a parallel disorder in man. The next decade should witness a tremendous growth in understanding of the genetic regulation of differentiation and of the molecules which mediate this process. With future research, perhaps treatment of antibody deficiency by replacement therapy, nearly unchanged for 30 years, can be replaced by vastly more effective therapies.

Acknowledgments

I particularly wish to thank my teacher, friend and collaborator, Max D. Cooper, whose germinal ideas and experiments permeate the field of B cell differentiation. I am very grateful to Ms. Carolyn Kosser for her expert assistance in preparing the manuscript.

References

Abney, E.R., Cooper, M.D., Kearney, J.F., Lawton, A.R., and Parkhouse, R.M.E. 1978. Sequential expression of immunoglobulin on developing mouse B lymphocytes. A systematic survey which suggests a model for the generation of immunoglobulin isotype diversity. J Immunol 120:2041–2049.

Atwater, J.D., and Tomasi, T.B., Jr. 1978. Suppressor cells and IgA deficiency. Clin Immunol Immunopath 9:379–384.

Blaese, R.M., Muchmore, A.V., Koski, I.R., and Dooley, N.J. 1977. Immunoglobulin class of specific suppressor T cells. In: Regulatory Mechanisms in Lymphocyte Activation, ed. D.O. Lucas, pp. 776–778. Academic Press; New York.

Blaese, R.M., Weiden, P.L., Koski, I., and Dooley N. 1974. Infectious agammaglobulinemia: Transmission of immunodeficiency with grafts of agammaglobulinemic cells. J Exp Med 140:1097–1101.

Bona, C.A., Heber-Katz, E., and Paul, W.E. 1981. Idiotype-antiidiotype regulation. I. Immunization with a levan-binding meyloma protein leads to appearance of auto-anti-(anti-idiotype) antibodies and to the activation of silent clones. J Exp Med 153:951–967.

Brooks, D.A., Beckman, I.G.R., Bradley, S., McNamara, P.J., Thomas, M.E. and Zola, H. 1981. Human lymphocyte markers defined by antibodies derived from somatic cell hybrids. IV. A monoclonal antibody reacting specifically with a subpopulation of human B lymphocytes. J Immunol 126:1373–1389.

Broom, B.C., De La Concha, E.G., Webster, A.D.B., Janossy, G. J., and Asherson, G.L. 1976. Intracellular immunoglobulin production *in vitro* by lymphocytes from patients with hypogammaglobulinemia and their effects on normal lymphocytes. Clin Exp Immunol 23:73–77.

Burnet, F.M. 1959. The Clonal Selection Theory of Acquired Immunity. Vanderbilt University Press; Nashville.

Burrows, P.B., LeJeune, M., and Kearney, J.F. 1979. Evidence that murine pre-B cells synthesize μ heavy chains but no light chains. Nature 280:838–841.

Cassidy, J.T., Oldham, G., and Platt-Mills, T.A.E. 1979. Functional assessment of a B cell defect in patients with selective IgA deficiency. Clin Exp Immunol 35:296–305.

Ciccimara, F., Rosen, F.S., and Schneeberger, E. 1976. Failure of heavy chain gylcosylation of IgG in some patients with common variable agammaglobulinemia. J Clin Invest 57:1386–1390.

Claman, H.N., Chaperon, E.A., and Triplett, R.F. 1966. Thymus-marrow cell combinations—synergism in antibody production. Proc Soc Exper Biol Med 122:1167–1171.

Coleclough, C., Perry, R.P., Karjalainen, K., and Weigert, M. 1981. Aberrant rearrangements contribute significantly to the allelic exclusion of immunoglobulin gene expression. Nature 290:372–378.

Conley, M.E., and Cooper, M.D. 1981. Immature IgA B cells in IgA-deficient patients. New Engl J Med 295:495–497.

Cooper, M.D., Conley, M.E., Levitt, D., and Lawton, A.R. In press. Cellular and molecular aspects of IgA deficiency. In: The Menarini Series on Immunopathology, vol. 3, Symposium on Immunogenetics. Schwab & Co.; Basel.

Cooper, M.D., Gabrielson, A.E., and Good, R.A. 1967. Role of the thymus and other central lymphoid tissues in immunological disease. Ann Rev Med 18:113–138.

Cooper, M.D., Kearney, J.F., and Lawton, A.R., III. 1978. The life history of antibody producing B cells. Presented at the Fifth International Congress on Birth Defects, Montreal, Canada, August 22–27, 1977. In: Birth Defects. Proceedings of the Fifth International Conference, Montreal, 21–27 August, 1977, eds. J.W. Littlefield and J. deGrouchy, pp. 178–195. Excerpta Medica; Oxford.

Cooper, M.D., Kearney, J.F., Lydyard, P.M., Grossi, C.E., and Lawton, A.R. 1977. Studies of generation of B cell diversity in mouse, man and chicken. In: Cold Spring Harbor Symposia on Quantitative Biology/Origins of Lymphocyte Diversity, vol. XLI, pp. 139–145. Cold Spring Harbor Laboratory; New York.

Cooper, M.D., Keightley, R.G., Wu, L.Y.F., and Lawton, A.R. 1973. Developmental defects of T and B cell lines in humans. Transplant Rev 16:51.

Cooper, M.D., Lawton, A.R., Preud'homme, J.L., and Seligmann, M. 1979. Primary antibody deficiencies. In: Immune Deficiency, eds. M.D. Cooper, A.R. Lawton, P.A. Miescher, and H.J. Meuller-Eberhard, pp. 31–47. Springer-Verlag; New York.

Cooper, M.D., Peterson, R.D., South, M.A., and Good, R.A. 1966. The functions of the thymus system and bursa system in the chicken. J Exp Med 123:75–102.

De La Concha, E.G., Oldham, G. Webster, A.D.B., Asherson, G.L., and Platt-Mills, T.A.E. 1977. Quantitative measurements of T and B cell functions in "variable" primary hypogammaglobulinemia: Evidence for a consistent B cell defect. Clin Exp Immunol 27:208–215.

Delespesse, G., Grausset, P., Cauchie, C., and Grovaerts, A. 1976. Cellular aspects of selective IgA deficiency. Clin Exp Immunol 24:273–279.

Early, P., and Hood, L. 1981. Mouse immunoglobulin genes. In: Genetic Engineering, vol. 3, eds. J. Setlow and A. Hollaender. Plenum Press, N.Y. p. 157–188.

Erlich, P. 1900. On immunity with special reference to cell life. Proc R Soc 66:424.

Fauci, A.S., Pratt, K.R., and Whalen, G. 1976. Activation of human B lymphocytes. II. Cellular interactions in the PFC response of human tonsillar and peripheral blood B lymphocytes to polyclonal activation by pokeweed mitogen. J Immunol 117:2100–2104.

Fu, S.M., Hurley, M.H., McCune, J.M., Kunkel, H.G., and Good, R.A. 1981. Pre-B cell and other precursor lines derived from patients with x-linked agammaglobulinemia. Clin Res 28:502A.

Gandini, M., Kubagawa, H., Gathings, W.E., and Lawton, A.R. 1981. Expression of 3 immunoglobulin isotypes by individual B cells during development: Implications for heavy chain switching. Am J Repro Immunol. 1:161–163.

Gathings, W.E., Lawton, A.R., and Cooper, M.D. 1977. Immunoflourescent studies of the development of pre-B cells, B lymphocytes and immunoglobulin isotype diversity in humans. Eur J Immunol 7:804.

Gathings, W.E., Mage, R.G., Cooper, M.D., Lawton, A.R., and Young-Cooper, G.O. 1981. Immunoflourescence studies on the expression of V_Ha rabbits. Eur J Immunol 11:200–205.

Gearhart, P.J., Sigal, N.H. and Klinman, N.R. 1975. Production of antibodies of identical idiotype but diverse immunoglobulin classes by cells from a single stimulated B cell. Proc Natl Acad Sci USA 72:1707–1711.

Geha, R.S., Schneeberger, E., Merler, E., and Rosen, F.S. 1974. Heterogeneity of "acquired" or common variable agammaglobulinemia. N Engl J Med 291:1–6

Gelfand, E.W., Dosch, H. – M., Shore, A., Limatibul, S., and Lee, J.W.W. 1980. Role of the thymus in human T cell differentiation. In: Biological Bases of Immunodeficiency, eds. E.W. Gelfand and H.M. Dosch, pp. 39–56. Raven Press; New York.

Gupta, S., Good, R.A., and Siegal, F.P. 1976. Rosette formation with mouse erythrocytes. II. A marker for human B and non-T lymphocytes. Clin Exp Immunol 25:319–327.

Hayward, A.R., and Lawton, A.R. 1977. Induction of plasma cell differentiation of human fetal lymphocytes: Evidence for functional immaturity of T and B cells. J Immunol 119:1213–1217.

Heiter, P.A., Korsmeyer, S.J., Waldmann, T.A., and Leder, P. 1981. Human immunoglobulin κ light-chain genes are deleted or rearranged in λ-producing B cells. Nature 290:368–378.

Herzenberg, L.A., Black, S.J., Tokukisa, T., and Herzenberg, L.A. 1980. Memory B cells at successive stages of differentiation. Affinity maturation and the role of IgD receptors. J Exp Med 151:1071–1087.

Hong, R., Santosham, M., Schulte-Wissermann, Horowitz, S., Hsu, S.H. and Winkelstein, J.A. 1976. Reconstruction of B and T lymphocyte function in severe combined immunodeficiency disease after transplantation with thymic epithelium. Lancet II:1270–1272.

Hong, R., Schulte-Wissermann, H., Horowitz, S., Borzy, M., and Finlay, J. 1978. Cultured thymic epithelium in severe combined immunodeficiency. Transplant Proc 10:201–202.

Huang, H.V., and Dreyer, W.J. 1978. Bursectomy *in ovo* blocks the generation of immunoglobulin diversity. J Immunol 121:1738–1747.

Janossy, G., and Greaves, M. 1975. Functional analysis of murine and human B lymphocytes subsets. Transplant Rev 24:177–236.

Jerne, N.K. 1955. The natural selection theory of antibody formation. Proc Nat Acad Sci USA 41:849–857.

Jerne, N.K. 1974. Towards a network theory of the immune response. Ann Immunol (Paris) 125C:373.

Jeunet, F.S., and Good, R.A. 1968. Thymoma, immunologic deficiencies and hematological abnormalities. In: Immunologic Deficiency Diseases in Man/Birth Defects Original Article Series, vol. IV, eds. D. Bergsma and R.A. Good, p. 192. The National Foundation; New York.

Kearney, J.F., Cooper, M.D., Klein, J., Abney, E.R., Parkhouse, R.M.E., and Lawton, A.R. 1977. Ontogeny of Ia and IgD on IgM-bearing B lymphocytes in mice. J Exp Med 146:297–301.

Keightley, R.G., Cooper, M.D., and Lawton, A.R. 1976. The T cell dependence of B cell differentiation induced by pokeweed mitogen. J Immunol 117:1538–1544.

Kincade, P.W., Self, K.S., and Cooper, M.D. 1973. Survival and function of bursa-derived cells in bursectomized chickens. Cell Immunol 8:93–102.

Klinman, N.R. 1972. The mechanism of antigenic stimulation of primary and secondary clonal precursor cells. J Exp Med 136:241–260.

Kubagawa, H., Vogler, L.B., Capra, J.D., Conrad, M.E., Lawton, A.R., and Cooper, M.D. 1979. Studies on the clonal origin of multiple myeloma. Use of individually specific (idiotypic) antibodies to trace the oncogenic event to its earliest point of expression in B cell differentiation. J Exp Med 150:792–807.

Lawton, A.R., and Cooper, M.D. 1974. Modification of B-lymphocyte differentiation by anti-immunoglobulins. In: Contemporary Topics in Immunobiology, vol. 3, eds. M.D. Cooper and N.L. Warner, pp. 193–225. Plenum Press; New York.

Lawton, A.R., Royal, S.A., Self, K.S., and Cooper, M.D. 1972. IgA determinants on B lymphocytes in patients with deficiency of circulating IgA. J Lab Clin Med 80:26–33.

Lawton, A.R., Wu, L.Y.F., and Cooper, M.D. 1975. A spectrum of B cell differentiation defects. In: Immunodeficiency in Man and Animals/Birth Defects Original Article Series, vol. XI, ed. D. Bergsma, pp. 28–32. Sinauer Associates; Sunderland, Mass.

Lischner, H.W., and Huff, D.S. 1975. T cell deficiency in DiGeorge syndrome. In: Immunodeficiency in Man and Animals/Birth Defects Original Article Series, vol. XII, eds. D. Bergsma, R.A. Good, J. Finstad, and N.W. Paul, pp. 16–21. Sinauer Associates; Sunderland, Mass.

Litwin, S.D., and Zanjani, E.D. 1977. Lymphocytes suppressing both immunoglobulin production and erythroid differentiation in hypogammaglobulin. Nature 266:57–58.

Lucivero, G., Lawton, A.R., and Cooper, M.D., 1981. Rosette formation with mouse erythrocytes defines a population of human B lymphocytes unresponsive to pokeweed mitogen. Clin Exp Immunol 45:185–190.

Maki, R., Kearney, J., Paige, C., and Tonegawa, S. 1980. Immunoglobulin gene rearrangement in immature B cells. Science 209:1366–1369.

McCune, J.M., Fu, S.M., and Kunkel, H.G. 1981. J chain biosynthesis in pre-B cells and other possible precursor B cells. J Exp Med 154:138–145

Metcalf, E.S., and Klinman, N.R. 1976. *In vitro* tolerance induction of neonatal murine B cells. J Exp Med 143:1327.

Metcalf, E.S., and Klinman, N.R. 1977. *In vitro* tolerance induction of bone marrow cells: A marker for B cell maturation. J Immunol 118:2111.

Mitchell, G.F., and Miller, J.F.A.P. 1968. Cell to cell interaction in the immune response. II. The source of hemolysin-forming cells in irradiated mice given bone marrow and thymus or thoracic duct lymphocytes. J Exp Med 128:821–837.

Moretta, L., Mingari, M.C., Webb, S.R., Pearl, E.R., Lydyard, P.M., Grossi, C.E., Lawton, A.R., and Cooper, M.D. 1977. Imbalances in T cell subpopulation associated with immunodeficiency and autoimmune syndromes. Eur J Immunol 7:696.

Nossal, G.J.V., and Pike, B.L. 1975. Evidence for the clonal abortion theory of B lymphocytes. J Exp Med 141:904–917.

Pearl, E.R., Lawton, A.R., and Cooper, M.D. 1979. Informative defects of B lymphocyte differentiation in human antibody deficiency disorders. In: Proceedings of an International Conference on B Lymphocytes in the Immune Response, eds. M.D. Cooper, D. Mosier, I. Scher, and E. Vitetta, pp. 341–348. Elsevier/North-Holland; New York.

Pearl, E.R., Vogler, L.B., Okos, A.J., Crist, W.M., Lawton, A.R., and Cooper, M.D. 1978. B lymphocyte precursors in human bone marrow. An analysis of normal individuals and patients with antibody deficiency states. J Immunol 120:1169–1175.

Preud'homme, J.L., Griscelli, C., and Seligmann, M. 1973. Immunoglobulins on the surface of lymphocytes in fifty patients with primary immunodeficiencies. Clin Immunol Immunopath 1:241–256.

Preud'homme, J.L., Brouet, J.C., and Seligmann, M. 1977. Membrane-bound IgD on human lymphoid cells, with special reference to immunodeficiency and immunoproliferative disease. Immunol Rev 37:127–151.

Raff, M.C., Megson, M., Owen, J.J.T., and Cooper, M.D. 1976. Early production of intracellular IgM by B lymphocyte precursors in mouse. Nature 259:224–226.

Raff, M.C., Owen, J.J.T., Cooper, M.D., Lawton, A.R., III, Megson, M. and Gathings, W.E. 1975. Differences in susceptibility of mature and immature mouse B lymphocytes to anti-immunoglobulin-induced immunoglobulin suppression *in vitro*: Possible implications for B cell tolerance to self. J Exp Med 142:1052–1064.

Reinherz, E.L., Geha, R.S., Wohl, M.E., Moumoto, C., Rosen, F.S., and Schlossman, S.F. 1981. Immunodeficiency resulting from loss of $T4^+$ inducer T cell function. N Engl J Med 304:811–816.

Reinherz, E.L., Rubenstein, A., Geha, R.S., Strelkauskas, A.J., Rosen, F.S., and Schlossman, S.F. 1979. Abnormalities of immunoregulatory T cells in disorders of immune function. N Engl J Med 301:1018–1022.

Reinherz, E.L., and Schlossman, S.F. 1980. The regulation of the immune response-inducer and suppressor T lymphocyte subsets in human beings. N Engl J Med 303:370–373.

Riley, S.C., Brock, E.J., and Kuehl, W.M. 1981. Induction of light chain expression in a pre-B cell line by fusion to myeloma cells. Nature 289:804–806.

Siegal, F.P., and Siegal, M. 1977. Enhancement by irradiated T cells of human plasma cell production. Dissection of helper and suppressor functions *in vitro*. J Immunol 118:642–647.

Siegal, F.P., Siegal, M., and Good, R.A. 1976. Suppression of B cell differentiation by leukocytes from hypogammaglobulinemic patients. J Clin Invest 58:109.

Waldmann, T.A., Broder, S., Blaese, R.M., Durm, M., Blackburn, M., and Strober, W. 1974. Role of suppressor T cells in the pathogenesis of common variable hypogammaglobulinemia. Lancet II:609–613.

Waldman, T.A., Broder, S., Krakauer, R., Durm, M., Meade, B., and Goldman, C. 1976a. Defect in IgA secretion and in IgA specific suppressor cells in patients with selective IgA deficiency. Trans Assoc Am Phys 89:215–244.

Waldmann, T.A., Broder, S., Krakauer, R., MacDermott, R.P., Dunn, M., Goldman, C., and Meade, B. 1976b. The role of suppressor cells in the pathogenesis of common variable hypogammaglobulinemia and the immunodeficiency associated with myeloma. Fed Proc 35:2067–2072.

Waldmann, T.A., Broder, W., Blaese, R.M., Durm, M., Goldman, C., and Muul, L. 1980. Role of suppressor cells in human disease. In: Biological Bases of Immunodeficiency, eds. E.W. Gelfand and H. –M. Dosch, pp. 223–239. Raven press; New York.

Warner, N.L., Szenberg, A., and Burnet, F.M. 1962. The immunological role of different lymphoid organs in the chicken. Aust J Exp Biol Med Sci 40:373–388.

Wu, L.Y.F., Blanco, A., Cooper, M.D., and Lawton, A.R. 1976. Ontogeny of B lymphocyte differentiation induced by pokeweed mitogen. Clin Immunol Immunopathol 5:208–217.

Wu, L.Y.F., Lawton, A.R., and Cooper, M.D. 1973. Differentiation capacity of cultured B lymphocytes from immunodeficient patients. J Clin Invest 52:3180–3189.

Zegers, B.J.M, Maertzdorf, V., Loghem, E., Mul, N.A.J., Stoop, J.W., Laag, J., van der Vossen, J.J., and Ballieux, R.E. 1976. Kappa chain deficiency. N Engl J Med 294:1026–1030.

Chapter 3

Disorders of Macrophages

Jeremiah J. Twomey

Introduction

Metchnikoff introduced the concept that cellular as well as humoral mechanisms contribute to host defense mechanisms. During the latter part of the nineteenth century, he presented the macrophage as a cell with an important role in host defenses. Little could he have imagined the complexity of functions that have subsequently been identified with the macrophage.

The idea of cellular immunity had to overcome considerable skepticism. Even the nomenclature for cells of the macrophage series has caused controversy. It seems inappropriate to combine macrophages with endothelial cells, as in the term "reticuloendothelial system," even though these cells share some antigenic determinants (Moreas and Stasney, 1977). However, the phrase draws attention to the fact that some vascular channels are partially lined with macrophages. The "mononuclear phagocyte system" has been proposed to include promonocytes, monocytes and tissue macrophages (van Furth et al., 1972). This nomenclature fails to recognize that, under certain circumstances, some macrophages become multinuclear. It has become customary to refer to most lymphocytes as belonging to the T or B series. The "monocyte-macrophage series" is in keeping with this line of terminology and would not impose upon diverging opinions as to whether monocytes are ancestors or precursors of all macrophages.

The macrophage is a complex structure as is the diversity of synthetic and other functions. A comprehensive treatise on macrophage physiology is beyond the scope of this chapter. Instead, attention is focused upon selected recent information dealing primarily with the human monocyte-macrophage series.

Origins of Monocytes and Macrophages

Monocytes are derived from hematopoietic precursors (Volkman and Gowans, 1965a). The local microenvironment, which may include inductive mediators (Lee and Wong, 1980), probably determines to which cell type early precursors mature. Monocytopoiesis is more closely linked to granulopoiesis than to the differentiation of other bone marrow elements. Both monocytes and granulocytes participate in host defenses; both are represented in some acute leukemias and share some membrane antigens (Breard et al., 1980). Promonocytes in the normal bone marrow divide actively (Meuret, 1974; van Furth et al., 1979). Unlike granulocytes, most mature monocytes are released rapidly from the bone marrow after maturation.

The monocyte is an intermediate resident of the blood stream between bone marrow precursors and tissue macrophages. Monocytes may remain in the circulation for up to a week. The nuclei of monocytes become more indented with cell age (Meuret, 1974), but rapidly become rounded and pyknotic once they become tissue macrophages. However, the maturation and migration of marrow precursors to sites of tissue inflammation can take as little as 18 hours (Volkman and Gowans, 1965b). The majority of macrophages in inflammed tissues are derived from monocytes (Volkman and Gowans, 1965b; Spector et al., 1965; Dannenberg et al., 1972).

Tissue macrophages are also capable of significant cell division. Up to 15% of liver macrophages can be induced into mitosis (Kelly et al., 1962) and there is about a 2% turnover rate among peritoneal macrophages (Roser, 1970). Mobile peritoneal macrophages can enter the blood stream through the thoracic duct and are, therefore, an alternative source of tissue macrophages to monocytes. The situation is probably different with macrophages that are fixed in tissues such as Kupffer cells. An unlikely degree of synchronization between Kupffer cell senescence and mitosis by a neighboring cell would be necessary, if local cell division was to contribute significantly to the orderly replacement of fixed tissue macrophages. Indeed, most Kupffer cells are probably replaced by circulating monocytes.

Two polarized views have emerged regarding the origin of tissue macrophages. The simplest view is that all tissue macrophages are derived from monocytes. Obviously, that cannot be entirely true, since tissue macrophages do have some capacity to replicate. The alternative hypothesis is that there are two types of macrophage; one is derived from monocytes that primarily serve an auxiliary function at sites of inflammation and a second is a self-sustaining series of tissue macrophages. Proponents of the second theory point out that monocytes and macrophages are histochemically different (Ogawa et al., 1978) and that colony-forming precursors of monocytes in the bone marrow and macrophages in the peritoneal cavity differ in phagocytic and flotational characteristics (Lin et al., 1977).

In man, these views appear to be too rigid. The bone marrow alone certainly can replace the alveolar air spaces after they are depleted of macrophages by irradiation (Thomas et al., 1976). Nevertheless, replication in situ is also an important source of tissue macrophages. The alveolar air spaces, at least, do not become depleted of macrophages after prolonged bone marrow failure (Golde et al., 1974), presumably because of macrophage mitosis within the alveoli. A schema whereby potential sources are combined to maintain the monocyte-macrophage series is proposed in Figure 3.1. Circulating monocytes, which are divided into central and marginal pools, occupy a central position. Monocytes are derived from bone marrow precursors and undergo negligible cell division themselves. Re-entry of peritoneal macrophages into the blood stream via the thoracic duct probably accounts for a small and often overlooked number of circulating mononuclear phagocytes. Their mobility makes it useful to consider free macrophages in body cavities (e.g., peritoneal and pulmonary alveolar macrophages) as being a special compartment of the tissue macrophage pool. Both mobile and fixed tissue macrophages can be replaced in the resting state by monocyte migration or macrophage replication in the tissues. The exact contribution by either mechanism is not known and is likely to be variable. When inflammation sets in, there is need for rapid mobilization of phagocytes. Monocytes are strategically located for rapid deployment to inflammed tissues, where their numbers are further expanded by an acquired capacity for cell division. The circulating monocyte pool can be regarded as the reserve troops of the monocyte-macrophage series. Since inflammatory macrophages are largely derived from migrated monocytes, it is not surprising that most or all multinucleated phagocytes are derived from monocytes.

Membrane Antigens and Receptors

Identification of membrane antigens has added considerably to our understanding of lym-

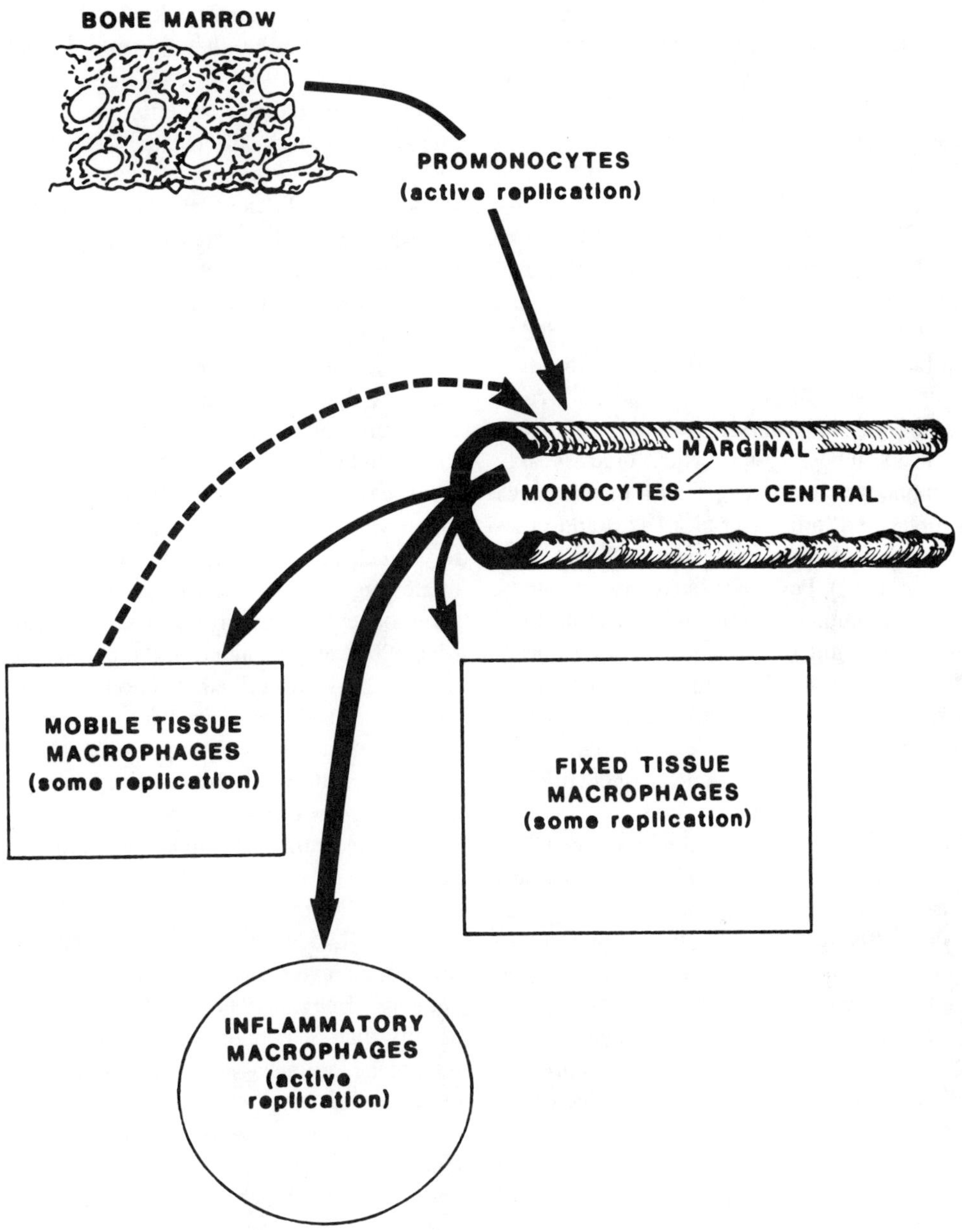

Fig. 3.1 A proposed schema of the compartments of the monocyte-macrophage series and how they are sustained.

phocyte subpopulations, their respective functions and changes in subpopulation mass with disease. Recent application of the hybridoma technique for developing monoclonal antibodies and use of cell sorters to separate subpopulations of lymphocytes have facilitated these studies. This approach appears equally applicable to the monocyte-macrophage series.

A monoclonal antibody, OKM-I, has been raised which reacts with about 80% of adherent mononuclear leukocytes and with granulocytes (Breard et al., 1980). It also reacts with null lymphoid cells engaged in natural killer cytotoxicity (Kay and Horowitz, 1980), but not with B or T lymphocytes or thymocytes. This is an IgG_{2_b} antibody which fixes complement and can eliminate monocytes involved in antigen presentation. However, it is distinct from membrane determinants that are related to immune response genes.

Capra's group have developed three monoclonal antibodies, 61-D3, 63-D2 and 63-D3, that also react with about 80% of adherent mononuclear leukocytes (Ugolini et al., 1980). Unlike OKM-I, these are IgG_1 antibodies and react weakly with granulocytes. They also react weakly with B lymphocytes. While they bind to most monocytes, they do not react with tissue macrophages (Capra, J.D., personal communication). This contrasts with the MI/70 antibody in the mouse system which binds weakly with monocytes but strongly with mouse tissue macrophages (Springer et al., 1979) and cross reacts with human monocytes (Ault and Springer, 1981). Perhaps these represent macrophage differentiation antigens analogous to T lymphocyte antigens that are expressed during different stages of their differentiation. Both 63-D2 and 63-D3 react with a 200,000-dalton membrane molecule, but it remains to be determined if they share the same antigen binding site.

Todd et al. (1981) recently introduced two additional monoclonal antibodies raised against normal adherent human mononuclear leukocytes. M0I reacted with null cells and granulocytes and as well as monocytes. Mϕ2 seemed to react only with monocytes. In the same issue of the Journal of Immunology, Haynes et al. (1981) described an IgG_{2_a} monoclonal antibody 4F2 to an antigen from a T cell culture line which reacted with monocytes, 70% of activated (but not resting) T lymphocytes and various cell lines; this seemed to be distinct from the DR system.

Mac-120 is yet another monoclonal antibody which reacts with slightly more than one-third of circulating monocytes (Raff et al., 1980). This may prove to have functional significance. Those monocytes that are Mac-120^+ stimulate in the autologous mixed leukocyte reaction, while those that are Mac-120^- stimulate in the allogenic mixed leukocyte reaction. The presence of Mac-120 is necessary for monocytes to initiate antigen-triggered T lymphocyte proliferation and lymphokine production, but not for the generation of interleukin I. This antibody reacts with a 105,000-dalton membrane antigen (Ugolini et al., 1980).

Obviously, antigenic determinants on macrophage membranes are the subject of intense investigation. The immediate goals are to find monoclonal antibodies that are reliably unique to macrophages and antisera that may subdivide macrophages into functionally distinct populations. Application of these reagents will facilitate macrophage isolation, quantitation and subpopulation analysis. Experience in related areas suggests that such antibodies will help chart membrane topography on macrophages. Since most studies employ circulating monocytes, these reagents will permit further comparison of monocytes with various tissue macrophages. So far, Mϕ2 and Mac-120 seem to be the most interesting probes. The former may be unique for monocytes, if not for macrophages, and Mac-120 seems to identify a subpopulation of monocytes with defined functional properties. There may soon be a need for a workshop in which the antigen specificity and the identity of cell types with which these various monoclonal antibodies react may be discussed.

The DR antigen group is believed to be a component of the human Ia complex. Both are products of immune response genes which comprise the HLA-D locus in man. (See Chapter 4.) Some monocytes and macrophages express Ia antigens (Engleman et al., 1980) at a lesser density than B lymphocytes. Expression of Ia membrane antigens is labile and can be regenerated, at least temporarily, through phagocytosis or exposure to antigens or mitogens (Beller et al., 1980). Macrophages bearing Ia antigens are attracted to specific locations through immunologic mechanisms, but not through simple inflammation (Beller et al., 1980). Homology at the HLA-D locus is crucial for optimal presentation of soluble antigens by macrophages to T lymphocytes (Rich et al., 1980). This homology may not be necessary for monocytes to mediate allogeneic mixed leukocyte reactions (Twomey et al., 1970). Indeed, disparity at the HLA-D locus is usually, but not consistently, necessary for stimulating mixed leukocyte reactions (Beller et al., 1980; Engleman et al., 1980).

Table 3.1 shows our experience with the frequency of five macrophage and two Ia antigens on normal monocyte membranes. Monocytes were concentrated to 80 to 90% purity by adherence to cold-insoluble globulin on gelatin-coated Petri dishes; antigens were demonstrated using monoclonal antibodies and ultraviolet microscopy. The majority expressed 61-D3, 63-D2, 63-D3 and OKM-I. Our experience with Mac-120 was similar to that of Raff et al. (1980). Ia heterogeneity is illustrated by the percentages of DR-3 and OKIa-positive monocytes. Flourescence was more brilliant with the OKIa than the DR-3 reagent. Only 20 to 50% of monocytes react with a third conjugate identified as p23, 30 (Breard et al., 1979).

Much remains to be learned about the relationship of Ia antigens to macrophage physiology. Do macrophages that lack these membrane markers but are similar in many other ways, such as the capacity for phagocytosis (Yamashita and Shevach, 1977), have relatively unique functions? It is known that masking DR antigens with antibody prevents macrophages from performing Ia-dependent functions (Breard et al., 1979). Do macrophages that no longer express Ia determinants differ from those that never express Ia antigens? What is unique about the mixed leukocyte reaction that makes macrophage-T lymphocyte homology unnecessary to provoke proliferative responses to alloantigens in contrast to other common antigens? What other determinants, if any, can substitute in part for membrane Ia in antigen presentation by macrophages?

Macrophage handling of foreign matter takes place within the cell. It has been known for a long time that antigen binding by opsonizing antibody enhances phagocytosis. Enhancement of phagocytosis is brought about by attachement of the Fc end of complexed antibodies to Fc receptors on macrophage membranes. There are at least three types of Fc receptor; one binds monomeric IgG_{2a}, a second binds complexed IgG_1, IgG_{2_a}, and IgG_{2_b} (Heusser et al., 1977) and a third, recently described, binds IgG_3 (Diamond and Yelton, 1981). Macrophages also bear complement receptors, components of which are likely to be bound to antigen-antibody complexes. One receptor binds the C_{3_c} end of C_{3_b} and a second binds the C_{3_d} fragment when cleaved from C_{3_b} (Ross and Polley, 1975). The former receptor also binds C_4. Both Fc and C_3 receptors appear at an early stage of monocyte differentiation (van Furth et al., 1979).

Material bound to macrophages through Fc receptors, but not through complement receptors, is rapidly ingested. The former, when presented to lymphocytes, triggers T cells to release a mediator which then promotes phagocytosis through complement attachment (Griffin and Griffin, 1980). This may have bearing upon why Fc and complement receptors are usually expressed on the same cells (Rabellino and Metcalf, 1975). Complement-mediated interiorization reduces by 100-fold the burden placed upon the Fc system to attain optimal phagocytosis (Ehlenberger and Nussenzweig, 1977). Macrophages are also capable of ingesting selected particles independent of receptor binding (Muschel et al., 1977).

Macrophages have receptors for cold-insoluble globulins which have also been termed fibronectin or $\alpha2$ surface binding glycoprotein (Doran et al., 1980; Bevilacqua et al., 1981). These trace plasma proteins also bind to collagen or fibrin, thereby forming bonds between macrophages and injured tissues. Cold-insoluble gobulins promote endocytosis, thus contributing to the clearing of extracellular particulate matter.

Activation, Endocytosis and Degradation

Macrophages exist in a resting or activated state. Activation is initiated experimentally by nonspecific substances such as glycogen, thioglycolate or phorbol myristic acetate, by microorganisms, including protozoa, bacteria or viruses and their products (most frequently *C. parvum* or mycobacterial products) or by mediators released by sensitized lymphocytes when challenged with antigens. There is variability in the functional expression of activation with different inducing agents (Moreland and Kaplan, 1977). Perhaps different subsets of

Table 3.1 Percentages of Cells in Concentrates of Human Blood Monocytes (84 ± 6% esterase positive) Bearing Monocyte-associated and Ia Antigens.

Marker Studied	Positive Monocytes, Mean ± SEM (%)
61-D3	84 ± 3
63-D2	85 ± 3
63-D3	83 ± 3
OKM-1	75 ± 3
Mac-120	35 ± 3
DR-3	77 ± 5
OKIa	58 ± 3

macrophages are induced selectively or responses are determined by the inducing agent. The reason for activation is to improve functional efficiency of the macrophage. Phagocytosis is enhanced and ingested microorganisms are disposed of more effectively (Ando et al., 1977). Yet, activation and phagocytosis are independent phenomena (Al-Ibrahim et al., 1978).

Macrophage activation involves a complex sequence of structural and metabolic events (Table 3.2). Membranes ready themselves for endocytosis by assuming a ruffled appearance and cannot refrain from ingesting surrounding body fluids through pinocytosis. These surface changes expose new membrane antigens (Kaplan and Mohanakumar, 1977) which, potentially, could be used to identify activated macrophages. The increased numbers of cytoplasmic mitochondria and lysosomes reflect the anticipated need for metabolic energy and degrading enzymes. At present, identification of macrophage activation is somewhat arbitrary and is quantitated histochemically, by increased ^{3}H-glucosamine uptake and oxidative metabolism, by reduced 5-nucleotidase or by chemiluminescence.

Endocytosis is the process whereby extracellular material is ingested by cells. Pinocytosis refers to the ingestion of liquid droplets and suspensions and phagocytosis denotes the interiorization of particles <100Å in diameter (Michl, 1980). Some particles, such as latex beads, are phagocytosed after simple contact with macrophage surfaces, while others, such as viable cells or encapsulated bacteria, first require attachment to receptors on macrophage membranes. For effective phagocytosis, it is necessary that the membranes of macrophages are flexible so that pseudopods can encircle particles and form vacuoles in which the particles are interiorized. Thus, there is considerable membrane loss and renewal by macrophages when they engage in active phagocytosis. The deformity at the surface is brought about through microfilaments that contain contractile proteins and requires metabolic energy. This energy is largely derived from adenosine triphosphate (ATP), which is generated through anaerobic glycolysis, the tricarboxylic cycle and creatine phosphate. Phagocytic activity is determined both by particle and receptor density and is modulated by lymphokines (A1-Ibrahim et al., 1978).

Inactivation and degradation of ingested microorganisms by macrophages and granulocytes are crucial to host defenses against infections. Prior immunity to the microorganism in question is probably irrelevant to this final intracellular step (McLeod and Remington, 1977), although the overall process whereby macrophages eliminate microorganisms is positively influenced by being immunologically sensitized (Luria, 1942). The process has two components: direct attack by lysosomal enzymes and generation of OH^- radicals which are powerful oxidants. The number of cytoplasmic lysosomes is increased with macrophage activation with or without phagocytosis (Dean et al., 1979). Lysosomal enzymes include lysozyme, hydrolases and neutral proteases. The latter two are released into the extracellular fluid during phagocytosis where they probably contribute to local inflammation and are exemplified clinically by gout.

Oxidation involves the generation of superoxide, that is, oxygen doublets minus one electron (O_2^-, and hydrogen peroxide (H_2O_2). Like lysosomal enzyme release, O_2^- production is triggered by macrophage activation and does not require phagocytosis (Johnston et al., 1976). Superoxide is unstable and its dissociation is registered by chemiluminescence. Thus, chemiluminescence is used to identify macrophage activation. Superoxide is needed for H_2O_2 generation, which in turn produces OH^- radicals the oxidant capacity of which is toxic to micro-

Table 3.2 Structural and Functional Changes Associated with Macrophage Activation.

Morphological Changes	Metabolic Changes
1. Membrane ruffling	1. Acelerated oxidative metabolism
2. Spreading	2. Superoxide (O_2^-) generation
3. Increased pinocytosis	3. H_2O_2 production
4. More mitochondria	4. Lysosomal enzyme release
5. More phagosomes, lysosomes and phagolysosomes	5. 5-Nucleotidase depletion

organisms (Johnston et al., 1975; Sagone et al., 1976). The capcity to generate both O_2^- and H_2O_2 is crucial to microbicidal competence.

Secretory Products of the Macrophage

Macrophages have a remarkable repertoire of secretory products (Nathan et al., 1980). These include lysosomal enzymes, enzyme inhibitors, cold-insoluble globulin, many complement components, mediators, interferon and products of arachidonic acid, metabolism such as prostaglandins. It remains to be determined whether all or only subpopulations of macrophages generate each of these products. Certainly, only some monocytes seem capable of prostaglandin synthesis (Picker et al., 1980). A treatise on this subject is beyond the scope of this chapter.

Prostaglandins

The polyunsaturated fatty acid, arachidonic acid is substrate for both the cyclo-oxygenase and lipoxygenase biosynthetic pathways. The former generates thromboxanes and prostaglandins (Pg) and the latter generates HETE which may be chemotactic for granulocytes. The monocyte-macrophage series is an important, but not the only, source of Pg, the most important of which are PgE_1, PgE_2 and $PgF_2\alpha$. It appears that membrane lipid, once interiorized, is a major source of substrate of Pg synthesis, provided it has access to lysosomal enzymes that effect the cyclo-oxygenase sequence (Brune et al., 1978). Thus, nonspecific (Farzad et al., 1977) or mediator (Friedman et al., 1979) provoked activation of macrophages increases their subsequent release of Pg.

In general, Pg of the E series and $PgF_2\alpha$ have opposing actions which are influenced by Pg concentrations. PgE tends to suppress a broad range of immune responses both in vivo and in vitro (Goldyne, 1977). This suppressor system, which involves cyclic AMP generation and inhibition of DNA synthesis, is discussed further in Chapter 8. $PgF_2\alpha$ amplifies immune responses in association with cyclic GMP generation, except at high concentrations, when it is also inhibitory.

These prostaglandins modulate inflammatory responses directly. PgE causes vasodilation, increased vascular permeability and increased sensitivity of pain receptors (Westurek, 1979; Tyers and Haywood, 1979). This serves as a rationale for treating chronic inflammatory disorders with drugs that inhibit cyclo-oxygenase (e.g., indomethacin). On the other hand, $PgF_2\alpha$ has the opposite effect and promotes wound healing. The augmentation of Pg synthesis that accompanies macrophage activation produces more $PgF_2\alpha$ than PgE. Since macrophages arrive relatively late at sites of tissue inflammation, the net effect of the Pg they release could be beneficial.

Interferons

These are glycoproteins made by cells in response to various stimuli including viruses. Classical interferon Type I is made by the monocyte-macrophage series, but only when stimulated to do so. The more potent immune interferon, Type II, is made by lymphocytes but requires macrophage participation (Roberts et al., 1979). This interaction probably does not involve Ia antigens, since allogeneic and syngeneic monocytes are equally effective (Epstein, 1976). However, the target cells for the effects of interferon are relatively species specific.

Interferon has attracted considerable attention because of its therapeutic potential in such important areas as cancer and viral infections, yet its net biologic effect remains uncertain. We know that interferon inactivates viruses, but it does so indirectly through cellular mechanisms and has some antitumor activity. The latter could result from inactivation of viral material needed to perpetuate the neoplastic process or from inhibition of DNA synthesis by the malignant cells. Conversely, cell division is crucial for many immune responses that may be important to host defenses, including resistance to neoplasms. The effects of interferon upon macrophages are complex and include activation and enhanced phagocytosis (Huang, 1977), but also include reduction of macrophage spreading on plastic and release of lysosomal enzymes (Lee and Epstein, 1980). It seems paradoxical that virus infection stimulates monocytes to release interferon, which then helps overcome the infection but may impair other parameters of macrophage function such as those that participate in immune responses (vide infra). Macrophages are also capable of inhibiting viral infections through a second poorly understood mechanism, that involves direct contact between macrophages and infected cells but does not involve interferon (Morse and Monahan, 1981).

Interleukins

These mediators act in sequence to bring about T lymphocyte responses. Interleukin I, or lymphocyte activating factor, is a molecule of about 14,000 daltons (Koopman et al., 1977) that is released by monocytes and macrophages. It is spontaneously released in small quantitites and in much larger amounts when macrophages are activated by such agents as lipopolysaccharide or phorbol myristic acetate. This monokine is also generated by immunologically activated T cells (Mizel et al., 1978). This stimulus by activated T cells requires cell-cell contact and, therefore, cannot be ascribed simply to macrophage activation by a factor released from T cells, such as macrophage activating factor. It has been observed that macrophages release unusually large amounts of interleukin I when derived from nude athymic mice (Meltzer and Oppenheim, 1977). Perhaps T lymphocytes also exercise negative regulatory control over the release of interleukin I.

Interleukin I, together with lectin or antigen, stimulates a subset of T lymphocytes to release interleukin II, which was previously called T cell growth factor (Smith et al., 1980). The generation of interleukin II may be the site at which antigen specificity is determined (Farrar et al., 1980) and operates late in the sequence that ends with effector T cell activation. However, other agents, such as phorbol myristic acetate, or 6-mercaptoethanol in some systems, can activate effector T lymphocytes directly and thus bypass the interleukin sequence. It is not known if these agents operate through similar receptors or mechanisms to activate macrophages and the final effector T cells, activate effector T cells similarly to interleukin II or have a counterpart in vivo. Such a direct form of T cell activation would obviate the need for macrophages or interleukin II-generating T cells, but would be unlikely to impose specificity upon T lymphocyte activation. The latter could be germane to autoimmunity.

Macrophage-Lymphocyte Interactions

The macrophage has an essential role in the effector limb of the immune response. It imposes stringent genetic restrictions through DR determinants upon critical macrophage interactions with lymphocytes, but leaves it to clonal selection of lymphocytes to give specificity to immune responses. Interactions between macrophages and lymphocytes are complex and involve both cell-cell contact and remote interchanges brought about through mediators. This section deals with antigen presentation by macrophages and signals transmitted between macrophages and lymphocytes through mediators. An intricate sequence emerges which is not yet completely understood.

Only a small fraction of available antigen is taken up by macrophages. Antigen that remains in the vicinity of the macrophage membrane is relatively stable, but most cytoplasmic antigen is rapidly degraded by lysosomal enzymes, causing it to lose immunogenicity (Rosenthal et al., 1976). Yet, macrophage-associated antigen is considerably more immunogenic than cell-free antigen (Unanue, 1980).

Both T and B lymphocytes make direct membrane contact with macrophages (Lipsky and Rosenthal, 1975). Contact can take place in the absence of antigen and when macrophages and lymphocytes differ at the major histocompatibility locus (Albrecht et al., 1978). However, lymphocyte clones that recognize specific antigens selectively attach to macrophages bearing the antigen in question (Todd et al., 1980) and only syngeneic attached lymphocytes migrate over macrophage membranes to form clusters. Perhaps surface interactions between macrophages and lymphocytes take two forms. One requires the presence of macrophage-associated antigen, a clone of lymphocytes that recognize that particular antigen and syngeny at the immune response gene locus. Alternatively, macrophages and lymphocytes may interact to a limited extent in a nonspecific fashion, the significance of which is presently not known.

The delivery of antigenic signals to responsive lymphocytes is a major responsibility of macrophages. Is this an unique property of macrophages or do macrophages simply serve to immobilize antigen? Antigen bound to fibroblasts is also capable of transferring the antigenic challenge (Katz and Unanue, 1973). However, lymphocyte preparations used in these experiments also included macrophages which could have served as intermediaries between carrier fibroblasts and reactive lymphocytes. Antigen immobilized on plastic does not activate lymphocytes. Oppenheim and Seeger (1976) concluded that lymphocyte activation generally required the presentation of antigen by macrophages.

The topography of antigen presentation remains uncertain. The presence of antigen seems to be essential to maintain membrane contact between macrophages and lymphocytes (Ben-Sasson et al., 1978). Yet, coating of membrane-associated antigen with antibody or its removal with trypsin does not interfere with subsequent macrophage-lymphocyte membrane interactions. The simplest explanation is that cytoplasmic antigen relocates and takes the place of the original membrane antigen. Alternatively, responsive lymphocytes receive the antigenic signal from trypsinized macrophages by means of cytoplasmic channels that open up between contacting macrophages and lymphocytes (Schoenberg et al., 1964).

This issue is crucial to understanding the mooring of lymphocytes to macrophages. If cell contact is maintained in the absence of surface antigen, then other membrane determinants such as Ia are what bind macrophages to lymphocytes. In that case, macrophage-associated antigen would participate only in attracting and activating responsive clones of lymphocytes. However, it seems more likely that membrane-associated antigen, perhaps supplemented by cytoplasmic antigen, does participate in macrophage-lymphocyte binding. Macrophage-associated antigen and macrophage Ia determinants may serve as covalent but distinct bonds for lymphocyte attachment. Alternatively, a complex of immunogen and Ia determinants may form a new structure on the surface of macrophages that promotes attachment and activation of lymphocytes. The latter possibility is favored by the ability to inhibit lymphocyte activation by macrophage-associated antigen when antibody to DR determinants is added late during the antigen determination process (Thomas et al., 1980).

The presentation of antigen by macrophages is clearly essential to initiate T lymphocyte responses (Twomey et al., 1970; Todd et al., 1980). This is illustrated using the mixed leukocyte reaction in Figure 3.2. Using lymphocytes that were severely depleted of monocytes by incubation in cotton-packed syringes, irradiated lymphocytes from one donor were unable to stimulate ^{3}H-thymidine incorporation by lymphocytes from an allogeneic donor. A small number of monocytes adherent to a glass cover slip (Mϕ slip) were not themselves stimulatory but did mediate a brisk response between the paired lymphocyte preparations. Our tech-

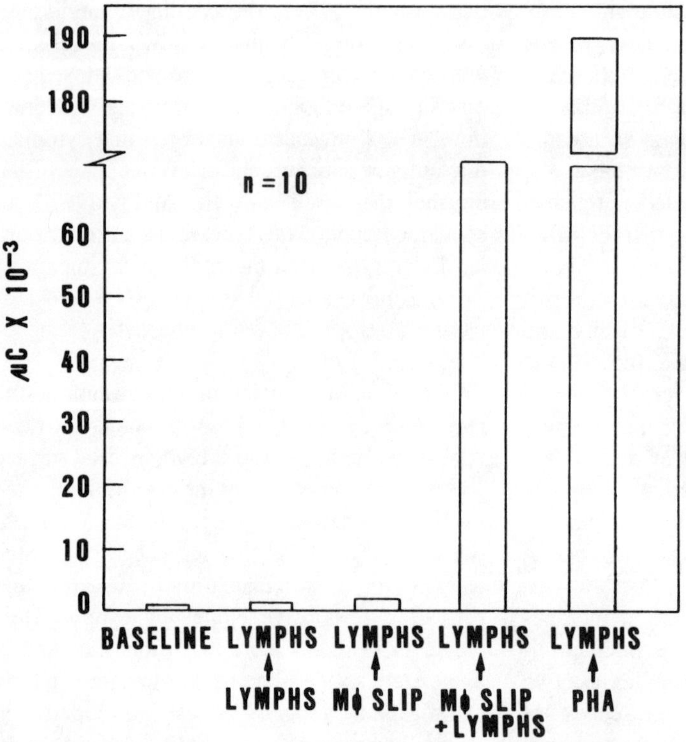

Fig. 3.2 Evidence that help from monocytes is needed for a mixed leukocyte reaction. Since responses occurred, the paired donors were obviously not compatible, which illustrates the absence of HLA-D restriction of macrophage participation. Mϕ slip: monocytes adherent to a glass coverslip.

nique did not deplete monocytes sufficiently to eliminate PHA-stimulated T cell proliferation.

Most antibody responses require a variable degree of T cell participation. Figure 3.3 illustrates the cell interactions needed for an antibody response to a hapten-protein antigen. For simplicity, the antigen is arbitrarily located on top of the DR determinant. Current evidence suggests that the hapten is presented to the B cell and the carrier protein to the T cell (Kunin et al., 1972). The T cell is then activated and releases T cell replacing factor (TRF) or interleukin II, which is needed for the B cell to release antibody. The literature remains inconsistent on the need for macrophage presentation of antigen to B cells in T cell-independent antibody responses. It has been reported that macrophages are not needed (Mosier et al., 1974), are needed at lower concentrations (Gorczynski, 1976) or are needed at comparable concentrations (Chused et al., 1976) to what is necessary for T cell responses. Obviously, the efficiency of macrophage depletion of B lymphocyte preparations and the use of different antigens and culture systems could account for this variable experience. It does seem that greater ''processing'' of antigen by macrophages is needed to render antigen immunogenic to T cells than to B cells (Pearson and Raffel, 1971).

A number of events have been identified during the course of immune responses. A sequence for these events is proposed herein. This sequence includes three phases: Phase A) presentation of immunogenic antigen by macrophages, Phase B) expansion of macrophage participation by activated lymphocytes and Phase C) mediator plus antigen initiation of the immune response. No doubt this outline, parts of which are still poorly understood, will need further modification.

Phase A commences with the attachment and phagocytosis of foreign matter by macrophages (Fig. 3.4). This is accomplished through direct contact or through various receptors on macrophage membranes. At this stage, complement receptors attach antigen but do not mediate interiorization. Once ingested, microorganisms are inactivated, particles are broken down and im-

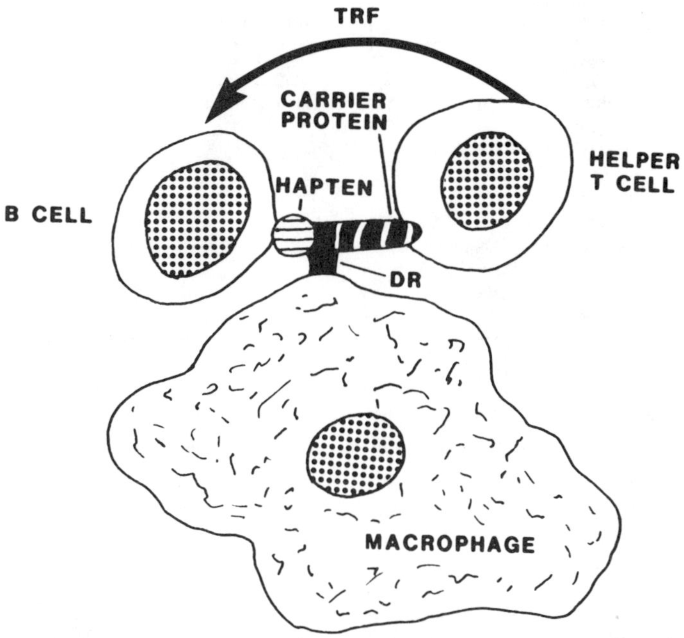

Fig. 3.3 A schematic outline of all interactions involved in antibody responses to hapten-protein antigens. The antigen is arbitrarily placed on top of a DR determinant on the macrophage membrane. TRF: T cell replacing factor (which probably equates with interleukin-2).

munogenic antigen is produced. Macrophage participation does not require prior sensitization, but does call for genetic similarity at the HLA-D locus for contact interactions to take place with lymphocytes. This phase ends with activation of antigen-specific clones of lymphocytes.

Phase B primarily involves mobilization of further macrophage participation in immune responses through mediators released from lymphocytes activated during Phase A. Certain anatomical locations, such as the peritoneal cavity, are relatively deficient in macrophages bearing Ia antigens (Beller et al., 1980), which are crucial for antigen presentation to lymphocytes. Activated T cells recruit additional Ia^+ macrophages to sites of immune reactivity (Beller et al., 1980). Secondly, T cells activated by antigen that are ingested by macrophages through Fc receptor attachment release a mediator that permits ingestion of antigen that is otherwise marooned on the surface of macrophages attached through complement receptors. As a result, the efficiency of phagocytosis and antigen presentation is improved (Ehlenberger and Nussenzweig, 1977). Looking forward, T cells activated during Phase A of the immune response probably prime macrophages to take part in Phase C of the immune response. Activated T cells attract macrophages to sites of immune reactions through the release of macrophage chemotactic factor (MCF). Once macrophages reach the desired location, further ambulation is halted by macrophage migration inhibitory factor (MIF). The net effect is an accumulation of macrophages for further involvement in the immune response. In addition, activated lymphocytes release macrophage activation factor (MAF).

It is known that the presence of macrophages is necessary for T cells to proliferate and release MIF (Twomey et al., 1970; Wahl et al., 1975). Since many events are taking place at the same time, that does not necessarily mean that proliferation as well as contact with antigen-bearing macrophages is needed for T cells to produce at least some lymphokines. However, it does seem that membrane interaction between macrophages and T cells is needed to get macrophages to release interleukin I in response to antigens (Mizel et al., 1978). That is included at the end of Phase A in Figure 3.4.

Antigen-activated T lymphocytes induce macrophages to release interleukin I, thereby initiating Phase C of the immune response (Hoffman, 1980). In the presence of antigen, interleukin I activates a responsive group of T lym-

Table 3.3 Evidence for Heterogeneity among Macrophages.

Evidence	References
1. Quantity, quality and location of cytoplasmic enzymes	Gordon et al., 1974; Ogawa et al., 1978; Fishman and Weinberg, 1979; Allen et al., 1980
2. Prostaglandin E secretion	Picker et al., 1980
3. Phagocytic potential	Wisse, 1974
4. Membrane Fc receptors	Muschel et al., 1977; Norris et al., 1979
5. Presentation of carbohydrate-hapten carriers	Gorczynski et al., 1979
6. Capacity to express Ia antigen	Beller and Unanue, 1980, 1981
7. Expression of Mac-120 antigen	Raff et al., 1980
8. Separate participation in helping or suppressing immune responses	Lee et al., 1979; Twomey et al., unpublished

phocytes (Farrar et al., 1980) and expands the pool of antibody producing B cells. T lymphocytes thus activated induce final expression of preactivated T cell immunity through the release of interleukin II (Smith et al., 1980) and support antibody responses through the release of T cell replacing factor which is probably identical to interleukin II. Thus, the final step in various T cell responses results from signals from a different set of T cells and does not involve macrophages. The proliferation that follows is needed for the final expression of T cell immunity (Maryanski et al., 1980).

Macrophage Heterogeneity

It has been established that lymphocytes belong in discrete subpopulations with distinct functions. Evidence that quantitative changes in these lymphocyte subpopulations occur with various disorders has attracted considerable interest. Functions ascribed to the monocyte-macrophage series are also complex. The possibility that these cells belong to separate subpopulations with individual sets of functions and that the distribution of cells among these populations may be distorted with disease deserves consideration.

Heterogeneity among macrophages could result from their origination from bone marrow or tissue precursors, the anatomical location of the cells, whether macrophages are in a resting or activated state and if the latter is triggered through immune or nonspecific mechanisms or intrinsic clonal differences within the overall series. Earlier sections discussed apparent differences between monocyte and tissue macrophages and changes that take place when macrophages are activated. There is no doubt that macrophages from various anatomical locations differ in their enzyme content (Fishman and Weinberg, 1979) and in membrane expression of Ia (Beller and Unanue, 1980) and macrophage-associated (Springer et al., 1979) antigens. This could reflect local environmental influences or homing patterns of discrete macrophage subpopulations.

There is more peroxidase in relatively dense than in more buoyant macrophages (Fishman and Weinberg, 1979) (Table 3.3). This enzyme is also richer in tissue macrophages than in macrophages derived from monocytes (Ogawa et al., 1978). The isozymes of dipeptidyl aminopeptidase differ in peritoneal and pulmonary alveolar macrophages (Allen et al., 1980). It is possible to separate monocytes that do and do not secrete PgE according to their buoyant density (Picker et al., 1980). The capacity for phagocytosis varies in different anatomical locations (Wisse, 1974) and with the degree of macrophage activation. The membranes of larger monocytes contain a greater density of Fc receptors than do the smaller monocytes (Norris et al., 1979), but that may be a product of cell size rather than a marker for discrete subpopulations (Muschel et al., 1977). While macrophage specificity has not been observed with hapten-protein antigens, different subsets of macrophages may be needed to present haptens complexed with various carbohydrate carriers (Gorczynski et al., 1979). Percentages of macrophages displaying surface Ia antigen vary

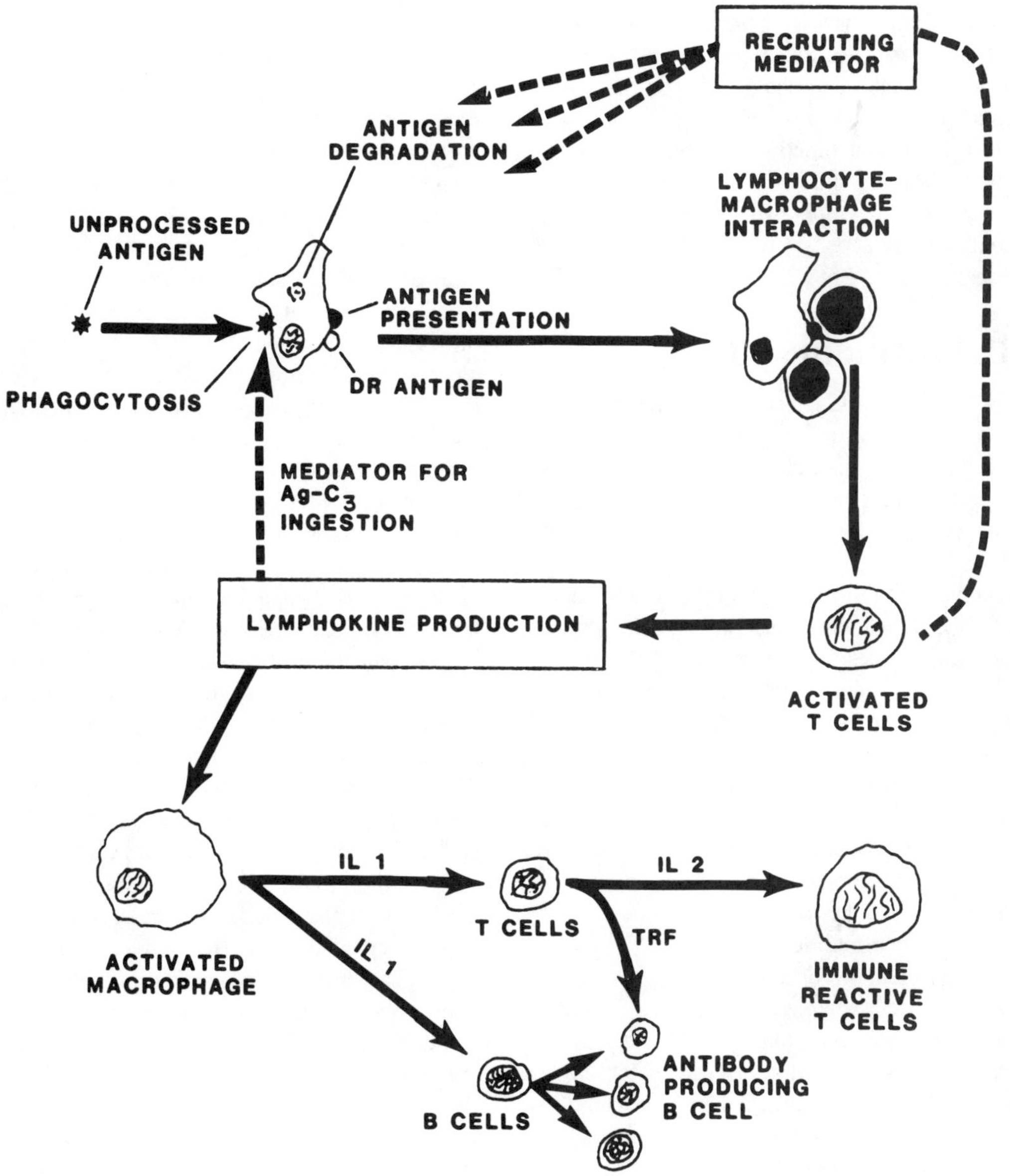

Fig. 3.4 A proposed sequence of cell-cell interactions and mediator production for T or B cell immune responses.

from tissue to tissue (Beller and Unanue, 1980). In addition, the capacity to express Ia antigen is limited to selected subpopulations of macrophages (Beller and Unanue, 1980). Recent evidence that Mac-120$^+$ macrophages have unique functional characteristics (Raff et al., 1980) raises hope that future application of hybridoma technique can separate important subpopulations within the monocyte-macrophage series incisively.

Macrophages exercise powerful regulatory influence over immune responses both in the form of help and suppression. On the surface, this appears contradictory if individual cells can provide both opposing effects. Recent evidence suggests that help and suppression are exercised by different macrophage populations. It is possible to separate macrophages that support and inhibit T lymphocytotoxicity using velocity sedimentation (Lee et al., 1979). Using expansion of human bone marrow colonies in agar into a liquid phase, we have produced preliminary evidence that macrophages of specified lineage either help or suppress. However, this may not be a permanent functional commitment in that those lines that initially helped changed to being inhibitory to lymphocyte responses after prolonged culture.

Impairments of Antimicrobial Function

Macrophages participate in host defenses through direct inactivation of microorganisms and participation in immune responses. The antimicrobial capacity of macrophages can be compromised in a number of ways. Attachment of foreign matter to macrophage membranes, which precedes ingestion, may be impaired. Phagocytosis and subsequent degradation by lysosomal contents is reduced by reticuloendothelial blockade caused by prior engorgement of macrophages by ingested material. Macrophages may be unable to inactivate ingested microorganisms because of defective oxidative metabolism. Degradation of ingested material may be hindered by structural lysosomal abnormalities.

Attachment of opsonized foreign matter is compromised when serum levels of immune complexes are elevated (Fig. 3.5). Presumably, this results in saturation of Fc receptor sites on macrophages by complexed immunoglobulins. This is found with systemic lupus erythematosus (Frank et al., 1979), rheumatoid arthritis (Williams et al., 1979) and other diseases. Here, clearance of foreign matter via Fc receptors is compromised to a degree that is proportional to the level of circulating immune complexes. Attachment of foreign matter to macrophages by $C3_b$ receptors is impaired with primary biliary cirrhosis (Jaffe et al., 1978). Reticuloendothelial clearance is reduced when serum levels of cold-insoluble globulin are reduced, as occurs with hemorrhage, tissue damage or cancer (Doran et al., 1980). The biologic significance of cold-insoluble globulin deficiency is not known. The efficiency of the reticuloendothelial system is further compromised with cancer by elevated levels of immune complexes and other substances produced by tumor cells that inhibit phagocytosis (Saito and Tomioka, 1980). Thus, phagocytosis and inactivation of *C. pseudotropicalis,* and probably other agents, is defective with Hodgkin's disease (van Loon et al., 1979). It has been well established that, with clinical conditions such as those outlined above, where attachment of particulate matter to macrophages is reduced, reticuloendothelial clearance is also impaired. The degree to which these conditions compromise overall host defense mechanisms is less clearly defined.

Reticuloendothelial blockade occurs after macrophages become engorged with ingested material. This is well illustrated by the various storage diseases. These stuffed macrophages have a reduced capacity for phagocytosis and lack specific enzymes needed to degrade the ingested substances because demand exceeds the capacity of the cell to generate additional enzyme (Kolodny, 1972). Thus, there are at least two components to reticuloendothelial blockade. Reticuloendothelial clearance is reduced with hyperlipidemic states such as myxedema and the Kimmelstein-Wilson syndrome (Drivas and Wardle, 1978). Reticuloendothelial blockade has been postulated as the underlying pathophysiology. However, reversible coating of macrophage membrane receptors with lipids may also compromise macrophage function (Waddell et al., 1976). Pulmonary alveolar proteinosis is an interesting example of reticuloendothelial blockade that is localized to involved pulmonary tissues (Harris, 1979). With reticuloendothelial blockade, the ingested material impairs further phagocytosis by the engorged macrophages. In addition, the lysosomal system is overburdened by the work at hand, causing degranulation and depletion of degrading enzymes. It can, therefore, be considered as an overburdening of the reticuloendothelial system except when there are specific enzyme deficiencies as found with storage disorders.

Normally, phagocytosed material appears in vacuoles which fuse with lysosomes. Lysosomal enzymes then degrade the ingested material. Storage disorders exemplify faulty phagolysosome degradation due to specific enzyme deficiencies. Phagolysosomal degradation is also impaired when there is faulty fusion of phagocytic vacuoles and lysosomes, as occurs with the Chediak-Higachi syndrome (Root et al., 1972). The primary defect involves lysosome structure; these organelles are greatly enlarged, have double membranes and fuse poorly with phagosomes (White and Clawson, 1979). Both monocytes and granulocytes are affected.

The importance of oxidative metabolism to inactivating ingested microorganisms has been emphasized. At least two distinct impairments of oxidation exist which compromise host defenses. The hexose monophosphate shunt has a crucial role in oxidative metabolism and is regulated in part by the lysosomal enzyme myeloperoxidase. Myeloperoxidase deficiency occurs as a rare autosomal recessive congenital defect involving monocytes and granulocytes, but not eosinophils (Lehner and Cline, 1969). Occasionally, as an acquired abnormality, it may accompany myelomonocytic leukemia (Kitahara and Kushner, 1979). Phagocytic cells from these patients (who clinically manifest susceptibility to infections) kill candida species, staphylococci, *S. marcescens* and probably other microorganisms poorly. Defective oxidative metabolism involving the hexose monophosphate shunt is also the basis for impaired intra-

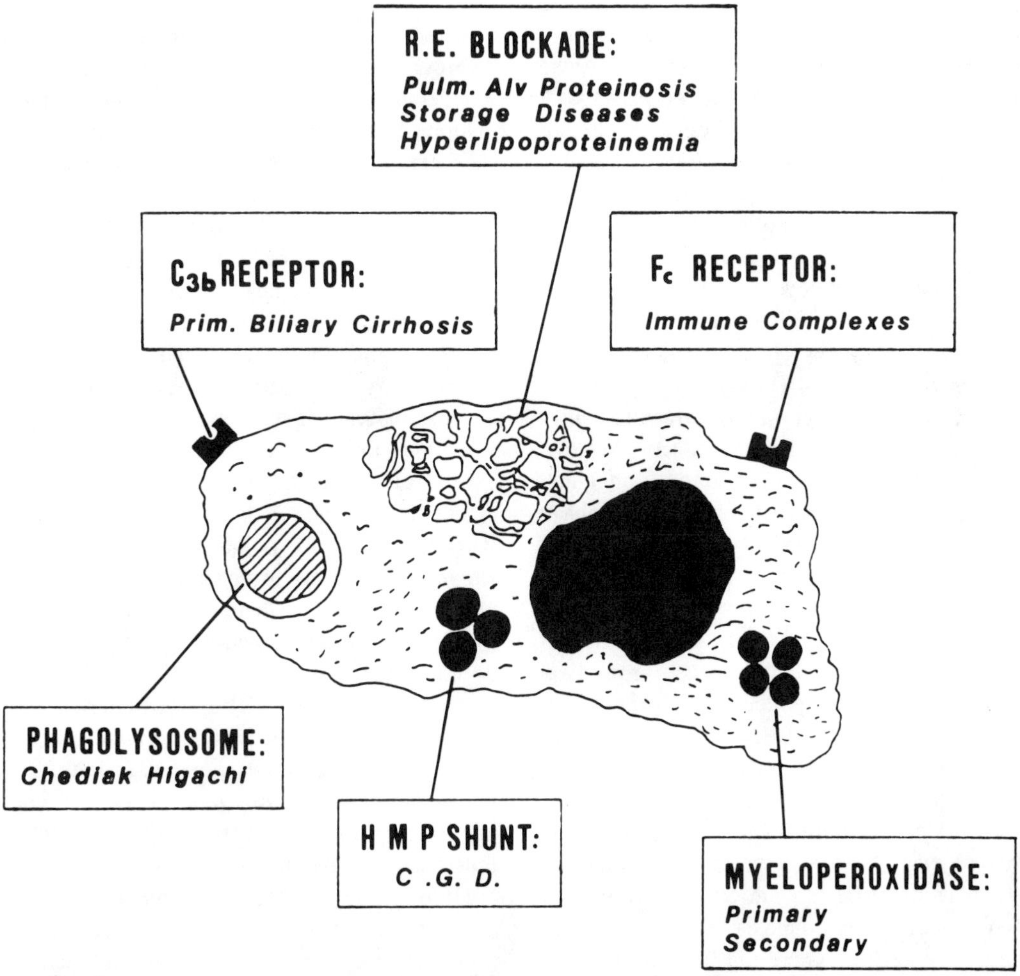

Fig. 3.5 An outline of various defined sites of macrophage dysfunction that could compare the ability of macrophages to resist microbial invasion.

cellular killing of microorganisms with fatal granulomatous disease of children (Rodey et al., 1969). This is clearly a distinct syndrome from myeloperoxidase deficiency (Pegram et al., 1978). Obviously, alternative mechanisms, such as degradation of microorganisms by hydrolytic enzymes or inactivation by cationic proteins, are not sufficient to compensate for defective oxidation.

Impairments in the Effector Limb of the Immune Response

The macrophage plays a crucial role in antigen presentation and lymphocyte activation. The complexity of this participation and its propensity to ingest cytopathic pathogens leaves the macrophage vulnerable. When compared with the long list of known lymphocyte disorders, there are remarkably few disease states that can be ascribed directly to macrophages. These disorders can be divided into defective helper participation in lymphocyte activation, excessive suppresion of lymphocyte responses and malignant proliferation. This section deals primarily with impaired macrophage participation in lymphocyte responses. The issue of suppression is addressed in Chapter 8 and histiocytic malignancies are discussed in Chapter 12.

Surprisingly, I am unaware of any congenital immunodeficiency caused by a macrophage disorder. Acquired deficits could be quantitative, as occurs with reduced monocytopoiesis due to bone marrow failure, or functional due to inactivation or cell injury. Ideally, such abnormalities are identified and placed in clinical perspective when the patient demonstrates susceptibility to infection, delayed cutaneous responses are impaired and macrophage participation in lymphocyte responses in vitro is defective. Unfortunately, these criteria are rarely met. Perhaps, the biggest problem involves extrapolating from laboratory data. Monocyte yields in blood mononuclear cell preparations vary considerably. There may be considerable monocyte loss through adherence to containers, if cells are left at room temperature for considerable periods. Most culture systems employ fixed numbers of lymphocytes per unit volume. Thus, relatively large numbers of monocytes are added to cultures with lymphopenia and their concentration is greatly lowered through dilution by lymphocytes with lymphocytosis or lymphocytic leukemia (Twomey and Douglass, 1974). Finally, tests of monocyte function are usually limited to one reaction, with lymphoproliferation being employed most frequently. These studies could overlook more circumscribed impairments involving other responses.

As might be expected, blood from patients with severe aplastic anemia is monocytopenic (Twomey et al., 1973). This monocytopenic blood contains insufficient monocyte concentrations to mediate mixed lymphocyte reactions in culture. Since this is an absolute monocyte deficiency, this could also compromise host defenses in vivo, especially when monocyte mobilization is needed at sites of tissue inflammation. Those macrophages that persist in tissues after replinishment from the bone marrow is interrupted remain functionally intact (Gales and Morley, 1980), but contribute little toward the increased numbers needed when inflammation sets in. While some anatomical sites seem capable of maintaining a normal macrophage mass through replication in situ (Golde et al., 1974), other tissues are not and mobilization of additional macrophages to these sites is reduced with bone marrow failure (Gales and Morley, 1980). This may have bearing upon the increased prevalence of anergy among patients with bone marrow failure (Libansky, 1969). However, the overall impact of monocytopenia upon host defenses is hard to determine. Monocytopenia is accompanied by granulocytopenia of comparable severity with aplastic anemia (Twomey et al., 1973). Thus, the high risk from infections with aplastic anemia could result from granulocytopenia, monocytopenia or both. The monocyte series remains intact with fatal congenital neutropenia (L'Esperance et al., 1975), indicating that neutropenia per se can severely compromise resistance to infections. Unfortunately, we have no counterpart for the monocyte-macrophage series. Perhaps such abnormalities are determined by lethal genetic defects.

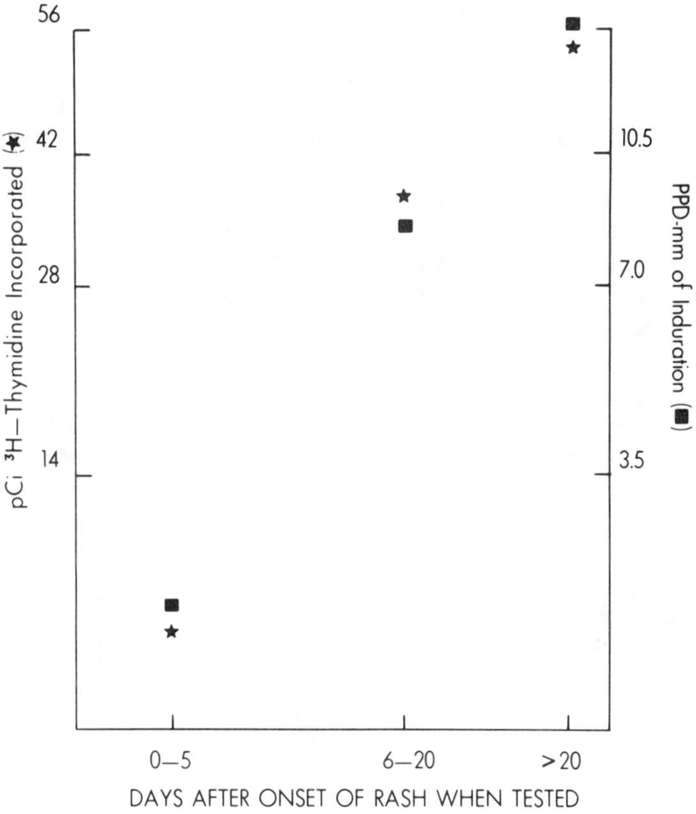

Fig. 3.6 The ability of monocytes from patients with idiopathic herpes zoster to mediate mixed lymphocyte reactions. (N = 4) and the magnitude of delayed hypersensitivity responses in vivo by tuberculous patients with measles (N = 10). Period of observation dates from the first recognition of rash. The close temporal relationship between recovery of in vitro and in vivo responses during convalescence is evident.

The concept that a battle of uncertain outcome takes place between macrophages and ingested virulent microorganisms helps understand the pathophysiology of intracellular infections. Macrophages that are killed by tubercle bacilli disintegrate forming the basis for caseation. Less injured cells assume the morphology of "epitheloid" cells. Thus, granulomatous responses to intracellular bacteria give considerable bulk to the lesions of these infections.

Viral infections often cause reversible blunting of immune responses. Transient cutaneous anergy has been observed during influenza (Reed et al., 1972), measles (Bentzon, 1953) and infectious mononucleosis (Haider et al., 1973). Lymphoproliferative responses to mitogens and antigens in culture are temporarily reduced with various viral illnesses. These include rubella (Montgomery et al., 1967), herpes zoster (Twomey et al., 1974), infectious mononucleosis (Twomey, 1974) and measles (Coovadia et al., 1977). Proliferative responses by normal leukocytes are also impaired when cultures are infected with virus (Sullivan et al., 1975; van Loon et al., 1979). Chemotoxic responsiveness of monocytes is impaired during influenza infections (Kleinerman et al., 1975). Macrophage dysfunction contributes to the proliferative hyporesponsiveness of cultured lymphocytes during viral illnesses (Twomey et al., 1974; Twomey, 1974). This has been related to the presence of virus within cultured monocytes. Probably, cytopathic virus interferes with normal monocyte function. Perhaps, suppressor, as well as helper, macrophage function is impaired by ingested viruses. Impaired macrophage-related suppression could contribute to various autoimmune epiphenomena that sometimes accompany viral illnesses.

Figure 3.6 examines the relationship between macrophage dysfunction in vitro and cutaneous anergy during convalescence from viral infections. The capacity of monocytes from four patients with herpes zoster to mediate mixed leukocyte responses by normal allogenic lymphocytes was compared with delayed cutaneous responses to tuberculin by 10 tuberculous patients with measles. It is evident that both cell culture and skin test responses were severely impaired when tested within the first 5 days after rash was noticed. Both responses improved, but did not normalize until the fourth week. The close relationship between in vitro and in vivo data is apparent. It is also noteworthy that the clinical setting was provided by two different viral infections. However, that might not be generally applicable, since viruses can survive and replicate with variable ease within macrophages (Drew et al., 1979). That, too, is clinically relevant in that tissues are most susceptible to infection with viruses that macrophages eliminate poorly. Thus, transient macrophage dysfunction is a major factor in the cause of immunologic impairment with virus infections. However, other factors, such as lymphocyte abnormalities and circulating immune inhibitors, may also contribute (Coovadia et al., 1977; Whittle et al., 1978).

Summary

Metchnikoff experienced difficulty in getting the macrophage recognized as a cell of importance to host defense mechanisms. A century later, it is no longer possible to do justice to all the contributions made by the macrophage to host defenses within the confines of a single chapter. The capacity of macrophages to attack other cells directly is found in Chapter 12, in which its potential importance to cellular resistance to neoplasms is discussed. The negative effect of macrophages upon immune responses is dealt with in Chapter 8, in which immunodeficiencies associated with excessive suppression are reviewed. The macrophage crops up repeatedly elsewhere in this book where lymphocyte responses are examined, indicating the pervasive impact of this cell upon immunity.

This chapter has focused upon new and unresolved issues that seem to keep pace with our rapidly increasing knowledge of this cell. A comprehensive schema dealing with the origins of the monocyte-macrophage series was presented. An attempt was made to bring many known facets of macrophage physiology into a cohesive sequence of immune responses. A relatively short section has been devoted to clinical immunodeficiencies that can be ascribed to macrophage disorders. Are most severe macrophage deficiencies incompatible with life? Are we overlooking subtle macrophage disorders, perhaps because they are overshadowed by other coexistent defects, especially lymphocyte impairments? Are there alternative measures that compensate for macrophage impairments? How great are reserves of the monocyte-macrophage series themselves? Obviously, much more is known about the physiology than the pathophysiology of these cells.

Recent discoveries have opened doors for incisive fundamental research on the monocyte-macrophage series. The development of monoclonal antibodies with relative macrophage specificity may permit studying the functional characteristics of subpopulations, as has recently been done successfully with the T lymphocyte series. Perhaps disorders associated with maldistribution of macrophage subpopulations will be identified. The elucidation of immune response gene products should shed considerable light on the molecular arrangement of antigen presentation. Clarification of the interleukin sequence solidly establishes the macrophage in the mediator network of the effector limb of the immune response. Finally, the glamour recently bestowed upon the macrophage by those interested in cellular immune reactions must not overshadow its other important secretory and defensive duties.

References

Albrecht, R.M., Hinsdell, R.D., Sandok, P.L., and Horowitz, S.D. 1978. Murine macrophage-lymphocyte interactions; Scanning election microscopic study. Infect Immunol 2:254–268.

Al-Ibrahim, M.S., Valentine, F.T., and Lawrence, H.S. 1978. Activated lymphocytes depress phagocytosis of latex particles by human monocyte-macrophages. Cell Immunol 41:217–230.

Allen, R.C., Sannes, P.L., Spicer, S.S., and Hong, C.C. 1980. Comparison of alveolar and peritoneal macrophages. J Histochem Cytochem 29:947–952.

Ando, M., Dannenberg, A.M., Sugimoto, M., and Tepper, B.S. 1977. Histochemical studies relating the activation of macrophages to the intracellular destruction of tubercle bacilli. Am J Path 86:623–633.

Ault, K.A., and Springer, T.A. 1981. Cross reaction of a rat-antimouse phagocyte-specific monoclonal antibody (anti-MacI) with human monocytes and natural killer cells. J Immunol 126:359–364.

Bash, J.A., and Vago, J.R. 1980. Carrageenan-induced suppression of T lymphocyte proliferation in the rat: In vivo suppression induced by oral administration. J Retic Soc 28:213–221.

Beller, D.I., Kiely, J.M., and Unanue, E.R. 1980. Regulation of macrophage populations. J Immunol 124:1426–1432.

Beller, D.I., and Unanue, E.R. 1980. Ia antigens and antigen-presenting function of thymic macrophages. J Immunol 124:1433.

Beller, D.I., and Unanue, E.R. 1981. Regulation of macrophage populations. J Immunol 126:263–268.

Ben-Sasson, S.Z., Lipscomb, M.F., Tucker, T.F., and Uhr, J.W. 1978. Specific binding of T lymphocytes to macrophages. J Immunol 120: 1902–1906.

Bentzon, J.W. 1953. The effect of certain infectious diseases on tuberculin allergy. Tubercle 34:34–41.

Bevilacqua, M.P., Amrani, D., Mosesson, M.W., and Bianco, C. 1981. Receptors for cold-insoluble globulin on human monocytes. J Exp Med 153: 42–60.

Breard, J., Fuks, A., Friedman, S.M., Schlossman, S.F., and Chess, L. 1979. The role of p23,30-bearing human macrophages in antigen induced T lymphocyte responses. Cell Immunol 45:108–119.

Breard, J., Reinberg, E.L., Kung, P.C., Goldstein, G., and Schlossman, S.F. 1980. A monoclonal antibody reactive with peripheral blood monocytes. J Immunol 124:1943–1948.

Brune, K., Glatt, M., Kalin, H., and Pesker, B.A. 1978. Pharmacological control of prostaglandin and thromboxane release from macrophages. Nature 274:261–263.

Chused, T.M., Kassan, S.S., and Mosier, D.E. 1976. Macrophage requirements for the in vitro response to TNP ficol: A thymic independent antigen. J Immunol 116:1579–1581.

Coovadia, H.M., Brain, P., Hallett, A.F., Wesley, A., Henderson, L.G., and Vos, G.H. 1977. Immunoparesis and outcome in measles. Lancet 1:619–621.

Dannenberg, A.M., Ando, M., and Shima, K. 1972. Mϕ accumulation, division, maturation and digestive and microbidical capacities in tuberculous lesions. J Immunol 109:1109–1121.

Dean, R.T., Hylton, W., and Allison, A.C. 1979. Induction of macrophage lysosomal enzyme secretion by agent acting at the plasma membrane. Exp Cell Biol 47:454–462.

Diamond, B.A., and Yelton, D.F. 1981. A new Fc receptor on mouse macrophages binding IgG_3. J Exp Med 153:514–519.

Doran, J.E., Mansberger, A.R., and Reese, A.C. 1980. Cold insoluble globulin-enhanced phagocytosis of gelatinized targets by macrophage monolayers: A model system. J Retic Soc 27:471–483.

Drew, W.L., Mintz, L., Hoo, R., and Finley, T.N. 1979. Growth of herpes simplex and cytomegalovirus in cultured human alveolar macrophages. Am Rev Resp Dis 119:287–291.

Drivas, G., and Wardle, N. 1978. Reticuloendothelial cell dysfunction in diabetes and hyperlipidemia. Metabolism 27:1533–1538.

Ehlenberger, A.G., and Nussenzweig, V. 1977. The role of membrane receptors for C3b and C3d in phagocytosis. J Exp Med 145:357–371.

Engleman, E.G., Charron, D.J., Benike, C., and Stewart, G.J. 1980. Ia antigen on peripheral blood mononuclear leukocytes in man. J Exp Med 99:1135.

Epstein, L.B. 1976. Immunology of the Macrophage, ed. D.S. Nelson, 1st ed., p. 201. Academic Press; New York.

Farrar, W.L., Mizel, S.B., and Farrer, J.J. 1980. Participation of lymphocyte activating factor (interleukin I) in the induction of cytotoxic T cell responses. J Immunol 124:1371–1377.

Farzad, A., Penneys, N.S., Ghaffar, A., Ziboh, V.A., and Schlossberg, J. 1977. PGE_2 and $PGE_{2\alpha}$ biosynthesis in stimulated and nonstimulated peritoneal preparations containing macrophages. Prostaglandins 14:829–837.

Fishman, M., and Weinberg, D.S. 1979. Functional heterogeneity among peritoneal macrophages. Cell Immunol 45:437–445.

Frank, M.M., Hamburger, M.I., Lawley, T.J., Kimberly, R.P., and Plotz, P.H. 1979. Defective reticuloendothelial system Fc-receptor function in systemic lupus erythematosus. N Engl J Med 300: 518–523.

Friedman, S.A., Remold-O'Donnell, E., and Piessens, W.F. 1979. Enhanced PGE production by MAF-treated peritoneal exudate macrophages. Cell Immunol 42:213–218.

Gales, R.J., and Morley, A.A. 1980. The mono-

nuclear phagocyte system in experimental chronic bone marrows failure. Exp Hemat 8:16–24.
Golde, D.W., Finley, T.N., and Cline, M.J. 1974. The pulmonary macrophage in acute leukemia. N Engl J Med 290:875–878.
Goldyne, M.E. 1977. Prostaglandins and the modulations of immunological responses. Int J Derm 16:701–712.
Gorczynski, R.M. 1976. Control of the immune response role of macrophages in regulaton of antibody and cell-mediated immune responses. Scand J Immunol 5:1031–1047.
Gorczynski, R.M., MacRae, S., and Jennings, J.J. 1979. A novel role for macrophage antigen discrimination of distinct carbohydrate bonds. Cell Immunol 45:276–294.
Gordon, S., Todd, J., and Cohn, Z.A. 1974. In vitro synthesis and secretion of lysozymes by mononuclear phagocytes. J Exper Med 139:1228–1248.
Griffin, F.M., and Griffin, J.A. 1980. Augmentation of macrophage complement receptor function in vitro. J Immunol 125:844–849.
Haider, S., Coutinho, M.deL., Emond, R.T.D., and Sutton, R.N.P. 1973. Tuberculin anergy and infectious mononucleosis. Lancet 2:74.
Harris, J.O. 1979. Pulmonary alveolar proteinosis: Abnormal in vitro function of alveolar macrophages. Chest 76:156–159.
Haynes, B.F., Hemler, M.E., Mann, D.L., Eisenbarth, G.S., Shelhamer, J., Mostowski, H.S., Thomas, C.A., Strominger, J.L., and Fauci, A.S. 1981. Characterization of monoclonal antibody (4F2) that binds to human monocytes and to a subset of activated lymphocytes. J Immunol 126:1409–1414.
Heusser, C.H., Anderson, C.L., and Grey, H.M. 1977. Receptors for IgG: Subclass specificity of receptors on different mouse cell types and the definition of two distinct receptors on a macrophage cell line. J Exp Med 145:1316–1327.
Hoffman, M.K. 1980. Macrophages and T cells control distinct phases of B cell differentiation in the humoral immune response. J Immunol 125: 2076–2081.
Hoffman, M.K., Koenig, S., Mittler, R.S., Oettgen, H.F., Ralph, P., Galanos, C., and Hammerling, U. 1978. Macrophage factor controlling differentiation of B cells. J Immunol 122:497–502.
Huang, K. 1977. Effect of interferon on phagocytosis. Texas Report Biol Med 35:350–356.
Jaffe, C.J., Vierling, J.M., Jones, E.A., and Lawley, J.J. 1978. Receptor specific clearance by the reticuloendothelial system in chronic liver disease. J Clin Invest 62:1069–1077.
Johnston, R.B., Keele, B.B., Mirsa, H.P., Lehmeyer, J.E., Webb, L.S., Baehner, R.L., and Rajagopalan, K.V. 1975. The role of superoxide anion generation in phagocytocytic bacterial activity. Studies with normal and chronic granulomatous disease leukocytes. J Clin Invest 55:1357–1372.
Johnston, R.B., Lehmeyer, J.E., and Guthrie, L.A. 1976. Generation of superoxide anion and chemilumines by human monocytes during phagocytosis and on contact with surface-bound immunoglobulin G. J Exper Med 143:1551–1556.
Kaplan, A.M., and Mohanakumar, T. 1977. Expression of a new cell surface antigen on activated murine macrophages. J Exp Med 146:1461–1466.
Katz, D.H., and Unanue, E.R., 1973. Critical role of determinant presentation in the induction of specific responses in immunocompetent lymphocytes. J Exp Med 137:967–990.
Kay, H.D., and Horowitz, D.A. 1980. Evidence by reactivity with hybridoma antibodies for a probable myeloid origen of peripheral blood cells active in natural cytotoxicity and antibody-dependent cell-mediated cytotoxicity. J Clin Invest 66:847–851.
Kelly, L.S., Brown, B.A., and Dobson, E.L. 1962. Cell division and phagocytic activity in liver reticuloendothelial cells. Proc Soc Exp Biol Med 110:555–559.
Kitahara, M., and Kushner, J.P. 1979. Acquired myeloperoxidase deficiency and recurrent infections in a patient with acute myelomonocytic leukemia. Cancer 44:2244–2248.
Kleinerman, E.S., Snyderman, R., and Daniels, C.A. 1975. Depressed monocyte chemotaxis during acute influenza. Lancet 2:1063–1066.
Kolodny, E.H. 1972. Clinical and biochemical genetics of the lipidoses. Seminars Hemat 9:251–271.
Koopman, W.J., Farrar, J.J., Oppenheim, J.J., Fuller-Bonar, J., and Dougherty, S. 1977. Association of a low molecular weight helper factor(s) with thymocyte proliferative activity. J Immunol 119:55–60.
Kunin, S., Shearer, G.M., Globerson, A., and Feldman, M. 1972. Immunologic function of macrophages: In vitro production of antibodies to a hepten-carrier conjugate. Cell Immunol 5: 288–295.
Lee, K.C., Kay, J., and Wong, M. 1979. Separation of functionally distinct subpopulations of Corynebacterium parvum-activated macrophages with predominantly stimulatory or suppressive effect on the cell-mediated cytotoxic T cell response. Cell Immunol 42:28–41.
Lee, K.C., and Wong, M. 1980. Functional heterogeneity of culture grown bone marrow derived macrophages. J Immunol 125:86–95.
Lee, S.H., and Epstein, L.B. 1980. Reversible inhibition by interferon of the maturation of human peripheral blood monocytes and macrophages. Cell Immunol 50:177–190.
Lehner, R.I., and Cline, M.J. 1969. Leukocyte myeloperoxidase deficiency and disseminated candidiasis. J Clin Inves 48:1478–1488.
L'Esperance, P., Brunning, R., Deinard, A.S., Park,

B.H., Bigger, D., and Good, R.A. 1975. Congenital neutropenia: Impaired maturation with diminished stem cell input. Birth Defects, Original Article Series 11:59–65.

Libansky, J. 1969. The investigation of the cellular type of immunity in patients with lymphoproliferative and myeloproliferative diseases. Int J Cancer 4:288:293.

Lin, H.S., and Freeman, P.G. 1977. Peritoneal exudate cells. IV. Characterization of colony forming cells. J Cell Physiol 90:407–414.

Lipsky, P.E., and Rosenthal, A.S. 1975. Macrophage-lymphocyte interaction: Antigen-independent binding of guinea pig lymph node lymphocytes and macrophages. J Immunol 115: 440–445.

Luria, M.D. 1942. Studies on the mechanism of immunity in tuberculosis. J Exp Med 75:247–267.

Maryanski, J.L., Cerottini, J.C., and Brunner, K.T. 1980. Susceptibility of proliferating cytolytic T lymphocytes to 33258 Hoechst-modified BUdR and light treatment. J Immunol 124:839–845.

McLeod, R., and Remington, J.S. 1977. Studies on the specificity of killing of intracellular pathogens by macrophages. Cell Immunol 34:156–174.

Meltzer, M.S., and Oppenheim, J.J. 1977. Bidirectional amplification of macrophage-lymphocyte interactions. J Immunol 118:77–87.

Meuret, G. 1974. Human monocytopoiesis. Exp Hemat 2:238–249.

Michl, J. 1980. Receptor mediated endocytosis. Am J Clin Nutr 33:2462–2471.

Mizel, S.B., Oppenheim, J.J., and Rosenstreich, D.L. 1978. Characterization of lymphocyte-activating factor (LAF) produced by the macrophage cell line P388D. J Immunol 120:1497–1508.

Montgomery, J.R., South, M.A., Rawls, W.E., Melnick, J.L., Olson, G.B., Dent, P.B., and Good, R.A. 1967. Viral inhibition of lymphocyte response to phytohemagglutinin. Science 157:1068–1070.

Moreas, J.R., and Stasney, P. 1977. A new antigen system expressed in human endothelial cells. J Clin Invest 60:449–454.

Moreland, B., and Kaplan, G. 1977. Macrophage activation in vivo and in vitro. Exp Cell Res 108:279–288.

Morse, S.S., and Monahan, P.S. 1981. Activated macrophages mediate interferon independent inhibition of herpes simplex virus. Cell Immunol 58:72–84.

Mosier, D.E., Johnson, B.M., Paul, W.E., and McMaster, P.R.B. 1974. Cellular requirements for the primary in vitro antibody response to DNP-ficoll. J Exp Med 139:1354–1360.

Muschel, R.J., Rosen, N., and Bloom, B.R. 1977. Isolation of variants in phagocytosis of a macrophage-like continuous cell line. J Exp Med 145:175–186.

Nathan, C.F., Murray, H.W., and Cohn Z.A. 1980. The macrophage as an effector cell. N Engl J Med 303:622–626.

Norris, D.A., Morris, R.M., Sandorson, R.J., and Kohler, P.F. 1979. Isolation of functional subsets human peripheral blood monocytes. J Immunol 123:166–172.

Ogawa, T. Koerten, H.K., and Daems, W.T. 1978. Peroxidatic activity in monocytes and tissue macrophages of mice. Cell Tis Res 188:361–373.

Oppenheim, J.J., and Seeger, R.C. 1976. The role of macrophages in the induction of cell-mediated immunity in vivo. In: Immunobiology of the Macrophage, eds. D.S. Nelson, pp. 111–130. Academic Press; New York.

Pearson, M.N., and Raffel, S. 1971. Macrophage digested antigen as inducer of delayed hypersensitivity. J Exp Med 133:494–505.

Pegram, P.S., DeChatelet, L.R. and McCall, C.E. 1978. Comparison of myeloperoxidase activity in leukocytes from normal subjects and patients with chronic granulomatous disease. J Infec Dis 138:699–702.

Picker, L.J., Raff, H.V., Goldyne, M.E., and Stobo, J.D. 1980. Metabolic heterogeneity among human monocytes and its modulation by PGE_2. J Immunol 124:2557–2562.

Rabellino, E., and Metcalf, D. 1975. Receptors for C_3 and Ig on macrophages, neutrophils and eosinophil colony cells grown in vitro. J Immunol 115:688–692.

Raff, H.V., Picker, L.J., and Stobo, J.D. 1980. Macrophage heterogeneity in man. J Exp Med 152:581–593.

Reed, W.P., Olds, J.W., and Kisch, A.L. 1972. Decreased skin-test reactivity associated wth influenza. J Infec Dis 125:398–402.

Rich, R.R., Abramson, S.L., Seldin, M.F., Puck, J.M., and Levy, R. 1980. Role of Ia positive cells in induction of secondary human immune responses to haptens in vitro. J Exp Med 152:218–234s.

Roberts, N.J., Douglas, R.G., Simons, R.M., and Diamond, M.E. 1979. Virus-induced interferon production by human macrophages. J Immunol 123:365–369.

Rodey, G.E., Park, B.H., Windhorst, D.B., and Ford, R.A. 1969. Defective bactericidal activity of monocytes in fatal granulomatous disease. Blood 33:813–820.

Root, R.K., Rosenthal, A.S., and Balestra, D.J. 1972. Abnormal bactericidal, metabolic and lysosomal function of Chediak-Higashi syndrome leukocytes. J Clin Invest 51:649–656.

Rosenthal, A.S., Blake, J.T., Ellner, J.J., Greineder, D.K., and Lipsky, P.E. 1976. Macrophage function in antigen recognition by T lymphocytes. In: Immunobiology of the Macrophage, ed., D.S. Nelson, pp. 131–160. Academic Press; New York.

Roser, B., 1970. The origins, kinetics and fate of

macrophage populations. J Retic Soc 8:139–161.

Ross, G.D., and Polley, M.J. 1975. Specificity of human lymphocyte complement receptors. J Exp Med 141:1163–1180.

Sagone, A.L., King, G.W., and Metz, E.N. 1976. A comparison of the metabolic response to phagocytosis in human granulocytes and monocytes. J Clin Invest 57:1352–1358.

Saito, H., and Tomioka, H. 1980. Suppressive factor of tumor origin against macrophage phagocytosis of staphylococcus aureus. Br J Cancer 41:259–267.

Schoenberg, M.D., Mumaw, V.R., Moore, R.D., and Weisberger, A.S. 1964. Cytoplasmic interactions between macrophages and lymphocytic cells in antibody synthesis. Science 143:964–965.

Smith, K.A., Gillis, S., Ruscetti, F.W., Baker, P.E., and McKenzie, D. 1979. T cell growth factor: The second signal in the T cell immune response. Proc NY Acad Sci 332:423–429.

Smith, K.A., Lachman, L.B., Oppenheim, J.J., and Favata, M.F. 1980. The functional relationship of the interleukins. J Exp Med 151:1551–1556.

Spector, W.G., Walters, M.N., and Willoughby, D.A. 1965. The origins of the mononuclear cells in inflammatory exudates induced by fibrinogen. J Path Bact 90:181–192.

Springer, T., Galfré, G., Secher, D.S., and Milstein, C. 1979. Mac-I: A macrophage differentiation antigen identified by monoclonal antibody. Eur J Immunol 9:301–306.

Sullivan, J.L., Barry, E.W., Albrecht, P., and Lucas, S.J. 1975. Inhibition of lymphocyte stimulation by measles virus. J Immunol 114:1458–1463.

Thomas, D.W., Schauster, J.L., Meltz, S.K., and Wilner, G.D. 1980. Nature of T lymphocyte recognition of macrophage-associated antigens. Cell Immunol 55:476–484.

Thomas, E.D., Ramberg, R.E., Sale, G.E., Sparkes, R.S., and Golde, D.W. 1976. Direct evidence for a bone marrow origin of the alveolar macrophage in man. Science 192:1016–1017.

Todd, R.F., III, Nadler, L.M., and Schlossman, S.F. 1981. Antigens on human monocytes identified by monoclonal antibodies. J Immunol 126:1435-1442.

Todd, R.F., Reinherz, E.L., and Schlossman, S.F. 1980. Human macrophage lymphocyte interaction in proliferation to soluble antigen I. Cell Immunol 55:114–123.

Twomey, J.J. 1974. Abnormalities in the mixed leukocyte reaction during infectious mononucleosis. J Immunol 112:2278–2281.

Twomey, J.J., and Douglass, C.C. 1974. An in vitro study of lymphocyte and macrophage function with lymphoproliferative disorders. Cancer 33: 1034–1038.

Twomey, J.J., Douglass, C.C., and Sharkey, O. 1973. The monocytopenia of aplasticanemia. Blood 44:187–195.

Twomey, J.J., Gyorkey, F., and Norris, S.M. 1974. The monocyte disorder with herpes zoster. J Lab Clin Med 83:768–777.

Twomey, J.J., Sharkey, O., Brown, J.A., and Jordan, P.H. 1970. Cellular requirements for the mitotic response in allogeneic mixed leukocyte cultures. J Immunol 108:984–990.

Tyers, M.B., and Haywood, H. 1979. Effects of prostaglandins on peripheral nociceptors in acute inflammation. Agents Actions (suppl 6): 6:65–78.

Ugolini, V., Nunez, G., Smith, R.G., Stasney, P., and Capra, J.D. 1980. Initial characterization of monoclonal antibodies against human monocytes. Proc Nat Acad Sci USA 77:6764–6768.

Unanue, E.R. 1980. Cooperation between mononuclear phagocytes and lymphocytes in immunity. New Engl J Med 303:977–985.

van Furth, R., Cohn, Z.A., Hirsch, J.G., Humphrey, J.H., Spector, W.G., and Langevoort, H.L. 1972. The mononuclear phagocyte system: A new classification of macrophages, monocytes and their precursor cells. Bull WHO 46:845–852.

van Furth, R., Raeburn, J.A., and van Zwet, T.L. 1979. Characteristics of human mononuclear phagocytes. Blood 54:485–500.

van Loon, A.M., van der Logt, J.T., and van der Veen, J. 1979. Poliovirus-induced suppression of lymphocyte stimulation: A macrophage-mediated effect. Immunology 37:135–143.

Volkman, A., and Gowans, J.L. 1965a. The origin of MΦ from BM in the rat. Br J Exp Pathol 46:62–70.

Volkman, A., and Gowans, J.L. 1965b. The production of MΦ in the rat. Br J Exp Pathol 46:50–61.

Waddell, C.C., Taunton, O.D., and Twomey, J.J. 1976. Inhibition of lymphoproliferation by hyperlipoproteinemic plasma. J Clin Invest 58:950–954.

Wahl, S.M., Wilton, J.M., Rosentreich, D.L., and Oppenheim, J.J. 1975. The role of macrophages in the production of lymphokines by T and B lymphocytes. J Immunol 114:1296–1301.

Westurick, J. 1979. Prostaglandins as mediators of inflammation-vascular aspects. Agents Actions (Suppl)6:59–63.

White, J.G., and Clawson, C.C. 1979. The Chediak-Higashi Syndrome. Am J Pathol 96:781–798.

Whittle, H.C., Dorsetor, J., Odulojii, A., Bryceson, A.D.M., and Greenwood, B.M. 1978. Cell-mediated immunity during natural measles infection. J Clin Invest 62:678–684.

Williams, B.D., Russell, B.A., Lockwood, C.M., and Cotton, C. 1979. Defective reticuloendothelial system function in rheumatoid arthritis. Lancet 1:1311–1314.

Wisse, E. 1974. Kupffer cell reactions in rat liver under various conditions as observed in the electron microscope. J Ultrastruct Res 46:499–520.

Yamashita, U.U., and Shevach, E.M. 1977. The expression of Ia antigens on immunocompetent cells in the guinea pig. J Immunol 119:1584–1588.

Chapter 4

Histocompatibility Antigens and Disease Susceptibility

James T. Rosenbaum
and Edgar G. Engleman

The genes of the major histocompatibility complex (MHC) influence susceptibility to a wide range of human diseases. Although in most instances the mechanisms responsible for MHC and disease associations are unknown, a knowledge of the MHC and its functions permits insight into the pathophysiology of many immunologically mediated diseases. In order to understand the premises on which these insights are based, we need to review some essential concepts concerning the MHC. Since the histocompatibility complex of the mouse is far better defined than the comparable human genetic region, we will begin with a description of the MHC in that species and then utilize the information gained from studies of that system to analyze associations between the human MHC and diseases such as rheumatoid arthritis, diabetes, mellitus, multiple sclerosis, myasthenia gravis and Graves' disease.

Historical Background

The realization that the immune system determines tissue histocompatibility originated in the 1940's with the work of Medawar. With his colleagues, Medawar performed a series of experiments to study the acceptance of tissue transplanted from one individual to another member of the same species. Mice of one genetic background rejected transplanted skin from mice of another genetic background and the rapidity of that rejection increased if the identical transplant was attempted a second time, but not if a second transplant was attempted with tissue originating from a third mouse strain. Medawar interpreted this accelerated rejection of foreign tissue as an example of immunologic memory.

The mechanism responsible for this phenomenon was clarified greatly by work of Snell later that same decade. Snell patiently bred strains of mice that were genetically identical except for the genes in one particular region. Such strains are called congenic; their production can be achieved by a series of backcrosses, which are matings between an offspring and a parental strain. If the offspring are selected for a trait present in one of the parental lines, for example, strain A, and then these offspring are repeatedly backcrossed to the other parental line, for example, strain B, eventually one can produce a strain that resembles strain B in every way except for the one trait from strain A which has been selected. Snell used these congenic strains of mice to show that the same genetic region that seemed to be responsible for tissue histocompatibility (that is, the ability of one strain to accept transplanted tissue from another strain) was also responsible for a red blood cell antigen that had been previously named H-2. Snell therefore designated a group of genes in the mouse as H-2 and showed that they represented the major histocompatibility complex. Minor histocompatibility complexes also exist but are less influential in determining graft acceptability. The achievement of Snell is even more remarkable when one considers that years of his painstaking breeding experiments were destroyed by fire before he succeeded in producing the inbred strains critical for his success.

The achievements of Snell, Medawar and other pioneers in the field of tissue transplantation took on added importance from two developments; these were the realization that genes within the MHC control immune responses as well as graft acceptance and the identification of MHC gene products in man. In the 1960's, McDevitt and Benacerraf (1969) as well as Sela had noted that antibody responses to certain synthetic polypeptides were genetically controlled in the mouse and the guinea pig. Utilizing the congenic strains of Snell, these investigators showed that the ability of a mouse to make an immune response to these repetitive amino acid sequences was controlled by genes that mapped to H-2, the mouse MHC. Ten years previously Dausset (1954) and Payne (1957) had begun independently to investigate transfusion reactions in individuals who had received properly crossmatched red cells. They demonstrated that these reactions could be accounted for by white cell surface proteins that differed between individuals even if the red cell types were identical. Because these gene products were first detected on white cells, they were designated human leukocyte antigens (HLA). The demonstration that HLA bear many structural and functional similarities to the mouse MHC products has added greatly to interest in mouse genetics. Since breeding experiments can be done in mice but not in humans, knowledge of the murine MHC is more complete than for the human system. A discussion of the mouse MHC is useful in understanding the role that histocompatibility complex gene products might play in the pathophysiology of human disease.

The Mouse MHC: H-2

A schematic map of H-2 is shown in Figure 4.1 (Klein, 1979). Three classes of H-2 products have been identified. Class I antigens designate the products of the loci *K, D* and *L*. These are the classic transplantation antigens, the ones historically first identified as determinants of graft compatibility. K, D and L antigens consist of two chains, a heavy chain of molecular weight equal to 44,000 and a light chain known as β_2 microglobulin of molecular weight 12,000. The light chain is invariant and not encoded by the 17th chromosome which codes for the other MHC products. K, D and L antigens are found on essentially all nucleated cells in the body. The *L* locus has only been described recently and therefore the distribution of its antigen is less certain than K and D.

K and D antigens are extremely polymorphic; there are many different alleles or alternative gene products that are recognized for either K or D. A given allele is denoted by a small case superscript, for example, H-2K^b (read "H two k of b"). Since loci and alleles are both designated by

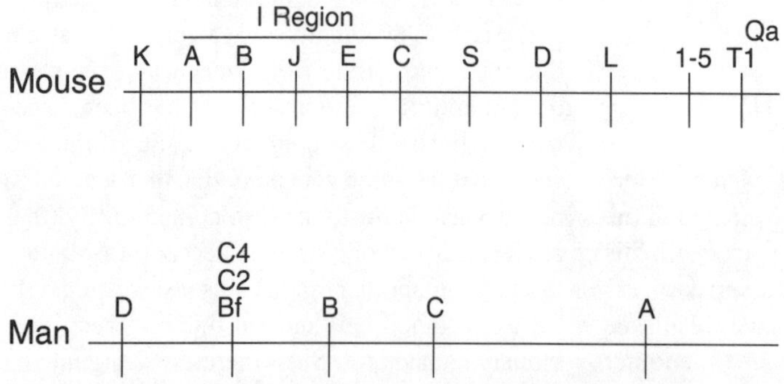

Fig. 4.1 The MHC in mouse and man.

letters, the nomenclature tends to become very confusing.

The products of the *I* region, a group of genes between *K* and *D*, are termed class II antigens. These glycoproteins have a much more restricted tissue distribution, expressed primarily on B lymphocytes, activated T cells and some macrophages. They too have a dimeric structure, with an α or heavy chain of molecular weight 33,000 and a light, or β chain, of molecular weight 28,000. Immunoprecipitations also show a third chain of invariant structure and molecular weight of 30,000 associated with class II antigens. The *I* region is subdivided into five subloci or subregions, *A, B, J, E* and *C*. At least three protein products have been ascribed to the *A* subregion; there is one for the *E* subregion. No products for *B, J* or *C* have been isolated. *I* region products are sometimes termed Ia, for *I* region associated. Through mechanisms not yet completely understood, *I* region genes control the ability to mount a humoral or cellular immune response to most, if not all, protein antigens. Ia antigens participate directly in the presentation of antigens by macrophages to T cells and the cooperation between T cells and B cells. Also, Ia antigens are major components of soluble factors that can either help or suppress specific immune responses. Ia antigens seem to be the strongest stimuli for an in vitro proliferative response between cultured lymphocytes of two individuals, known as a mixed lymphocyte reaction (MLR). Ia antigens determine whether graft versus host disease will develop after bone marrow is transplanted between individuals of the same species and Ia antigens are perhaps the strongest determinant for tissue histocompatibility.

Although the biochemical product of *I-J* has not been characterized, products of this subregion are thought to be present on subsets of T cells and macrophages (Murphy et al., 1981). These subsets play a critical role in helping or suppressing immune responses. For example, most T cells that suppress immunity express I-J determinants on their surface.

In some cases the expression of an Ia antigen on the cell surface can depend on what allele is present for two different subregions. This phenomenon is known as two-gene complementation (Jones et al., 1978). For example, the *A* subregion codes for a chain of molecular weight 33,000 and the *E* subregion codes for a chain with a molecular weight of 28,000. These two chains are expressed together on the cell surface as a dimer if certain alleles are present for the *E* subregion (see Fig. 4.2). In the absence of one of these alleles, neither product is expressed on the cell surface. This two-gene complementation has functional as well as structural significance in that the capacity to generate an immune response to certain antigens is determined by the allele present at both loci, *A* and *E*.

The glycoprotein encoded by the *S* region is known as a class III antigen. It has a molecular weight of approximately 200,000, displays limited polymorphism and seems to be identical to the fourth component of the complement cascade.

In addition to the classic transplantation anti-

Table 4.1 Similarities between the Major Histocompatibility Complexes of Mouse and Man.

Antigen Class	Locus	Biochemistry of Product	Tissue Distribution	Function
I	K,D and L in mouse A,B and C in man	Heavy chain mw = 44,000; extremely polymorphic Light chain (β_2 microglobulin) mw = 12,000; invariant; coded outside the MHC	Wide	Allograft acceptance Cell-mediated cytotoxicity
II	I-A and I-E in mouse D in man	Glycoprotein dimers; α chain mw = 33,000; β chain mw = 28,000 Associated, third invariant chain; mw = 30,000	Limited	Mixed lymphocyte reaction; Graft vs. host disease; T cell help; macrophage antigen presentation
III	S in mouse C4 in man	mw = 209,000	Fluids	Fourth component of complement

gens, Ia antigens and complement components, a series of other proteins encoded by loci just outside the mouse MHC also have immunologic significance. These include Qa1, Qa2, Qa3, Qa4, Qa5 and T1. The products of several of these genes have been identified. They seem to be cell surface dimers with a heavy chain of similar molecular weight to K and D antigens and a light chain identical to β_2 microglobulin. Some of these proteins appear to have a functional role in the immune system because their expression is limited to functionally specific subsets of lymphocytes.

In addition to their role in transplantation and immune responses, H-2 products might also be involved in a number of other functions that are not normally considered immune in nature (Klein, 1975). H-2 seems to influence smell, mating preference, testis size and testosterone serum levels, the binding of glucagon to cellular receptors and basal liver cyclic adenosine monophosphate levels. Some of these nonimmunologic functions might be relevant to an understanding of HLA and disease associations.

HLA: The Products of the Human MHC

The human MHC is still known as the HLA region, although its products are more widely distributed than simply on leukocytes. As in the mouse, there are three classes of protein encoded for by the MHC region. The class I products are encoded by the *A*, *B* and *C* loci. These glycoproteins have a similar structure, the same distribution and apparently the same functional significance as the products of the loci *K*, *D* and *L* in the mouse. These analogies are summarized in Table 4.1. The *D* region codes for class II products which are termed DR for *D r*elated. Again, in terms of size, distribution and function, DR antigens appear to be analogous to Ia. And in parallel with the mouse system, certain complement components including properdin factor B, C2 and C4 appear to be coded in or near the human MHC. The existence of products analogous to Qa, T1 or I-J is less certain, but evidence is increasing that at least some of these antigens do exist in the human system (Gazit et al., 1980).

HLA typing can be performed for the alleles of four loci, *A*, *B*, *C* and *D*. As in the mouse, these alleles are extremely polymorphic. The *B* locus, for example, has nearly 40 alternative products. These alleles and their relative frequencies are given in Table 4.2. Every individual inherits genes from each parent. A set of genes from a single parent makes up a haplotype and two haplotypes define a genotype. Therefore, each individual has two A alleles, two B alleles, etc. Some of these alleles demonstrate a phenomenon known as linkage disequilibrium, defined as the inheritance of one allele in a haplotype along with another allele on the same chromosome more frequently than one could expect from chance alone. For example, the frequency of A1 among Caucasians is approximately 0.14 and the frequency of B8 is 0.10. If A1 and B8 are inherited independently, then they should occur together at a frequency of 0.014 ($0.1 \times 0.14 = 1.4\%$). Instead, A1 and B8 are found together 6.4% of the time, much more frequently than the 1.4% one would predict. The explanation for this linkage disequilibrium is unknown, but, as shown below, it is relevant to an understanding of HLA and disease associations.

Typing for A, B and C antigens is accomplished by a technique known as lymphocytotoxicity. Certain individuals who have been ''immunized'' with foreign HLA antigens will develop antibodies against them. These immunizations are usually in the form of transfusions or pregnancy. Sera from these immunized individuals can then be used to lyse lymphocytes that bear the same HLA type as the immunizing cells. Through a series of international collaborative workshops, the specificities of these various typing sera have been defined and nomenclature has been agreed upon. Tentative designations are preceded by a W for workshop. Thus, W27 was the original designation for B27. The typing has become increasingly refined and specific. For example, two new antigens, B38 and B39, have recently been recognized. Previously, both were designated B16 because many sera crossreacted with both B38 and B39. When it was realized

Table 4.2 Frequency[a] of HLA Antigens in Caucasians.

Antigen	<1%	1–10%	Frequency 10–20%	20–30%	30–40%	40–50%
	34	23 28 31				
A	36	25 29 32	11 24	3 1		2
	43	26 30 33				
	42	13 41 55				
		14 45 54	18 7			
	47	27 48 57				
B						
	54	37 49 58	51 8	44		
		38 50 60				
	59	39 52 61	62 35			
		53 63				
C		C1 C2 C8	C5 C6	C3 C4 C7		

[a]One characteristic of HLA antigens is that each specificity is relatively rare in the random population. The most common specificity is HLA-A2, with a frequency of about 45%. Other specificities, such as HLA-A1 and A3, are between 20 and 30%, but the majority of the specificities are in the range of 1 to 10% frequency in the random population. Taken from Terasaki, P.I., 1980, Histocompatibility Testing 1980, U.C.L.A. Tissue Typing Laboratory, Los Angeles, Ca., p. 9, Fig. 23.

that some typing sera would react only with a subset of B16 and other sera reacted only with another B16 subset, the allele was split into B38 and B39. Even B27 has now been split into two subtypes with monoclonal antibodies (Grumet et al., 1982).

Since DR antigens are restricted to B lymphocytes and monocytes among normal peripheral blood mononuclear cells, typing for DR antigens must be done on a purified population of B cells and/or monocytes, thus adding to the complexity of the assay. One can also perform a functional assay for the D antigens with the mixed lymphocyte reaction (MLR) test. Lymphocytes that differ by at least one D antigen will stimulate each other when cultured together. This stimulation can be quantitated by measuring the amount of newly synthesized DNA with a radioactive marker. One can select stimulator lymphocytes that are known to be homozygous for D antigens. These stimulator cells can then be metabolically inhibited by, for example, x-irradiation so that they are incapable of synthesizing new DNA. If irradiated stimulator cells homozygous for a known D type fail to stimulate lymphocytes of an unknown D type, the lymphocytes of the unknown D type must share a common D type with the homozygous stimulator cells. With a panel of stimulator cells representing all possible D alleles, one can perform multiple MLR and thus effectively D type an individual. This typing is cumbersome and time-consuming. The correlation between D typing by MLR and DR typing by B lymphocyte cytotoxicity is not perfect, probably because antigens in addition to DR stimulate in the MLR (Engleman et al., 1981).

While several Ia antigen loci have been recognized in the mouse, as yet only one such locus, HLA-DR, has been identified in man. The evidence for additional Ia loci is not conclusive, but it is certainly suggestive. Realizing that a phenomenon such as two-gene complementation occurs in the mouse, one could hardly hope to understand HLA and disease associations fully if other loci exist but cannot be identified.

HLA and Disease Associations

With this background of mouse and human immunogenetics in mind, a critical look at the numerous associations that exist between particular HLA alleles and disease susceptibility is possible. These associations include over 60 diseases, many of which are listed in Table 4.3. These diseases include examples from virtually every medical subspecialty. In general, the mechanism of the associations remains speculative, but certain explanations are especially plausible. Diseases with an HLA association can be grouped into three categories: diseases for which the actual susceptibility gene may lie outside the MHC but is linked to a particular

Table 4.3 HLA and Disease Associations.[1]

Subspeciality	Disease	Associated Allele	Relative Risk
Infectious Disease	Tuberculosis	B8	5.07
	Leprosy	DR2	3.30
	Paralytic poliomyelitis	Bw16	4.28
	Recurrent herpes labialis	A29	3.11
	Healthy hepatitis surface antigen carriers	Bw41	11.16
Oncology	Hodgkin's disease	A1	1.37
	Mycosis fungoides	Cw1	3.15
	Multiple myeloma	B5	1.93
	Acute lymphatic leukemia	A2	1.39
Endocrinology	Graves' disease	Dw3	3.66
	Subacute thyroiditis	Bw35	13.73
	Hashimoto's thyroiditis	DR3	3.40
	Insulin-dependent diabetes	DR3	5.69
		DR4	2.84
	Idiopathic Addison's disease	Dw3	6.30
	Congenital Adrenal hyperplasia	B5	3.64
Hematology	Von Willebrand's disease	Bw35	2.58
	Idiopathic thrombocytopenic purpura	DR2	10.00
	Pernicious anemia	A10	1.78
	Glucose-6-phosphate dehydrogenase deficiency	A2	3.03
Gastroenterology	Coeliac disease	DR3	21.12
	Hemochromatosis	A3	8.24
	Duodenal ulcer	B5	2.92
Gastroenterology	Crohn's disease	B15	1.53
	Ulcerative colitis	B27	1.88
	Alcoholic liver disease	B40	2.53
	Chronic active hepatitis (autoimmune subset	DR3	13.90

[1]The data in this table have been abstracted from the HLA and Disease Registry (Ryder et al., 1979). The strength of each association is estimated by the relative risk, calculated as:

$$\frac{\text{\% patients with specific HLA antigen}}{\text{\% patients without specific antigen}} \times \frac{\text{frequency of antigen negativity in controls}}{\text{frequency of antigen positivity in controls}}$$

For a few of the diseases (idiopathic thrombocytopenic purpura, juvenile rheumatoid arthritis and systemic lupus,) data from more recent studies than those in the Registry are given so that D allele associations are provided. The table is not intended to include all diseases with a claimed HLA association. However, it should provide some concept of the range of these associations and their relative strengths. For diseases for which multiple alleles bear an association, usually only the strongest association is given. The lack of a D association in many cases may merely reflect the lack of D typing for that particular disease. In some cases, associations have not been confirmed by subsequent studies, which may be due to methodologic error in the initial report. The variability of associations depending on the ethnic group or the disease subset studied or the artifact of finding some associations when multiple statistical tests are performed.

HLA allele, diseases with a primarily D or DR association and diseases with an association primarily with a B locus antigen. Each category deserves separate discussion because the mechanisms pertinent to one may not be relevant to the other categories.

The first category, diseases for which the HLA association derives from linkage to the recognized susceptibility locus which may be outside the MHC, is exemplified by hemochromatosis and a form of congenital adrenal hyperplasia due to 21-hydroxylase deficiency. In both cases the disease is not considered immunologic in nature and the association exists only because a particular HLA allele (A3 for hemochromatosis or certain B alleles for 21-hydroxylase deficiency) is inherited in linkage disequilibrium with the actual susceptibility gene.

The second category, diseases with a primarily D or DR association, is the largest group of diseases associated with HLA. This grouping includes some diseases, such as rheumatoid arthritis, with no recognized A or B association and other diseases, such as Graves' disease and

Table 4.3 *(cont.)*

Subspeciality	Disease	Associated Allele	Relative Risk
Rheumatology	Juvenile rheumatoid arthritis	DR5	8.0
	Rheumatoid arthritis	DR4	5.8
	Ankylosing spondylitis	B27	87.44
	Systemic lupus erythematosus	DR2	3.8
	Sjogren's syndrome	Dw3	9.72
	Reiter's syndrome	B27	36.97
	Behcet's disease	B5	6.26
	Kawasaki's disease	Bw22	2.41
Neurology/Psychiatry	Multiple sclerosis	DR2	4.80
	Myasthenia gravis	B8	5.50
	Optic neuritis	Dw2	2.36
	Schizophrenia	Cw4	3.70
	Manic depressive disorder	Bw39	6.84
	Subacute sclerosing panencephalitis	A29	3.62
Ophthalmoloty	Acute anterior uveitis	B27	10.36
	Scleritis	B15	4.08
Pulmonary	Goodpasture's	DR2	13.10
	Asbestosis	B27	2.66
Allergy	Ragweed	B7	3.57
	Grass pollinosis	DR3	4.7
Cardiology	Mitral valve prolapse	Bw35	3.39
	Rheumatic heart disease	A2	1.68
	Essential hypertension	Bw21	3.83
	Congenital heart disease	A2	1.80
Nephrology	Acute poststreptococcal glomerulonephritis	B12	3.44
	Polycystic kidneys	B5	2.64
Dermatology	Psoriasis	Cw6	13.25
	Dermatitis herpetiformis	DR3	56.40
	Lichen planus	A3	1.75
	Balanitis	B27	37.40
	Vitiligo	B12	1.82

insulin-dependent diabetes mellitus, with a weak B allele association and a much stronger D association. In these instances, the presumption is that the D allele is the true susceptibility gene and an A or B association is secondary to linkage disequilibrium with the D allele. This occurs commonly for A1, B8, D3 and DR3. Most of the diseases within this category are putatively autoimmune, including systemic lupus erythematosus, Sjögren's syndrome, Goodpasture's syndrome, idiopathic thrombocytopenic purpura, rheumatoid arthritis, Graves' disease, insulin-dependent diabetes and myasthenia gravis. In some of these diseases, especially diabetes and multiple sclerosis, a viral etiology seems likely at least in some cases. Since DR is so analogous to Ia, the presumption that seems most plausible is that the mechanism by which DR predisposes to disease in these instances is due to either a heightened or lessened immune response to a viral and/or a self antigen.

To clarify this DR/autoimmune hypothesis, we will consider two diseases in some detail. These are myasthenia gravis as the prototype of disease resulting from antibody against self and diabetes as the prototype for autoimmune disease that can develop subsequent to a viral illness.

Since an antibody against the acetylcholine receptor may be causally related to the development of myasthenia gravis, the hypothesis that an immune response (*Ir*) gene controls the ability to respond immunologically to this receptor is plausible. A causal role for these antibodies is supported by the observation that the antibody can be detected in over 90% of myasthenics and that, at least on occasion, infants born to mothers with myasthenia gravis will develop transient weakness presumably due to transplacental passage of the autoantibody. In experimental animals a syndrome resembling myasthenia gravis can be induced by immunizations with acetylcholine receptors from the electric eel (Patrick and Berman, 1980). In the mouse the susceptibility to this disease is under the control of H-2, as is the T cell proliferative response to the receptor. But other genes, especially those that control immunoglobulin allotypes, also influence disease susceptibility and many animals will develop a high titer of anti-acetylcholine receptor antibody without developing disease. The presence of autoantibodies without disease may result from the complexity of the acetylcholine receptor as an antigen. Because the receptor probably has more than one antigen site (epitope), a heightened response to one site might be the most critical in disease development but not be detected by an assay that measures antibodies to all acetylcholine receptor antignic sites. Thus, a plausible hypothesis is that an Ir gene product, DR3, is causally related to the development of myasthenia gravis by virtue of its influence on the immune response to the acetylcholine receptor.

A discussion of insulin-dependent (juvenile onset) diabetes mellitus (IDDM) is useful in illustrating how HLA might influence the development of an autoimmune disease following a viral illness. Glucose intolerance or diabetes mellitus clearly is a heterogeneous disease (Rotter and Rimoin, 1981). It is often broadly subdivided into insulin-dependent and insulin-nondependent varieties, but even further subdivisions can be made. For example, the insulin-dependent group can be subdivided into those patients who develop autoantibodies such as antithyroid, antipancreatic islet cell and antiparietal cell and those who lack these antibodies. Among the latter category are many whose illness appears to have been triggered by a viral infection such as mumps or coxsackie. DR3 is strongly associated with the group marked by autoantibodies, while DR4 is increased primarily in the group that lacks detectable autoantibodies except against insulin itself. The association of an HLA-D allele with a particlar disease subset also occurs in both rheumatoid and juvenile rheumatoid arthritis, Sjögren's syndrome, chronic active hepatitis and polymyositis. HLA typing can thus confirm the heterogeneity of a disease entity for which several different pathogenic events can result in phenotypically similar disease.

The association of IDDM with DR4 is especially marked in those whose disease begins during the months October through December. This observation is compatible with the hypothesis that DR4 influences disease susceptibility by virtue of its effect on a prodromal viral illness. MHC gene products appear to be capable of influencing viral or microbial infections on a number of levels. First, in some instances, the MHC determines the magnitude of a humoral or cellular immune response to a viral antigen. This mechanism might be critical in resistance to several viral-induced leukemias in mice. Second, H-2 gene products, in particular K and D, rather than Ia antigens appear to determine the ability to mount a cytotoxic response against virally infected cells. Third, the Radiation Leukemia virus can induce an increased synthesis of cell surface H-2D antigens and susceptibility to the leukemia appears to vary inversely with the increased expression of the MHC surface antigen (Meruelo et al., 1978). Any of these observations might be relevant to a mechanism by which DR4 determines the course of a viral infection and ultimately the development of diabetes. Interestingly, diabetes can be induced in mice either by immunization with autologous pancreas or by certain viral infections. While the former disease is H-2-controlled, the latter is not. DR4 might predispose to IDDM because it alters the course of a viral prodrome or because it determines an immune response to a by-product of this infection, such as a self antigen.

Despite the attractiveness of the hypothesis that DR antigens determine disease susceptibility by controlling immune response to a self or viral antigen, several objections can be raised. First, the function of DR antigens as immune response region gene products is less well proven in man than mouse. The strong biochemical and distributional analogies between Ia and DR suggest that immune response (*Ir*) genes do exist in man, but the proof of their existence is much more difficult than in mice because of the absence of inbred strains and the ethical constraints that limit immunizations solely for the purpose of studying immune response genes.

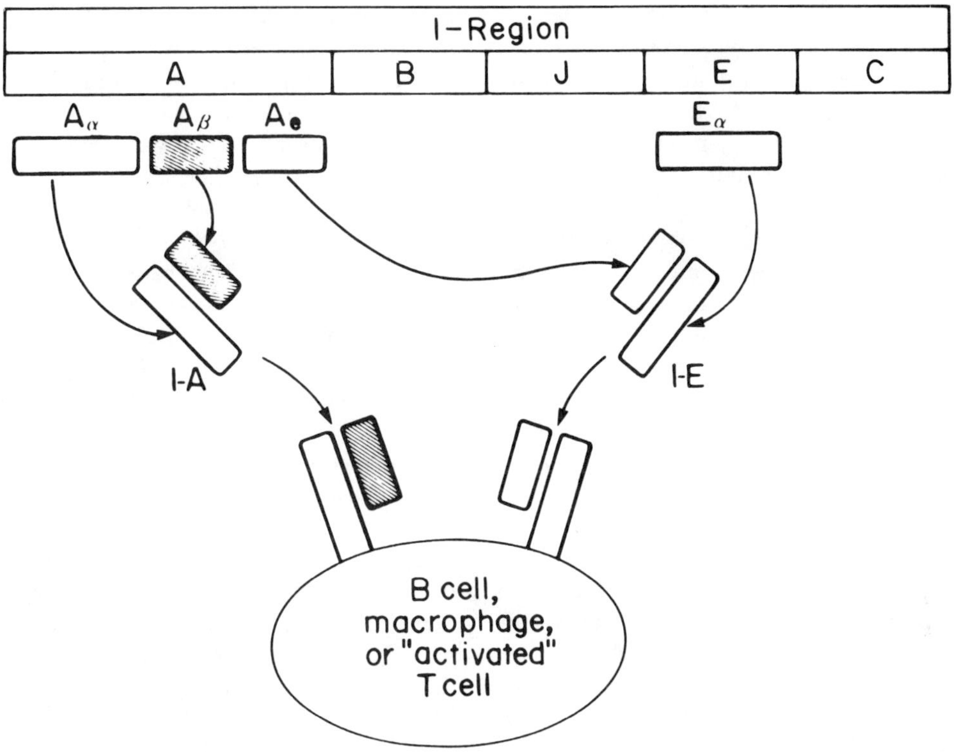

Fig. 4.2 Diagrammatic illustration of two-gene complementation. Two *Ir* gene products have been identified in the mouse. One is coded entirely by the *A* subregion. The expression of the second is dependent on a light chain (Ae) from the *A* subregion and a heavy chain from the *E* subregion. Adapted from Uhr, J.W., et al., 1979, Science, 295:296: Copyright 1979 by the American Association for the Advancement of Science.

Despite these difficulties, evidence supports the existence of immune response genes in man for at least four antigens: tetanus toxoid, collagen, native DNA and schistosomal cell wall (see, for example, Sasazuki et al., 1980). The second objection to this immune response gene hypothesis is that, although the diseases are considered autoimmune, in most instances the actual pathogenic role of autoantibodies is still in dispute.

Even in myasthenia gravis the role of autoantibodies as the cause of disease is debatable. If anti-acetylcholine receptor antibodies are solely responsible for myasthenia gravis, how can disease develop without detectable antibodies and why are infants born to mothers with myasthenia gravis not always affected? In diseases such as sytemic lupus, rheumatoid arthritis and multiple sclerosis, the proof that autoantibodies are causally related to disease development is even more suspect. The evidence that DR4 appears to determine an immune response to collagen is intriguing in this respect (Solinger et al., 1981). The data to support this are based on an increased production of a lymphokine, leuckocyte inhibitory factor, when DR4- positive lymphocytes are incubated with collagen in vitro. While anti-collagen antibodies might not be sufficient by themselves to induce rheumatoid arthritis, the production of an immune response to collagen along with other genetic and/or environmental factors might predispose to joint disease.

Finally, if a DR antigen predisposes to disease by determining an immune response to a pathogenic organism or a self antigen, it is difficult to explain why similar associations are not found in all ethnic groups. For example, DR4 is markedly increased among rheumatoid arthritis patients in most ethnic groups, but not among Jews. Dw3 is increased among Caucasians with Graves' disease, but not among Japanese. Dw3 is an extremely rare antigen in Japan, but Graves' disease does occur in Japan; there it is associated with Dw12, an antigen virtually unknown among Caucasians. Observations such as these suggest that the true susceptibility gene is not the D or DR antigen recognized by present typing methodology. Instead, the true susceptibility marker might be comparable to the mouse cell surface antigens such as T1, I-J or the elusive second Ia dimer. This possibility would also account for the imperfect correlation between a particular HLA allele and a disease. For example, while nearly 70% of multiple sclerosis (MS) patients are DR2-positive, many patients develop MS in the absence of DR2 and the vast majority of DR2 positive individuals do not develop MS. Either DR2 is one of several genes and/or environmental events responsible for the development of MS or DR2 itself is not the true susceptibility gene.

One particular haplotype, A1,B8,DR3, is associated with several diseases, including myasthenia gravis, diabetes, Graves' disease, Addison's disease, celiac disease, systemic lupus and Sjögren's syndrome. One recent report suggests that this haplotype is frequently characterized by reduced clearance of circulating immune complexes, even if no disease is present (Lawley et al., 1981). The HLA association helps to explain why these diseases may occur together in the same individual and why similar autoantibodies might be present in all. But why one DR3 individual develops thyroid disease and another develops Addison's disease remains unknown.

The third group of diseases associated with HLA are those that have primarily a *B* locus association with little or no relation to HLA-D. This category includes the spondylarthritides ankylosing spondylitis (AS) and Reiter's syndrome (RS), acute anterior uveitis and subacute thyroiditis. Since this latter disease is presumably viral in origin, the MHC/viral interactions previously discussed are relevant, especially those interactions which involve a classic transplantation antigen rather than DR or Ia products. A viral etiology, however, is less likely in the spondylarthritides. Of all the HLA/disease associations, the strongest is probably that between B27 and ankylosing spondylitis. Although B27 is present in only 6% of Caucasian blood bank donors, 90% of ankylosing spondylitis patients demonstrate this antigen. This means that a B27-positive individual is roughly one hundred times more likely to develop AS than a B27-negative individual.

Although several studies have searched for an association between AS and an HLA-D antigen, none has been found. This failure may simply reflect the limits of D typing, but an alternative explanation is that B27 predisposes to disease by a mechanism that does not involve a classic immune response gene. Reiter's syndrome, like AS, is strongly associated with B27 and shares many symptoms with AS. An immune response gene predisposing to RS would seem an attractive hypothesis when one considers that the disease is usually preceded by certain infections, either gram-negative dysentery or nongonococcal urethritis (NGU). An *Ir* gene determining an unusual immune response to the infectious agent might account for disease development. However, the organisms that can cause NGU are distinctly different from the organisms that cause the dysentery that may precede RS. Unless dysentery and urethritis result in an immune response to the same self antigen, it would seem unlikely that an *Ir* gene accounts for susceptibility to RS.

An alternative explanation is that B27 interacts with a bacterial or viral antigen such as Klebsiella. This hypothesis has been espoused primarily by an Australian group of investigators, who have demonstrated that antisera to certain Klebsiella isolates is cytotoxic to B27-positive lymphocytes from patients with AS, presumably because a Klebsiella product can bind to B27 as a receptor (Geczy et al., 1980). This hypothesis is intriguing, but it has not yet been confirmed. It is hoped that monoclonal antibodies to HLA-B27 (Grumet et al., 1981, 1982) will aid in studies of the B27 molecule and is role in disease.

Alternatively, either NGU or gram-negative dysentery may cause release of a similar inflammatory mediator such as prostaglandin; B27-positive individuals may be susceptible to disease because of sensitivity to this mediator (Rosenbaum, 1981). This hypothesis is reminiscent of the observation that H-2 plays a role in influencing nonimmunologic responses such as testosterone levels and the binding of glucagon to hepatocytes and it is supported by some recent findings that suggest that HLA antigens influence lymphocyte responses to histamine and prostaglandins (Staszak et al., 1980).

In rats, almost all the manifestations of Reiter's syndrome can be induced by injections of killed mycobacteria in mineral oil (Freund's adjuvant) into the footpad. Approximately 2 weeks later, susceptible strains of rats develop arthritis, spondylitis, conjunctivitis, uveitis, balanitis, urethritis, diarrhea and skin disease, all characteristic of Reiter's syndrome. The arthritogenic component of the mycobacterium appears to be a cell wall substance known as peptidoglycan. Endotoxin, a cell wall component of gram-negative bacteria, can induce uveitis in rats and rabbits after intravenous injection and it may be arthritogenic after direct synovial injection. Both the endotoxin- and the peptidoglycan-induced diseases can be prevented by prostaglandin synthetase inhibitors. Thus, animal syndromes that resemble Reiter's can be induced by at least two different bacterial cell wall substances; in both instances, prostaglandins may be involved in the mechanism. If prostaglandins or another inflammatory mediator determine the development of Reiter's syndrome in man, then B27 might be influencing disease development by an effect on the response to this mediator.

Clearly the mechanism whereby a particular HLA allele influences disease susceptibility will be clarified by a greater understanding of the cause of any given disease. Conversely, the cause of a disease might be clarified by virtue of its HLA association.

Summary

With the exceptions of the nonimmunologic diseases hemochromatosis and 21 hydroxylase deficiency, the mechanisms of HLA and disease associations remain speculative. Despite this limitation, HLA typing often offers clues that may eventually be useful in unraveling the pathogenesis of a vast array of diseases. The list of diseases with an HLA association is rapidly expanding due to greater availability of *D* locus typing, greater precision in the specificity of typing antisera and the realization that many diseases have discrete subsets because a variety of causes can result in similar pathologic manifestations. Recently, a variety of drug toxicities have been added to the list of disorders associated with a particular HLA allele, including reactions to penicillamine, gold, levamisole and hydralazine. HLA type might also influence disease prognosis.

Our future understanding of the human MHC will depend on greater sophistication of serologic methods and on attempts to characterize the MHC on a molecular or DNA level. Equally important will be our ability to identify the infectious agents or self antigens responsible for disease initiation. The combination of an understanding of MHC functions at the molecular level and identification of pathogens should result eventually in new means of therapeutic intervention. For example, if myasthenia gravis is due to an immune response gene that predisposes to anti-acetylcholine receptor antibodies, then antibodies against the *Ir* gene products might be selectively immunosuppressive, inhibiting the development of autoantibodies without predisposing to the infections that afflict most immunocompromised hosts. Understanding the HLA system provides a means for investigating the pathophysiology of a wide range of human immunologic disorders.

References

Berman, P.W., and Patrick, J. 1980. Linkage between the frequency of muscular weakness and loci that regulate immune responsiveness in murine experimental myasthenia gravis. J Exp Med 152:507–520.

Dausset, J. 1954. Leuco-agglutinins. IV. Leuco-agglutinins and blood transfusion. Vox Sang 4:190–198.

Engleman, E.G., Benike, C.J., Grumet, F.C., and Evans, R.L. 1981. Activation of human T lymphocytes subsets: Helper and suppressor/cytotoxic T cells recognize and respond to distinct histocompatability antigens. J Immunol 127:2124–2129.

Gazit, E., Terhorst, C., and Yunis, E.J. 1980. The human 'T' genetic region of the HLA linkage group is a polymorphism detected on lectin activated lymphocytes. Nature 284:275–277.

Geczy, A.F., Alexander, K., Bashir, H.V., and Edmonds, J. 1980. A factor(s) in Klebsiella culture filtrates specifically modifies an HLA-B27 associated cell surface component. Nature 283:782–784.

Grumet, F.C., Fendly, B.M., Fish, L., Foung, S., and Engleman, E.G. 1982. A monoclonal antibody (B27M2) subdividing HLA-B27. Human Immunol. In press.

Jones, P.P., Murphy, D.B., and McDevitt, H.O. 1978. Two gene control of the expression of murine Ia. J Exp Med 148:925–939.

Klein, J. 1975. Biology of the Mouse Histocompatibility-2 Complex. Springer-Verlag; New York.

Klein, J. 1979. The major histocompatibility complex of the mouse. Science 203:516–521.

Lawley, T.J., Hall, R.P., Fauci, A.S., Katz, S.I., Hamburger, M.I., and Frank, M.M. 1981. Defective Fc-receptor functions associated with the HLA-B8/DRw3 haplotype: Studies in patients with dermatitis herpetiformis and normal subjects. New Engl J Med 304:185–187.

McDevitt, H.O., and Benacerraf, B. 1969. Genetic control of specific immune responses. Adv Immunol 11:31–74.

Meruelo, D., Nimelstein, S., Jones, P.P., Lieberman, M., and McDevitt, H.O. 1978. Increased synthesis and expression of H-2 antigens on thymocytes as a result of radiation leukemia virus infection: A possible mechanism for H-2 linked control of virus induced neoplasia. J Exp Med 147:470–487.

Murphy, D.B., Yanauchi, K., Habu, S., Eardley, D.D., and Gershon, R.K. 1981. T cells in suppressor circuit and Non-T: Non-B cells bear different I-J determinants. Immunogenetics. 13:205–213.

Payne, R. 1957. Leukocyte agglutinins in human sera. Correlation between blood transfusions and their development. Arch Int Med 99:587–606.

Rosenbaum, J.T. 1981. Why HLA B27: An analysis based on two animal models. Annals Int Med 94:261–263.

Rotter, J.I., and Rimoin, D.L. 1981. The genetics of the glucose intolerance disorders. Am J Med 70:116–126.

Ryder, L.P., Anderson, E., and Svejgaard, A. 1979. HLA and Disease Registry. Munksgaard; Copenhagen.

Sasazuki, T., Kaneoka, H., Nishimura, Y., Kaneoka, R., Hayama, M., and Ohkumi, M. 1980. An HLA linked immune suppression gene in man. J Exp Med 152:2975–3135.

Solinger, A.M., Bhatnagar, R., and Stobo, J.D. 1981. Cellular, molecular, and genetic characteristics of T cell reactivity to collagen in man. Proc Nat Acad Sci. 78:3877–3880

Staszak, C., Goodwin, J.S., Troup, G.M., Pathal, D.R., and Williams, R.C. 1980. Decreased sensitivity to prostaglandin and histamine in lymphocytes from normal HLA-B12 individuals and a possible role in autoimmunity. J Immunol 125: 181–185.

Terasaki, P. 1980. Histocompatibility Testing 1980. UCLA Histocompatibility Testing Laboratory; Los Angeles.

Uhr, J.W., Capra, J.D., Vitetta, E.S., and Cook, R.G. 1979. Organization of the immune response genes. Science 296:292–297.

Chapter 5

Age and the Immune System

Marc E. Weksler and Gregory W. Siskind

Introduction

This review attempts to place in perspective a body of knowledge concerning immune senescence. To a considerable extent, the chapter reflects our view of the immunobiology of aging, which has guided the research studies of our laboratory. Our working hypothesis is that the involution of the thymus after sexual maturity plays a crucial role in the age-associated changes in the immune system. We would certainly not disagree with the possibility that additional factors may contribute to immune senescence. We believe that immune senescence bears on the diseases of aging that have become epidemic in the industrialized countries of the world. There is little doubt that genetic or cellular engineering or immunotherapeutic approaches to immune senescence will be possible in the future. However, we feel it important to consider the real possibility that the immune deficiency associated with aging may be an adaptive mechanism to autoimmune reactions that develop with increasing age. Consequently, nonspecific immune potentiation may not be advantageous.

Thymic Involution and Aging

The involution of the thymus after puberty was recognized long before the immunologic function of the organ was discovered. In the early 1930's, careful anatomical studies showed that the mass of the human thymus, which is well maintained until 15 years of age, rapidly decreases after sexual maturity (Boyd, 1932). By the age of 45 or 50, the lymphoid mass of the human thymus is only 15% of its maximum. In the early 1960's, an immunological function of the thymus was first suggested. The crucial role of the thymus in the generation of mature peripheral lymphoid cells is now well established. The thymus is required for the normal differentiation of a subpopulation of lymphocytes, the so-called thymic-derived lymphocytes or T cells. Precursors of T lymphocytes arise in the bone marrow and migrate to the thymus, where their differentiation continues. Although the differentiation process is not completely understood, it is known that both the microenvironment of the thymus and hormones produced by the thymus are important. There is some evidence that the T cells exported from the thymus are not fully mature but must undergo an additional differentiation event in the peripheral lymphoid organs. In the absence of a normal thymus, the peripheral T cell system fails to develop; there are marked defects in delayed hypersensitivity, the development of cytotoxic T cells and helper and suppressor T cell activities which are important in regulating the immune response. After sexual maturity, the thymus begins to involute and presumably loses its capacity to facilitate the differentiation of prethymic T cell precursors. It is, therefore, logical to consider the contribution of thymic involution to the age-related changes in immune function.

Differentiation of Lymphoid Precursors

One marker of human T cell maturation which is acquired in the thymus is the receptor for sheep erythrocytes (SRBC). The presence of this receptor has offered a convenient method to enumerate T lymphocytes. Mature T lymphocytes form ''rosettes'' with SRBC. The age-associated decline in the capacity of the human thymus to stimulate the maturation of T lymphocytes is manifested by an age-related decrease in the percentage of cells in the thymus which can bind SRBC. At 20 years of age more than 90% of thymic lymphocytes bind SRBC, while at 50 years of age only 65% of thymic lymphocytes bind SRBC and at 80 years of age the incidence falls to 50% (Singh and Singh, 1979).

The progressive decline in the capacity of the thymus to mediate the differentiation of T cells has also been demonstrated by transplantation studies in experimental animals. Thymus glands from mice of different ages have been transplanted into young syngeneic thymectomized recipients (Hirokawa and Makinodan, 1975). Glands from newborn to 3-month-old mice were the most effective in mediating the differentiation of T cell precursors. Over the age of 3 months, there was a progressive age-dependent loss in the capactiy of the thymus to reconstitute irradiated mice to be capable of producing peripheral T cells and manifesting thymic-dependent immune function.

The influence of the thymus on lymphocyte maturation had been thought to be limited to the T lymphocyte subpopulation. Recently, however, the thymus has also been found to play a role in the differentiation of the B cell population (Sherr et al., 1978; Szewczuk et al., 1981). Using a cell transfer system, it was shown that, to be capable of generating a normal high-affinity heterogeneous response, the differentiation of the immature B cell population requires the presence of mature thymocytes. The age of the donor determines the capacity of the thymocytes to bring about this maturation of B cell population. Thus, thymocytes from mice over 6 months of age are severely impaired in their capacity to mediate B cell differentiation as compared with thymocytes from younger mice.

Endocrine Function of the Thymus during Aging

During the past 10 years, several putative thymic hormones (thymopoietin, α_1-thymosin, facteur thymique serique (FTS)) have been isolated and purified and the amino acid sequence of several determined. The serum concentration of each of these hormones has been shown to decline with age. Thymopoietin is a 49 amino acid polypeptide, isolated and sequenced by Gideon Goldstein and his associates. Thymopoietin activity in human serum is well maintained between birth and 30 years of age. Thereafter, a linear decline in serum thymopoietin activity occurs. After the age of 60, no thymopoietin activity can be detected (Lewis et al., 1978). FTS is an 11 amino acid polypeptide isolated from serum. The concentration of FTS in human serum begins to fall after the age of 20 and becomes undetectable after the age of 50 (Bach et al., 1972). The concentration of thymosin alpha-1 in human serum appears to decline even earlier (Alan Goldstein, personal communication, 1980). Thus, the decline in thymic mass is followed by a progressive decline in the serum concentration of thymic humoral factors.

Peripheral T Cell Populations

Despite the involution of the thymus gland, most studies have found that the relative and absolute number of T lymphocytes in the blood of humans does not change between the ages of 20 and 90 years (Gupta and Good, 1979). Studies in normal long-lived mice have also shown that the number of splenic T lymphocytes does not change with age (Stutman, 1972). However, in short-lived autoimmune-prone mice, an age-associated decrease in the number of T lymphocytes in the spleen has been reported. The maintenance of the number of T cells in aged humans and experimental animals, despite the involution of the thymus gland and the decline in the serum concentration of thymic hormone, appears superficially paradoxical. However, it is important to appreciate that the number of T cells present depends, not only on the rate of T cell production, but also on the rate of T cell destruction. Since many T cells are extremely long-lived cells, it is possible that the residual thymic function present during middle and old age is sufficient to replace the number that die. It is possible that some replication of post-thymic T cells might take place. It should also be remembered that the total T cell population has not been measured. Usually, only one (the blood or the spleen) of a number of distinct lymphoid compartments is sampled and the T cell complement in this compartment is found to be unchanged with age. It remains a definite possibility that the total number of T cells within the body of young and old individuals is actually different.

Senescence of the Immune Response

Humoral Immunity

An effect of age on the immune system was first noted more than 50 years ago when the serology of human blood group substances was being studied. The serum concentration of antibody to the erythrocyte A and B antigens was found to decline with age (Thomsen and Kettel, 1929). Subsequently, the concentration of "natural" anti-SRBC antibody (Paul and Bunnel, 1932) and "natural" antibody to salmonella (Roberts-Thompson et al., 1974) was shown to decline with age. In contrast to the age-related decline in the antibody response to foreign antigens, the incidence and concentration of autoantibodies increases with age.

A decrease in the antibody response to foreign antigens and an increase in autoantibodies has also been observed in old experimental animals. Thus, the response of mice to sheep erythrocytes decreases with age, while the level of antinuclear antibody rises (Singhal et al., 1978); the response of mice to trinitrophenylated (TNP) SRBC decreases with age while response to TNP mouse erythrocytes remains constant (Naor et al., 1976). These findings suggest that the characteristic age-associated changes in immune competence are the consequence, not only of a deficiency of thymic function, but also of an alteration in the regulation of the immune system.

Despite the decreased immune response to foreign antigens by aged subjects, there is little or no corresponding decline in serum immunoglobulin concentration (Hallgren et al., 1973). It is possible, although not proven, that the decreased antibody response to foreign antigens is balanced by the increased antibody response to autologous antigens, so that the total immunoglobin concentration remains essentially constant. To express the matter in somewhat different terms, over the course of life there may be a progressive shift in the quantitative distribution of elements (B and T cells) which normally exist, in a steady state, in a network of interacting idiotypes and anti-idiotypes. This shift in distribution within the network appears to be characterized by an increased number of self-reactive clones. In this manner, the total production of immunoglobulin would remain constant despite a shift in the types of antibodies being produced. It is also possible, although not proven, that repeated exposure to common environmental antigens results in a shift in the distribution of antibody specificities within the network.

Cell-mediated Immunity

The age-related decline in thymus-dependent immunity affects not only the antibody response to most antigens (that is, to T-dependent antigens), but also delayed hypersensitivity, tumor and graft rejection and T cell-mediated resistence to mycobacterial, viral and fungal infection. Delayed cutaneous hypersensitivity to a variety of antigens has been studied in humans of various ages (Roberts-Thompson et al., 1974). Subjects over the age of 60 are significantly impaired in reactivity. A lower percentage of humans over the age of 70 have positive skin reactions to tuberculin than do persons under 70 (Waldorf et al., 1968). The loss of T cell-mediated immunity to *Mycobacterium tuberculosis* probably contributes to the clinical observation that reactivation tuberculosis is more frequent among the elderly. The age-related decrease in delayed cutaneous hypersensitivity is not due simply to a decline in immunological memory resulting from a prolonged interval between sensitization and challenge. When young and old humans were exposed for the first time to dinitrochlorobenzene (DNCB) and were challenged shortly thereafter, only 5% of subjects under 70 years of age failed to manifest a contact sensitivity reaction, while 30% of the subjects over 70 were not sensitized (Waldorf et al., 1968). Thus, there is a defect in the capacity of many elderly persons to develop or manifest contact-type hypersensitivity.

Cellular Basis of Immune Senescence

The age-related impairment in antibody production and delayed hypersensitivity observed in the clinical studies summarized above could be due to either a primary defect in the immune system or the inability of a normal immune system to function in a defective internal environment. This question has been examined by studying the response of lymphocytes from old humans in vitro and by studying the behavior of lymphocytes from old experimental animals after transfer into young genetically identical recipients. Under these circumstances, the intrinsic function of lymphocytes can be evaluated in the absence of influences from other physiological changes that accompany aging and might compromise immune function. Data obtained by both experimental approaches are consistent with the view that the predominant defect in immune function of the aged is due to intrinsic defects in their peripheral lymphoid cell populations.

T lymphocytes from humans proliferate when cultured with an antigen to which they have been immunized. The in vitro proliferative response to tuberculin-purified protein derivative (PPD) by lymphocytes from patients with tuberculosis was studied by Nilsson (1971). Lymphocytes from old patients incorporate less thymidine when cultured with PPD than do lymphocytes from young patients. That is, the in vitro proliferative response of T lymphocytes to antigen is inversely correlated with age, suggesting an intrinsic defect in the function of T lymphocytes from elderly persons. Similarly, the proliferative responses of T lymphocytes from aged humans to the plant lectins, phytohemagglutinin (PHA) and pokeweed mitogen (PWM), and to allogeneic or autologous non-T lymphocytes are impaired (Weksler and Hutteroth, 1974; Fernandez and MacSween, 1980).

The basis for the age-associated defect in human T cell proliferation has been studied in detail (Inkeles et al., 1977). Although the total number of T cells is the same in old and young humans, there is only one-half the number of mitogen-responsive T cells in the blood of healthy old subjects as compared with young subjects. This conclusion is based upon the results from the three independent experimental approaches: limiting dilution analysis, susceptibility of dividing cells to viral infection and thymidine incorporation in the presence of colchicine. There is no demonstrable difference in the capacity of T cells from old and young subjects to bind PHA. That is, the number and affinity of lymphocyte receptors for PHA is the same in T cell preparations from young and old subjects. Not only is the number of mitogen-responsive T cells reduced in old donors, but the capacity of mitogen-responsive T cells to divide repeatedly in culture is impaired (Hefton et al., 1980). This was established by measuring the number of lymphocytes dividing for the first, second or third time after 72 hours in culture with PHA. At that time, although the number of T cells dividing for the first time is comparable in cultures of lymphocytes from old and young donors, the number of T cells from old donors dividing for a second or third time is only one-half and one-quarter, respectively, of that observed in cultures of lymphocytes from young donors. This defect in the proliferative capacity of lymphocytes from old subjects may be comparable to defects reported in the proliferative capacity of other types of cells from old subjects (Hayflick, 1965). Fibroblasts (Martin et al., 1970) and arterial smooth muscle cells (Bierman, 1978) from old humans have both been found to divide fewer times in culture than do cells of these types obtained from young persons.

The molecular basis of the proliferative defect observed in lymphocytes from old humans has been investigated. Recent studies have indicated that a T cell product, T cell growth factor (TCGF), which is secreted during culture, is necessary for T cell proliferation. The production of TCGF by lymphocytes from young and old humans has been compared (Gillis et al., 1981). Lymphocytes from old humans produce only half as much TCGF in culture as do lymphocytes from young donors. Not only do lymphocytes from old humans produce less TCGF, but they are also defective in their response to TCGF. That is, TCGF stimulates proliferation of T cells from young persons but does not stimulate the proliferation of T cells from old persons. This appears to be due, at least in part, to the inability of lymphocytes from old donors to bind TCGF. Whether this is the consequence of a decrease in the number and/or the affinity of TCGF receptors has not been determined.

Prostaglandins, which appear to be important cell regulatory molecules, have also been implicated as contributing to the impaired proliferative responses of lymphocytes from old persons. T lymphocytes from old donors are more sensitive to the inhibitory effects of prostaglandins of the E series which are produced in culture by blood monocytes (Goodwin and Messner, 1979). In addition, indomethacin, which blocks prostaglandin synthesis, often augments the proliferative response of T lymphocytes from old donors to a marked degree. The greatest degree of augmentation is observed in cultures of lymphocytes from donors whose lymphocyte proliferative responses are the most impaired in the absence of indomethacin. It has also been reported that macrophages from old mice secrete more prostaglandins of the E series than do macrophages from young animals (Rosenstein and Strausser, 1980).

Recently, techniques have been developed to study antibody production by human lymphocytes in culture. Both T-dependent and T-independent antibody synthesis can be stimulted in vitro by formalinized staphylococci. The staphylococci act as polyclonal activators of B cells and the response is generally assayed in terms of the number of plaque-forming cells (PFC) observed with SRBC as targets. Using this assay, an age-associated defect in antibody production by cultured unfractionated human lymphocytes is seen (Kim et al., 1981). However, when purified B cell preparations are studied, there is no significant difference between the responses of cells from old and young donors. With young subjects, more PFC are generated in cultures of unfractionated lymphocytes than in cultures of purified B lymphocytes. In contrast, with old subjects, more PFC are generated in cultures of purified B lymphocytes than in cultures of unfractionated lymphocytes. These results suggest that the age-associated changes in the peripheral lymphoid cell population are mainly the consequences of alterations in the non-B lymphocyte population. The non-B cell population appears to augment the B cell response in the young but to suppress the response in the aged. The conclusion that B lymphocytes from old humans are relatively unimpaired in the aged is supported by studies showing comparable proliferative responses by B lymphocytes from young and old donors. Thus, thymidine incorporation by purified B lymphocyte preparations incubated with either staphylococci or antihuman immunoglobulin antibody is comparable with preparations from young and old subjects.

Macrophages clearly play critical roles in the immune response. They appear to be involved in antigen processing and presentation and in the generation of factors which stimulate lymphoid cells. In addition to their role in the afferent limb of the immune response, macrophages are also involved as phagocytic cells in the effector limb of the immune response. These complex functions of macrophages have not as yet been defined in detail. Consequently, the role of macrophages in contributing to the age-associated changes in immune function has been difficult to evaluate. The recent observation that the addition of lipopolysaccharide to human macrophages stimulates the release of a factor which replaces murine T cells in the in vitro primary antibody response of murine lymphoid cells to SRBC offers a new approach to the assay of human macrophage function. The capacity of macrophages from old and young humans to produce this T cell replacing factor (TRF) has been measured and no difference has been detected (Kim et al., 1981). These studies suggest that macrophages from elderly humans are not impaired in their function, at least with respect to the production of TRF.

Thus, at the cellular level, the principle cause of the defective immune function of elderly humans appears to lie in the T cell population. Macrophage and B cell functions are relatively intact in the aged. However, only relatively crude assays of human macrophage and B cell function have been examined so far. It would not be surprising if further study revealed subtle age-associated deficits in the function of these cell types. In this regard, it is worth noting that evidence for defective B cell function in aged experimental animals has been reported (Dobken et al., 1980; DeKruyff et al., 1980b). The overall data thus suggest that in humans, T cell function is altered in two ways with age. These are a decreased responsiveness to appropriate stimuli, probably leading to decreased T helper activity and decreased delayed hypersensitivity responses, and an increased suppressor activity which affects B cell responses and possibly also T cell responses.

The availability of inbred strains has permitted genetic analysis of lifespan and immune senescence. Furthermore, cell transfer techniques not possible in the outbred human species can be carried on in bred mice. The fact that different species, and strains within a species, vary in their lifespan suggests a genetic control of aging. Until recently, little was known about the number or location of genes that regulate lifespan. Theoretical interpretation of paleontological evidence of changes in the lifespan of man suggests that less than a thousand genes are involved in regulating lifespan (Cutler, 1975). In mice, some of the genes that regulate lifespan are located in the major histocompatibility complex. This is relevant to immune senescence, since the major histocompatibility complex controls many immune functions. Congenic mice, identical except for small segments in the major histocompatibility complex, have different lifespans (Smith and Walford, 1977). The relationship between lifespan and immune function is supported by the fact that mouse strains with the longest lifespan maintain immune competence for the longest period. These findings suggest the possibility that genes within the major histocompatibility complex influence not only immune function, but also the rate of immune senescence and lifespan. Some data suggesting a relationship between HLA type and lifespan in man have been reported (Greenberg, 1979).

It has long been known that mice show an age-related decline in their antibody response to the T-dependent antigen, SRBC. These early observations have been extended recently by the use of hapten-protein conjugates, which permit a more detailed characterization of the immune defect. In studies using the T-dependent antigen dinitrophenylated bovine gamma globulin (DNP-BGG), it was found that, in addition to the age-related decline in total antibody production, there is a preferential loss of high affinity antibodies and of IgG antibodies (Goidl et al., 1976). The preferential loss of high affinity antibodies has implications both for the health of old animals and for the mechanism underlying immune senescence. High affinity antibody probably affords more effective protection against infection than does low affinity antibody. Thus, the increased susceptibility of old animals to infection may reflect, at least in part, the loss of high affinity antibody production. Since binding a number of cell surface antigen receptors is probably one of the signals required to activate lymphocytes, the affinity of antigen receptors must play a crucial role in the induction of the immune response. If the affinity of antigen receptors is low, a higher concentration of antigen would be required to activate the cell. The loss of high affinity lymphocytes may thus explain the observation that a higher dose of antigen is necessary to elicit a maximum immune response in old as compared to young animals (Makinodan and Adler, 1975). If a higher concentration of antigen were required to initiate an immune response, an infectious disease would progress further before an immune response began and host resistance developed. Loss of high affinity lymphocytes may also explain the observation that an increased dose of tolerogen is required to induce immunologic unresponsiveness in old animals (Dobken et al., 1980; DeKruyff et al., 1980a). As a consequence, it is possible that low concentrations of autologous antigens, which are sufficient to maintain self-tolerance in young animals, are not adequate to maintain self-tolerance in old animals. Such a defect in the maintenance of self-tolerance could be responsible for the increased frequency of auto-antibodies in the aged.

The production of high affinity antibody and the shift to IgG antibody production both depend upon normal T cell helper function (DeKruyff and Siskind, 1979). The preferential loss of high affinity and IgG antibody with age could thus be directly related to the involution of the thymus and the consequent decrease in helper T cells. This conclusion is supported by the findings that the age-related loss of high affinity and IgG antibodies is accelerated after thymectomy; that old mice given the thymic hormone thymopoietin regain their capacity to make IgG and high affinity antibodies (Weksler et al., 1978). The primacy of thymic involution in immune senescence is also suggested by the fact that, despite several reports of an age-related decrease in the response to T-independent antigens (Callard et al., 1977; Dobken et al., 1980; DeKryuff et al., 1980b), the response to T-dependent antigens is, in general, more depressed in old mice than is the response to T-independent antigens (Makinodan and Adler, 1975). Whether the reported age-related change in the response to T-independent antigens is due to an intrinsic defect in B cell function is secondary to increased suppressor T cell activity or is due to a failure of the thymus gland of old animals to mediate B cell differentiation has not been definitively established. However, in vitro and cell transfer studies, as discussed below, suggest that all three factors are probably involved.

The cellular basis for the age-associated defects in the immune response of experimental animals has been extensively investigated by in vitro cell culture methods. Such studies have usually employed mouse lymphocytes and have, in general, yielded results which are comparable to those obtained in studies with human subjects. For example, the response of T lymphocytes from old mice to plant lectins or allogeneic lymphocytes declines with age (Adler and Chrest, 1979). As was found in man, the decreased response to plant lectins was due to a decline in the number of mitogen-responsive T cells and to an impaired capacity of the mitogen-responsive cells to divide repeatedly in culture. Other in vitro parameters of T cell function, including the generation of cytotoxic T cells in mixed lymphocyte culture, also decline with age. A primary specific PFC response to either a T-dependent or a T-independent antigen can be generated in cultures of murine spleen cells. The in vitro PFC response to the T-dependent antigen SRBC was found to be markedly impaired with cells from aged animals (DeKruyff et al., 1980b). A reduced response already is seen at 12 months of age and, by 18 months of age, the response is reduced to less than 5% of the maximal PFC response which is observed between the ages of 3 and 6 months. Several distinct age-associated changes in the immune system contribute to the impaired response of aged mice to SRBC. A deficiency of helper T cells, excessive suppressor T cell activity and an intrinsic, age-associated defect in B cell function was the finding that the anti-DNP PFC response of spleen cells from aged mice to the T-independent antigen DNP-polyacrylamide beads (DNP-PAA) was impaired even after the spleen cell population was depleted of T cells. This implies that the reduced PFC response cannot be due solely to a suppressive effect of T lymphocytes but must be due, at least in part, to an intrinsic defect in the function of the peripheral B cell population (DeKruyff et al., 1980). These studies also demonstrated, by mixed cell culture experiments, an age-associated increase in suppressor T cell activity. It has been reported that the in vitro proliferative response of B lymphocytes to mitogen declines with age. However, it is important to note that the response of B cells to lipopolysaccharide (LPS) declines less with age than does the response of T cells to PHA (Gerbase-DeLima et al., 1974). It should be emphasized that, in most studies where the response to B cell mitogen such as LPS was impaired, the cellular basis of the defect remains uncertain, since T cells have generally not been removed from the cell preparations prior to culture. This is essential; T cell preparations from old mice have been shown to have increased nonspecific suppressor activity. Therefore, removal of T cells is necessary to distinguish an intrinsic defect in B cell function from T cell-mediated suppression of the B lymphocyte response.

Cell transfer studies with inbred mice have provided additional insights into the immune deficiency of aging. In such studies, the function of lymphocytes from old and young animals are compared after their transfer into lethally irradiated syngeneic young recipients. This technique permits a direct assessment of the in vivo function of lymphocytes from old and young mice in the absence of influence by the age-associated physiological or pathological changes that may exist in old animals. Thus, such studies can help distinguish between host effects on immune function (that is, defects arising from the internal environment of the old animals) and defects intrinsic to the cell population being studied. Classic studies by Makinodan and Adler (1975) established that 90% of the age-associated defect in the PFC response of mice to SRBC is due to defects intrinsic to the peripheral lymphoid cell population of the aged animals, while only 10% of the defective PFC response can be attributed to the internal environment of the old host. Subsequently, it was shown that the preferential loss of high affinity and IgG antibody production by old animals also results from intrinsic changes in the peripheral lymphoid cells (Goidl et al., 1976). These transfer studies have also shown that suppressor cell activity increases with age. Thus, the immune response of lethally irradiated recipients of a mixture of spleen cells from old and young donors is lower than the response of mice reconstituted with cells from young donors alone. Spleen cells from 12-, 24- or 34-month-old mice, when transferred together with spleen cells from 2- to 3-month-old mice, inhibit the response of recipients by 60, 80 and 90% respectively, as compared to the responses of recipients given only spleen cells from 2- to 3-month-old donors. It is interesting that the suppression induced by spleen cells from old mice does not preferentially affect high affinity antibody production. This suggests that increased suppressor activity, while probably contributing to the immune defect of aging, does not totally account for it. The results are thus comparable to those obtained in the in vitro studies described above, in which it was shown that deletion of suppressor T cells from the spleen cell population of old mice increased their response to a T-independent antigen but did not restore the response to the level achieved by cells from young mice (Dekruyff et al., 1980b).

The fact that lethally irradiated young mice reconstituted with spleen cells from old donors manifest the impairments in high affinity antibody production and IgG PFC response which are characteristic of old animals permitted us to carry out a series of studies which provide considerable insight into the cellular basis of immune senescence. The high affinity and IgG antibody responses of irradiated recipients of spleen cells from old donors are restored if thymocytes from young donors are transferred together with the spleen cells from old donors (Goidl et al., 1976). Furthermore, residence of spleen cells from old donors for 8 weeks in young irradiated recipients possessing an intact thymus gland results in a reversal of the age-associated defects in high affinity and IgG antibody production. No reversal of the age-associated immune defects is seen in thymectomized recipients of spleen cells from old donors. Finally, the age-associated defects of old spleen cells can be reversed by incubation with the thymic hormone thymopoietin prior to cell transfer (Weksler et al., 1978). The importance of thymic involution in leading to immune senescence is also suggested by the observation that adult thymectomy accelerates the appearance of age-associated immune defects (Weksler et al., 1978).

Taken together, available data support the view that the age-associated defects in immune function are mainly the result of changes in the T cell compartment of the immune system. Available results are consistent with the hypothesis that thymic involution plays a critical role in the sequence of events leading to immune senescence. The experiments demonstrating a reversal of certain of the age-associated defects in immune function following treatment with thymic hormone are of particular interest since they offer a potential therapeutic strategy for modifying the immune deficiency of aging.

Aging and the Regulation of the Immune Response

The involution of the thymus gland and the decline in the serum concentration of thymic hormone precede the age-associated loss of immune function. This temporal relationship suggests that immune senescence might be simply the result of a progressive deficiency in thymic function. Furthermore, the decrease in thymic mass and serum thymic hormone concentration is probably the most regularly occurring age-associated change in the immune system. When other parameters of immune function are examined, there is marked individual variability among aged subjects; some subjects exhibit profound immune defects and others have completely normal immune function. In fact, most physiological parameters studied in aged subjects show an increasing variability with age. In contrast, thymic involution and decrease in thymic hormone concentration occur in an exceeding regular fashion with relatively little individual variation. These findings support a primary role for thymic involution as a necessary but not sufficient cause of the age-associated changes in immune function. Defects in thymic function do not seem to fully account for the complexity of immune senescence. Thus far, it has not been possible to associate immune senescence with the loss of a specific lymphocyte subpopulation or immunoglobulin class. While one might view immune senescence as an immunodeficiency state (in fact, the most common immunodeficiency), the perturbations of immune functions observed in immune senescence tend to be more complex and varied than those seen in most other immunodeficiency states. This wide range of immunological perturbations (e.g., increased autoantibody formation, decreased ease of tolerance induction, increased monoclonal immunoglobulin production, increased incidence of circulating immune complexes) is not usually associated with the classical immune deficiency diseases. However, since the immune system is a network of interacting and countervailing elements, it is possible that thymic involution results, not only in immune deficiency, but also in alterations in immune regulation.

It has been known for some years that the incidence of autoantibodies in humans and experimental animals increases progressively with age. Less than 5% of healthy humans under 40 years of age have autoantibodies to thyroglobulin, DNA or immunoglobulin (rheumatoid factor). In contrast, 60 to 70% of healthy individuals over the age of 80 years have one or more of these autoantibodies (Hallgren et al., 1973). It is important to note that elderly persons with these autoantibodies do not have the typical clinical manifestations of autoimmune disease observed in young persons with autoantibodies. This is not to say that these autoantibodies do not have pathologic significance. An immunologic theory of aging has been proposed (Walford, 1969); it rests upon the thesis that autoimmune damage to cells and tissue contributes to the actual process of aging. Not only can autoantibodies directly damage cells and tissues, but, in addition, the coexistence of autoantibodies and the antigens with which they react can lead to the circulation of immune complexes. Recently, it has been found that nearly one-half of the healthy persons studied over the age of 65 have high levels of circulating immune complexes (Day, N., and Weksler, M.E., unpublished observation). The pathogenic role of circulating immune complexes in vascular and renal diseases is well documented. Whether healthy older subjects with high levels of immune complexes are at increased risk of developing such diseases as compared with age-matched subjects who do not have circulating immune complexes is not known. We believe that discovering the role of circulating immune complexes as potential factors leading to chronic tissue damage is an important area for future investigation. The possibility exists that such complexes might contribute to a variety of different types of chronic tissue damage, including atherosclerotic vascular disease.

The presence of autoantibodies in elderly humans is not the only evidence of impaired regulation of B cell function. Altered B cell regulation is also suggested by the increased prevalence of benign monoclonal gammapathies with age (Axelsson et al., 1966). In these patients the monoclonal proteins are not associated with the bony lesions or malignant transformation of plasma cells seen in myeloma; they thus appear to be manifestations of impaired B cell regulation rather than neoplastic disease. Studies in mice have also revealed an increase in the frequency of benign monoclonal immunoglobulins with age (Radl et al., 1980). Of particular interest was the finding that the prevalence of monoclonal proteins was very much greater in neonatally thymectomized mice. Thus, thymic involution may also contribute to the development of benign monoclonal gammapathies in elderly subjects.

Protection against autoantibodies presumably depends upon a number of mechanisms, including those involved in the induction and maintenance of self-tolerance. Autologous antigens which are present at low concentrations are believed to induce helper T cell tolerance and activate suppressor T cells. Since the activation of autoreactive B cells probably requires helper T cell activity, T cell tolerance presumably serves as a primary defense mechanism against autoantibody production. Suppressor T cells probably serve as a back-up system to control the expression of autoreactive B cells which might, at times, be activated by mechanisms which bypass the requirement of T cell help. Autologous antigens which are present at high concentrations may also induce a specific B cell tolerance. Other mechanisms, such as auto-anti-idiotype antibodies, are probably also involved in self-tolerance. All of these mechanisms for the induction and maintenance of self-tolerance are affected by age. It has been shown that both B and T cell tolerance is more difficult to induce in older animals (McIntosh and Segre, 1976; Fujiwara and Cinader, 1974; Dobken et al., 1980; DeKruyff et al., 1980a).

Administration of the B cell tolerogen, DNP-D-GL, prior to immunization with DNP-BGG dramatically reduces the anti-DNP PFC response in young mice. Far greater amounts of tolerogen are required to induce comparable degrees of unresponsiveness in older mice (Dobken et al., 1980). This resistance to tolerance induction was shown by cell transfer studies to be an intrinsic property of the peripheral B cell population of older mice. The detailed mechanism for the age-related decrease in the ease of B cell tolerance induction is not known. It is known, however, that B cell tolerance is more readily induced in high affinity than in low affinity B cells (Davie et al., 1972; Szewczuk and Siskind, 1977; DeKruyff and Siskind, 1980). The reduced affinity of the B cell population of aged mice may thus contribute to its lack of susceptibility to tolerance induction. A defect in the capping of the surface immunoglobulin of B cells from aged rats following treatment with anti-immunoglobulin antibody has been reported (Woda and Feldman, 1979). Such an age-related alteration in the behavior of B cell membrane immunoglobulin might also contribute to the age-related decrease in ease of B cell tolerance induction. It is interesting that, as with a number of other parameters of immune function, the decrease in ease of tolerance induction begins relatively early (at approximately 6 months) in the lifespan of long-lived BALB/c mice (Dobken et al., 1980).

The effect of age on the ease of induction of helper T cell tolerance has also been studied (DeKruyff et al., 1980a). The model employed was the induction of carrier-specific unresponsiveness by the injection of ultracentrifuged BGG followed by challenge with DNP-BGG. The reduction in the anti-DNP PFC response as a consequence of the prior injection of BGG tolerogen was taken as an assay of helper T cell tolerance. It was found that a higher dose of tolerogen is required to induce the same degree of T cell unresponsiveness in older mice. Cell transfer studies showed that the altered ease of tolerance induction is an intrinsic property of the peripheral T lymphocyte population of the aged mice. The relative resistance to T cell tolerance induction begins at about 6 months of age in long-lived BALB/c mice. The mechanism of the increased resistance of T cells from older mice to tolerance induction has not been elucidated. It was suggested above that a loss of high affinity antibody producing cells might contribute to the increased resistance of B cells to tolerance induction. Whether a similar mechanism might operate at the T cell level is not known. There is some evidence for an age-related loss of T cells with high affinity receptors for antigen. It has been reported that the affinity of cytotoxic T cells for target cells is lower in old mice than in young mice (Zharhary and Gershon, 1980).

Over the past 10 years it has become clear that suppressor cells play an important role in the regulation of the immune response. While most attention has been devoted to T lymphocytes with suppressor activity, there is evidence that non-T lymphocytes, including monocytes and B lymphocytes, can also regulate the immune response downward. Altered suppressor cell activity has been reported in several diseases characterized by immune deficiency or autoimmunity. In general, high levels of suppressor activity have been associated with immune deficiency and low levels of suppressor activity with autoimmunity. The alterations in the immunologic system which are associated with aging include both decreased immune responses to foreign antigens (immune deficiency) and the presence of autoantibodies (autoimmunity). It has been suggested that this paradox might result from different subpopulations of suppressor cells being involved in regulating immune responses to self and to foreign antigens. There is considerable evidence that spontaneous suppressor activity for foreign antigens is increased in old humans and old experimental animals. Thus, the human non-B lymphocyte population (monocytes and/or T lymphocytes) from old donors inhibits the in vitro synthesis of antibody by autologous B cells (Kim et al., 1981). Similarly, spleen cells from old mice suppress the in vitro antibody responses of syngeneic spleen cells from young mice (Goidl et al., 1976). In studies where more precise assessment of the age-related changes in suppressor activity was carried out, suppressor activity increases markedly after 12 months of age, approximately one-third the maximal lifespan for mice (DeKruyff et al., 1980). In contrast to the increase in spontaneous apparently nonspecific suppressor activity with age, mitogen-induced suppressor activity has been reported to remain constant or decrease with age (Hallgren and Yunis, 1977).

Exposure of lymphocytes to LPS in vivo or in vitro induces autoantibody formation. LPS bypasses the requirement for T cell helper function and directly activates B cells, including autoreactive ones. Spleen cells from old mice incubated in vitro with LPS produce more autoantibodies than do spleen cells from young mice (Meredith et al., 1979; Goidl, et al., 1981). This suggests an increased incidence of autoreactive B cells in aged animals.

It has generally been felt that the increased incidence of autoantibodies in the aged reflects abnormalities in the normal mechanisms of regulation of the immune system, such as a decrease in suppressor cell activity. However, most studies of aging in man and in long-lived mouse strains have revealed an age-related increase in suppressor activity. The possibility exists that a different subset of suppressor cells is involved in regulating responses to autologous and to foreign antigens (Naor et al., 1976): additional study is necessary to validate this interesting hypothesis.

The fact that two of the mechanisms (suppressor cell activity and auto-anti-idiotype antibody production) involved in regulating the immune system downward are both increased in aging suggests that a failure of these regulatory mechanisms is not the cause of autoantibody production in the aged. In fact, the age-related increase in the activity of mechanisms involved in regulating the immune response downward suggests that they might actually be activated as protective mechanisms in an effort to prevent or turn off autoantibody production. According to this hypothesis, the decreased immune response to foreign antigens that accompanies aging is actually an undesirable side effect of homeostatic mechanisms which protect the organism against the consequences of autoantibody production. A plausible hypothesis is that a decline in the capacity to induce B and T cell tolerance leads to a loss of self-tolerance and, in the face of constant stimulation by self-antigens, expansion of the number of autoreactive B cells and an increase in autoantibody production. The increased incidence of self-reactive B cells after LPS stimulation in vitro reflects this situation. The autoimmune responses which follow the loss of self tolerance may also result in the stimulation of suppressor cell activity and auto-anti-idiotype antibody production, both of which normally suppress these reactions. The situation is further complicated by the fact that certain autoantibodies may react with regulatory T cells and thereby contribute to the regulatory imbalance within the immune system. For example, some elderly humans have an autoantibody with specificity for a population of suppressor T cells (Strelkauskas, 1980). This could result in abnormalities of immune regulation leading to the perpetuation of the autoimmune state.

A set of autoantibodies are now recognized which play an important role in the normal regulation of the immune response. An idiotype is defined as the antigen-combining site of an antibody molecule when it is considered as an antigenic determinant. Anti-idiotype antibodies are antibodies specific for the antigen-combining site of another antibody molecule. Depending upon their class and concentration, anti-idiotype antibodies can act to depress or to augment an immune response. Thus, the idiotype and the anti-idiotype antibody form a mutually stimulatory and inhibitory pair. It has been shown that during a normal immune response an animal produces not only antibody specific for the foreign antigen, but also auto-anti-idiotype antibody specific for the idiotype of the antibody to the foreign antigen (Schrater et al., 1979; Goidl et al., 1979). It has further been shown that such auto-anti-idiotype antibodies can specifically inhibit secretion of antibody by interaction with idiotype on the surface of B lymphocytes (Goidl et al., 1979; Schrater et al., 1979). Jerne (1974) has suggested that the immune system exists as a steady-state network of interacting idiotypes and anti-idiotypes. It seems possible that in this way the immune system acts to regulate itself. It should be emphasized that idiotype-specific regulatory interactions probably operate on both T and B lymphocytes, as well on serum antibody. There is considerable evidence that some suppressor T cell activity is actually idiotype-specific (Sy et. al., 1980). Recent studies have shown that among the autoantibodies formed by old mice there is an increased production of auto-anti-idiotype antibody in old mice (Goidl et al., 1980). This regulation downward contributes to the apparent immune defect in aged mice. Finally, it has been shown that the repertoire of idiotypes on antibodies changes with age (Goidl et al., 1980). That is, the set DNP-specific idiotypes produced by mice in response to DNP-Ficoll changes with age. This represents an additional age-related change in B cell function and regulation.

In summary, a complex set of changes occurs with age in the mechanisms which are normally involved in regulating the immune system. These changes can explain both the immunodeficiency and enhanced autoreactivity that occur in old humans and experimental animals. It can be reasonably suggested that resistance to tolerance induction results in an increased susceptibility to the activation of autoreactive B lymphocytes to autoantibody formation. Increased suppressor cell activity and increased auto-anti-idiotype antibody production appear as a homeostatic mechanism to autoantibody formation and the immune response contributes to the immunodeficiency of aging. Thus, the activation of suppressor activity might be secondary to the autoimmune phenomena which occur in the aged. Such a view implies that the increased suppressor activity in the aged represents a defense mechanism against autoimmunity and that its effect on the immune response to extrinsic antigens is an undesirable side effect of a normal regulatory mechanism.

Biological Significance of Immune Senescence

It has been suggested that immune senescence plays an important role, not only in the development of diseases which prevent animals from reaching the maximal lifespan, but also in establishing the maximal lifespan of the species. The finding that genes of the major histocompatibility complex influence both the rate of immune senescence and lifespan suggests a close relationship between the immune system and aging. Furthermore, two procedures which increase the lifespan of animals, undernutrition and reduction in body temperature in poikilotherms, are associated with marked effects on the immune system. Among humans there is a wide variation in immune competence after middle age and preliminary evidence points to an association between immune competence and life expectancy. Thus, old humans with autoantibodies (MacKay, 1972), with low suppressor activity (Hallgren and Yunis, 1977) or with greatly impaired cutaneous delayed hypersensitivity (Roberts-Thompson et al., 1974) are at increased risk of death. Whether the loss of immune competence truly identifies individuals who are at high risk of early death requires confirmation by additional prospective study. Confirmation of a causal relationship between immune senescence and early death would require the demonstration that the maintenance of immunologic vigor prolongs survival.

Regardless of whether future work does or does not sustain an immunological theory of aging, it is almost certain that immune senescence plays an important part in the increased susceptibility of old humans to the diseases of aging. The increased incidence of infection clearly can be related to the loss of immune competence. It is also likely that immune senescence contributes to the increased incidence of neoplastic disease among the elderly. Finally, the disordered state of self-tolerance, the formation of autoantibodies and the circulation of immune complexes may contribute to or accelerate a variety of disease states, including atherosclerotic vascular disease, as a result of chronic low grade tissue damage. Thus, studies of the effects of age on the immune system offer strategies to influence the development of these diseases by therapeutic modification of the immune system. However, it is important to bear in mind that the progressive programmed decline in thymic function may well be an evolutionary developed protective mechanism against overwhelming autoimmune disease. If this hypothesis were true, then premature intervention to increase immune function might have greater negative than positive consequences. It is thus crucial to learn more about the changes in immune function which accompany aging and their biologic consequences and evolutionary significance.

Acknowledgments

Supported in part by grants AI 11694, CA 20075, CA 13339, CA 26344, AG 00239 and AG 00541. This manuscript is adapted from one published in the Annual Review of Gerontology and Geriatrics.

References

Adler, W.H., and Chrest, F.J. 1979. The mitogen response assay as a measure of immune deficiency of aging mice. In: Developmental Immunobiology, Ed. G.W. Siskind, S.D. Litwin, and M.E. Weksler, p. 233. Grune and Stratton; New York.

Axelsson, U., Bachmann, R., and Hallen, J. 1966. Frequency of pathological proteins (M-components) in 6,995 sera from an adult population. Act Med Scand 179:235.

Bach, J.F., Papiernick, M., Levasseur, P., Dardenne, M., Baros, A., and LeBrigand, H. 1972. Evidence for a serum-factor secreted by the human thymus. Lancet 2:1056.

Bierman, E.L. 1978. The effect of donor age on the in vitro life span of cultured human arterial smooth-muscle cells. In Vitro 14:951.

Boyd, E. 1932. The weight of the thymus gland in health and in disease. Amer J Dis Children 43:116.

Callard, R.E., Basten, A., and Waters, L.K. 1977. Immune function in aged mice. II. B cell function. Cell Immunol 31:26.

Cutler, R.G. 1975. Evolution of human longevity and the genetic complexity governing aging rate. Proc Natl Acad Sci USA 72:4664.

Davie, J.M., Paul, W.E., Katz, D.H., and Benacerraf, B., 1972. Hapten-specific tolerance. Preferential depression of the high affinity antibody response. J Exp Med 136:426.

DeKruyff, R.H., Rinnooy Kan, E.A., Weksler, M.E., and Siskind, G.W. 1980a. Effect of aging on T-cell tolerance induction. Cell Immunol 56:58.

DeKruyff, R., Kim, Y.T., Siskind, G.W., and Weksler, M.E. 1980b. Age related changes in the *in vitro* immune response: Increased suppressor activity in immature and aged mice. J Immunol 125:142.

DeKruyff, R., and Siskind, G.W. 1979. Studies on the control of antibody synthesis. XIV. Role of T cells in regulating antibody affinity. Cell Immunol 47:134.

DeKruyff, R.H., and Siskind, G.W. 1980. Studies on the control of antibody synthesis. XVI. Effect of immunodepression on antibody affinity. Cell Immunol 49:90.

Dobken, J., Weksler, M.E., and Siskind, G.W. 1980. Effect of age on ease of B-cell tolerance induction. Cell Immunol 55:66.

Fernandez, A., and MacSween, J. 1980. Decreased autologous mixed lymphocyte reaction with aging. Mechanisms of Ageing and Development 12:245.

Fujiwara, M., and Cinader, B. 1974. Cellular aspects of tolerance. V. The *in vivo* cooperative role of accessory and thymus derived cells in responsiveness and unresponsiveness in SJL mice. Cell Immunol 12:194.

Gerbase-DeLima, M., Wilkinson, J., Smith, G.S., and Walford, R.L. 1974. Age related decline in thymic independent immune function in a long-lived mouse strain. J Gerontol 29:261.

Gillis, S., Kozak, R., Durante, M., and Weksler, M.E. 1981. Immunological studies of aging. Decreased production of and response to T cell growth factor by lymphocytes from aged humans. J Clin Invest 67:937.

Goidl, E.A., Innes, J.B., and Weksler, M.E. 1976. Immunological studies of aging. II. Loss of IgG and high avidity plaque-forming cells and increased suppressor activity in aging mice. J Exp Med 1445:1037.

Goidl, E.A., Michelis, M.A., Siskind, G.W., and Weksler, M.E. 1981. Effect of age on the induction of autoantibodies. Clin Exp Immunol 44:24.

Goidl, E.A., Schrater, A.F., Thorbecke, G.J., and Siskind, G.W. 1979. Production of auto-anti-idiotype antibdy during the normal immune response to TNP-ficoll. II. Hapten-reversible inhibition of anti-TNP plaque-forming cells by immune serum as an assay for auto-anti-idiotypic antibody. J Exp Med 150:154.

Goidl, E.A., Thorbecke, G.J., Weksler, M.E., and Siskind, G.W. 1980. Production of auto-anti-idiotypic anti-body response and the idiotype repertoire associated with aging. Proc Natl Acad Sci USA 77:6788.

Goodwin, J.S. and Messner, R.P. 1979. Sensitivity of lymphocytes to prostaglandin E_2 increases in subjects over age 70. J Clin Invest 64:434.

Greenberg, L.J. 1979. Aging and immune function in man: Influence of sex and genetic background. In: Aging and Immunity, eds. S.K. Singhal and N.R. Sinclair, p. 43. Elsevier/North-Holland; New York.

Gupta, S., and Good, R.A. 1979. Subpopulation of human T lymphocytes X. Alterations in T, B, third population cells and T cell with receptors for immunoglobulin M or G in aging humans. J Immunol 122:1214.

Hallgren, H.M., and Yunis, E.J. 1977. Suppressor lymphocytes in young and aged humans. J Immunol 118:2004.

Hallgren, H.M., Buckley, C.E., Gilbertsen, V.A., and Yunis, E.J. 1973. Lymphocyte phytohemagglutinin responsiveness, immunoglobulins and autoantibodies in aging humans. J Immunol 111:1101.

Hallgren, H.M., Yunis, E.J. 1980. In: Immunological Aspects of Aging, eds. D. Segre and L. Smith, Marcell Dekker: New York.

Hayflick, L. 1965. The limited *in vitro* lifespan of human diploid strain. Exp Cell Res 37:164.

Hefton, J.M., Darlington, G., Casazza, B.A., and Weksler, M.E. 1980. Immunological studies of aging. V. Impaired proliferation of PHA responsive human lymphocytes in culture. J Immunol 125:1007.

Hirokawa, K., and Makinodan, T. 1975. Thymic involution: Effect on T cell differentiation. J Immunol 114:1659.

Inkeles, B., Innes, J.B., Kuntz, M.M., Kadish, A.S., and Weksler, M.E. 1977. Immunological studies of aging. III. Cytokinetic basis for the impaired response of lymphocytes from aged humans to plant lectins. J Exp Med 145:1176.

Jerne, N.K. 1974. Towards a network theory of the immune system. Ann Immunol (Paris) 125 (C):373.

Kim, Y.T., Siskind, G.W., and Weksler, M.E., 1981. Cellular basis of the impaired response of elderly humans. In: Human B Cell Functions: Activation and Immuno-regulation, eds. A.S. Fauci and R. Ballieux. Raven Press; New York.

Lewis, V.M., Twomey, J.J., Bealmear, P., Goldstein, G., and Good, R.A. 1978. Age, thymic involution and circulating thymic hormone activity. J Clin Endo Met 48:145.

MacKay, I. 1972. Aging and immunological function in man. Gerontologia 18:285.

Makinodan, T., and Adler, W.H., 1975. Effects of aging on the differentiation and proliferative potentials of cells of the immune system. Fed Proc 34:153.

Martin, G.M., Sprague, C.A., and Epstein, C.J. 1970. Replicative life span of cultivated human cells effects of donor's age, tissue and genotype. Lab Invest 23:86.

McIntosh, K.R., and Segre, D. 1976. B and T cell tolerance induction in young-adult and old mice. Cell Immunol 27:230.

Meredith, P.J., Kristie, J.A., and Walford, R.L. 1979. Age increases expression of LPS induced autoantibody-secreting B cells. J Immunol 123:87.

Naor, D., Bonavida, B., and Walford, R.L. 1976. Autoimmunity and aging: The age-related response of mice of a long-lived strain to trinitrophenylated syngeneic mouse red blood cells. J Immunol 117:2204.

Nilsson, B.S. 1971. Reactivity to PPD and phytohemagglutin in relation to PPD skin reactivity and age. Scand J Resp Dis 52:39.

Paul, J.R., and Bunnell, W.W. 1932. Anti-SRBC agglutinon with age. Am J Med Sci 183:90.

Radl, J., DeGlopper, E., Van den Berg, P., and Van Zwieten, M.J. 1980. Idiopathic paraproteinemia. III. Increased frequency of paraproteinemia in thymectomized aging C57BL/KaLwRij and CBA/BrRij mice. J Immunol 125:31.

Roberts-Thompson, I.C., Whittingham, S.I., Youngchayud, V., and MacKay, T.R. Aging, immune response and mortality. Lancet 2:368.

Rosenstein, M.M., and Strausser, H.R. 1980. Macrophage-induced T cell mitogen suppression with age. J Reticendothel Soc 27:159.

Schrater, A.F., Goidl, E.A., Thorbecke, G.J., and Siskind, G.W. 1979. Production of auto-anti-idiotypic antibody during the normal immune response to TNP-ficoll. I. Occurrence in AKR/j and BALB/c mice of hapten-augmentable, anti-TNP plaque-forming cells and their accelerated appearance in recipients of immune spleen cells. J Exp Med 150:138.

Sherr, D.H., Szewczuk, M.R., and Siskind, G.W. 1978. Ontogeny of B-lymphocyte function. V. Thymus cell involvement in the functional maturation of B-lymphocytes from fetal mice transferred into adult irradiated hosts. J Exp Med 142:196.

Singh, V., and Singh, A.K. 1979. Age-related changes in human thymus. Clin Exp Immunol 37:507.

Singhal, S.K., Roder, J.C., and Duwe, A.K. 1978. Suppressor cells in immunosenesence. Fed Proc 37:1245.

Smith, G.S., and Walford, R.L. 1977. Influence of the main histocompatability complex on aging in mice. Nature 270:727.

Strelkauskas, A. 1980. Autoantibodies to a regulatory T cell subset in human aging. In: Immunological Aspects of Aging, eds. D. Segre and L. Smith. Marcel Dekker: New York.

Stutman, O. 1972. Lymphocyte subpopulations in NZB mice: Deficit of thymus-dependent lymphocytes. J Immunol 109:602.

Sy, M.S., Dietz, M.H., Germain, R.N., Benacerraf, B., and Green, M.I. 1980. Antigen- and receptor-driven regulatory mechanisms. IV. Idiotype-bearing I−J+ suppressor T cell factors induce second-order suppressor T cells which express anti-idiotypic receptors. J Exp Med 151:1183.

Szewczuk, M., and Siskind, G.W. 1977. Ontogeny of B-lymphocyte function. III. *In vivo* and *in vitro* studies on the ease of tolerance induction in B lymphocytes from fetal, neonatal and adult mice. J Exp Med 145:1590.

Szewczuk, M.R., DeKruyff, R.H., Weksler, M.E., and Siskind, G.W. 1980. Ontogeny of B lymphocyte funtion. VIII. Failure of thymus cells from aged donors to induce the functional maturation of B lymphocytes from immature donors. Eur J Immunol 10:918

Szewczuk, M.R., Sherr, D.H., and Siskind, G.W. 1978. Ontogeny of B lymphocyte function. VI. Ontogeny of thymus cell capacity to facilitate the functional maturation of B lymphocytes. Eur J Immunol 8:370.

Thomsen, O., and Kettel, K. 1929. Die starke der menschlichen isoagglutinine und entsprechenden Blutkorper-chenrezeptoren in verschiendenen lebensaltern. Z Immunforsch 63:67.

Waldorf, D.S., Wilkens, R.F., and Decker, J.L. 1968. Impaired delayed hypersensitivity in an aging population. J Am Med Assoc 203:831.

Walford, R. 1969. The Immunologic Theory of Aging. Munksgaard; Copenhagen.

Weksler, M.E., and Hutteroth, T.H. 1974. Impaired lymphocyte function in aged humans. J Clin Invest 53:99.

Weksler, M.E., Innes, J.B., and Goldstein, G. 1978. Immunological studies of aging. IV. The contribution deficiencies of aging mice. J Exp Med 648:996.

Woda, B.A. and Feldman, J.D. 1979. Density of Surface Immunoglobulin and Capping on Rat B Lympcyle. I. Changes with Aging. J Exp Med 149:416.

Zharhary, D., and Gershon, H. 1980. T-cytotoxic reactivity of senescent mice. Fourth International Congress of Immunology, Paris. Abstract 3.8.37.

Chapter 6

Congenital Immunodeficiencies

Richard Hong

Introduction

In this chapter, various mechanisms by which immunodeficiency can occur are proposed. Over the years, my analysis of the immunodeficiency disorders has come to be somewhat at variance with standard dogma. In large part, my departure from tradition is based upon clinical observation and the effect of therapy.

A major advance in the understanding of immunodeficiency was made possible by the animal models created by thymectomy and bursectomy. This led to the concept of two immunities, T cell and B cell, each developing under separate control and each concerned with different kinds of protective capability. The concept of separate immunities gave rise to the three major classes of deficiency, isolated T deficiency, isolated B deficiency or combined T and B deficiencies. Animal models of the various kinds were created and clinical counterparts in man were discovered. A very neat classification which explained etiology, predicted clinical symptomatology and suggested appropriate therapy was proposed (Fudenberg et al., 1971). Further verification of the hypothesis appeared with the dramatic responses to fetal thymus transplantation and bone marrow transplantation (Good and Bach, 1974).

As the methodology for the study of patients improved and as more patients were studied, a number of inconsistencies appeared. However, observations not in keeping with the expected results, rather than stimulating re-examination of the hypothesis, were largely ignored.

The Stem Cell Defect

Original Observations

The concept of stem cell deficiency arose from two basic animal models, the bursectomized chicken and the neonatally thymectomized mouse. It is helpful to review these earlier observations to place them in proper perspective with more recent findings. Chicken studies were of signal importance in the early understanding of the anatomy of the immune system. The fact that removal of the bursa could render an animal essentially agammaglobulinemic while having no effect on T cell immunity was perfectly correlated with subsequent demonstration of intact T cell immunity in human agammaglobulinemic patients (Peterson et al., 1965). Similarly, neonatal thymectomy in a mouse led to marked deficiency of T cell-controlled immune responses, leaving an intact B cell system (Miller, 1961; Good et al., 1962; Waksman et al., 1962). The finding by DiGeorge (1967) that an embryological defect involving thymic primordia in the 3rd and 4th pharyngeal pouches which resulted in what was originally thought to be athymia was associated with normal B cell function provided further clinical verification for an independent two-cell system. If T cells could be eliminated by thymic ablation of dysplasia and B cells could be removed by bursal manipulation and in either case the other lymphoid system was unaffected, the only reasonably simple genetic cause of a combined T-B cell defect would be a stem cell fault. To postulate a genetic problem in two such different sites of differentiation as the thymus and the bursa was unnecessarily tedious. If the results of therapy [the complete correction of a combined T and B cell defect by an infusion of bone marrow (i.e., stem cells) and the correction of the DiGeorge syndrome by fetal thymus transplantation] were examined, then Koch's postulates were largely fulfilled.

The ultimate truth of a hypothesis depends upon its ability to withstand the test of time. Although exceptions to the general rule were found, refinements should have been basically confirmations of the general theme of the hypothesis. As more information accumulated, however, it became clear that a major revision was in order.

T Control of the B Cell System

The first modification was required when Claman et al. (1966) showed an intimate dependence of antibody production on T cells, challenging the concept of complete independence of the two systems. Although some antigens can bypass the T helper cell requirement, most are T-dependent for vigorous B cell responses. Further, complete isotype diversity (i.e., IgA and IgG responses) was shown to be T-dependent. The nude mouse, an animal which is congenitally athymic, showed some IgM responses, but poor IgG and IgA responses. Serum levels of IgG and IgA were markedly diminished in these animals. Thus, in the naturally occurring situation of congenital absence, in which the defect occurred much earlier than could be produced by surgical ablation, profound B cell defects were secondary to an absence of the thymus gland. Since nude mouse bone marrow could reconstitute lethally x-irradiated animals, there was no stem cell defect. In other words, combined B and T cell disease occurred in a mutant strain which clearly did not have a stem cell defect. The difference between thymectomy at birth and thymic dysplasia in utero was largely a matter of timing. The relative sparing of the B cells following neonatal thymectomy could be explained by the long life of peripheralized T cells which could exert their effects long after surgical extirpation. Too much peripheralization had occurred before surgery.

What of the human model, the DiGeorge syndrome? As more cases were studied, a normal B cell compartment was not a constant feature. Complete and incomplete forms of the DiGeorge syndrome occurred, with complete or incomplete absence of the thymus gland. Also, ectopic thymuses were discovered (sometimes in the middle ear), so one could never be absolutely certain that there was no thymus. Further, a thymus gland, originally of small size, could undergo gradual attrition and be virtually absent at examination, but peripheralized T cells could have fulfilled a helper function, allowing detectable B cell products and responses in the face of an absent post mortem thymus. Another largely ignored feature of the DiGeorge syndrome was the tendency for spontaneous cure. In addition to the recorded cases, we have personally observed three children who showed diminution of T cell function at birth which completely reverted to normal with time and without therapy. Thus, any reconstitution attributed to thymus transplantation must be viewed with skepticism. Indeed, in one of the early reported successes, normalization of lymphocyte count occurred within 24 hours (August et al., 1968).

The other classic example of B cell independence in man, the Nezelof syndrome, must also be viewed critically. The Nezelof analysis was made within the framework of the T cell-independent B cell system bias; presence of Ig was equated with full and competent B cell responses. We now know that presence of Ig is not the same as presence of antibody. As additional cases of the Nezelof variety have been examined with more extensive modern methodology, individuals cannot be found who have shown a normal intact B cell system [i.e., normal levels of all three major Ig's and normal antibody responses to a number of antigens when the basic fault is thymic dysplasia with onset in utero (reviewed in Horowitz and Hong, 1977a)].

It is particularly illustrative to examine cases of adenosine deaminase (ADA) deficiency. We have observed three cases in which thymic biopsy could be correlated with B cell function. In one, a lymphoid thymus, lacking Hassall's corpuscles but showing only modest involuntary changes, was seen. This patient had normal Ig levels and responded to several immunogens as well as naturally occurring viral infections. Although her total lymphocyte count was less than 600/mm^3, she had modest proliferative responses. Another patient had a completely alymphoid thymus. Ig synthesis was never observed, in vitro responses to T cell mitogens was nil and she died at 3 months of age despite attempts to provide enzyme through exchange transfusion. A third patient showed a thymus with a histologic picture of dysplasia between the two extremes. She had some, but not completely normal, Ig responses and showed modest T cell proliferation in vitro. It is known that with time B cell responses can disappear in ADA deficiency, but the initial defect involves the T cells. In ADA deficiency, it is thought that there is a gradual loss of T cells due to the accumulation of toxic metabolites as a result of the ADA deficiency. The toxic metabolite accumulation primarily affects T cell replication, leading to a progressively more severe T cell deficiency. It can be seen that ADA deficiency could produce variable degrees of T cell deficiency at various ages depending upon the severity of the enzyme defect and possibly the ability of the mother to correct the defect in utero (Cohen et al., 1978). In the cases cited above, one can use the thymic histology as an index of the severity of the T cell deficiency and see a definite dependence of the B cell deficiency upon the T cell mass. In my experience, no child with normal antibody production and a dysplastic thymus has been observed except in enzyme deficiency where the T cell loss is usually a postnatal event.

I believe these observations indicate a profound dependence of the B cell system upon intact T cells. There is, in fact, little evidence that a B cell system of any note will develop if the thymus never develops or is somehow destroyed early in fetal life. Four points deserve emphasis at this time.

Models of T cell deficiency created by thymus ablation are confounded by effects of T cells which peripheralize prior to the surgery and by the long lifespan of such cells. Preservation of B cell activity in such animal models cannot be taken as evidence of full B cell development in the absence of T cells.

In nude mice, where there is total absence of the thymus from the earliest time of immune system development, B cell deficiency is constant. This seems to me to be a most convincing argument for the role of the thymus in B cell development and avoids the problems inherent in interpreting the surgically produced thymic deficiency model. Nevertheless, immunoglobulins are readily measured in nude mice; I shall deal with that problem later.

In humans, the DiGeorge syndrome has been repeatedly presented as an example of isolated T deficiency. In so doing, one ignores the tremendous heterogeneity of B cell deficiency observed in the syndrome and also the tendency for DiGeorge syndrome patients to show spontaneous remission. These patients should not be used in the analysis of immune defects in man except to show how extreme variation can make extrapolation from clinical studies especially hazardous.

The overwhelming weight of evidence is in favor of a thymus control over B cell development and suggests that intrauterine thymus failure must result in associated B cell deficiency. Combined T and B cell deficiency then can result solely from a T cell defect.

What of the immunoglobulins which are found in the nude mouse or in the Nezelof syndrome? Examination of the immunoglobulins in such cases shows quite poor specific antibody responses. The phenomen of Ig response in the face of nonreactivity to antigen can be explained by polyclonal B cell activation. Certain materials, one of which is pokeweed mitogen (PWM), can trigger B cells to synthesize and secrete immunoglobulin. Following a PWM stimulus in vitro, all of the B cell clones in the culture are increased in number and are

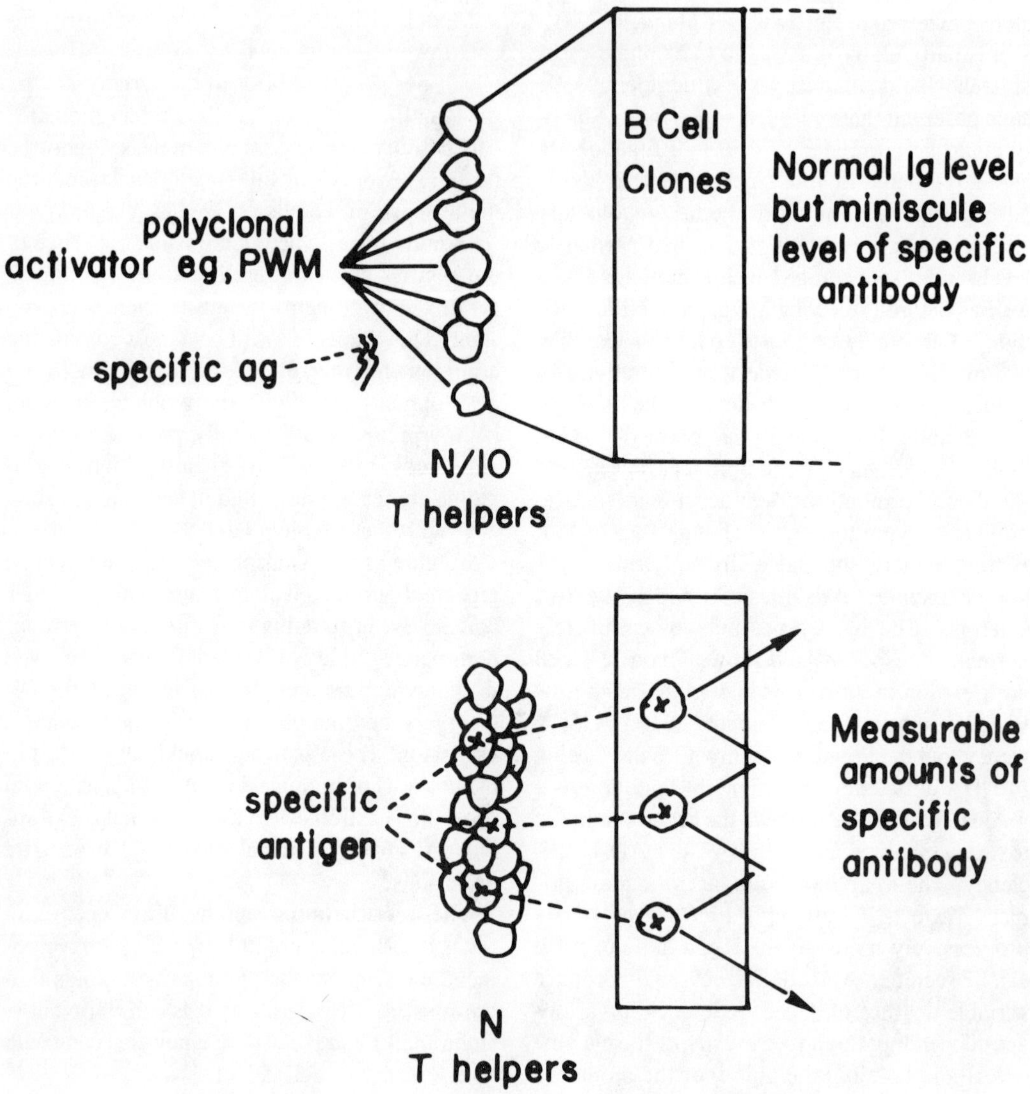

Fig. 6.1 Measurable Ig levels associated with T cell deficiency or normal T cell numbers. In the upper drawing, there is a paucity of T helper cells (N = 10). Since T-dependent polyclonal stimulators react nonselectively with helpers, there are sufficient T helper cells to stimulate Ig secretion by all of the B cell clones which proliferate, but only a small amount. However, specific antibody comprises only a small percent of the total Ig. A given antigen (specific ag) cannot initiate clonal B cell responses, because the probability of finding T helper cells for that antigen is only 10% of the usual situation.

In the lower drawing, there are sufficient T helpers to allow the antigen to "find" its relevant helper cell. This induces expansion of specific antibody-producing clones, which then produce measurable levels of antibody. The expansion of the few specific antibody-forming clones is shown to equal the total Ig production of all the stimulated clones in the upper drawing. These quantitative relationships are probably exaggerated as compared to the true in vivo situation; the basic principle seems reasonable, however.

caused to mature to a state where they can secrete immunoglobulin. Such a response will produce easily measurable levels of total immunoglobulin. However, because all clones are equally proliferating, a single clonal product is not disportionately produced. Therefore, except in a few special cases, levels of a given antibody are not present in amounts sufficient to be measured unless one uses very sensitive assays which measure at a cellular level. It requires stimulation of a clone by its unique relevant antigen to produce an expansion great enough to yield an easily detectable product. These points are diagrammatically shown in Figure 6.1. Often, the immunoglobulins of the Nezelof syndrome are visibly restricted in their electrophoretic heterogeneity, further suggesting an impaired B cell response. On this basis, it cannot be stated that the B cell system in the Nezelof syndrome is normal. In man, a truly or nearly normal B cell system in the face of demonstrated severe T cell deficiency has not been shown except for the secondary postnatal thymus defects such as ADA and nucleoside phosphorylase (NP) deficiency.

Another experience which demonstrates the thymus role on the B cell system is the result obtained with cultured thymus transplantation. We have achieved a correction of both T and B cell systems with thymus alone in nearly 20 instances and know of 3 instances in other institutions. We have never achieved only a T cell response, which is what would be predicted if T and B systems were truly independent. Also, correction by transplantation of thymus alone speaks against a stem cell defect.

Correction of T-B Defects by Bone Marrow

A final line of evidence for a stem cell defect as the cause of combined immunodeficiency (CID) is the observation that bone marrow transplantation can effect a cure of both T and B systems; the longest survivor has maintained normal T and B cell functions for over 10 years (Gatti et al., 1968). One must assume a replicating population. While this experience would appear to provide the most convincing support for a stem cell replacement as the mechanism of cure and hence a stem cell deficiency as the cause of CID, certain unexplained factors and some new information require further examination of the older data.

First, direct proof that the dysplastic thymus of the patient becomes filled with the infused stem cells and generates new competent T cells is lacking. In fact, in one case autopsied 1 month after transplant, the thymus was still empty of lymphocytes (Lawton et al., 1973). On the contrary, we have shown that cultured thymus transplants show infusion of cells as early as 2 weeks after transplant. Secondly, it is now known that most patients with CID have B cells; these B cells appear to be capable of antibody synthesis and secretion (Pearl et al., 1979; Gelfand and Dosch, 1981). Furthermore, following bone marrow transplantation, the T cells of the donor are engrafted and the B cells of the host remain and are reconstituted fully functionally (Seligmann et al., 1974). Lastly, it is now known that a factor produced by stimulated T cells (interleukin 2) can further mature other T cells in the absence of a thymus gland (Wagner et al., 1980). In view of the above, one could explain the success of bone marrow transplantation without invoking processing of a donor stem cell population by the host thymus. Proof of this last point is required to use bone marrow transplantation results as evidence for a stem cell defect.

Assessment of T and B Cells in Combined T-B Disease

As there is as yet no morphologic or serologic marker of the lymphoid stem cell, we cannot directly assay for its presence. On the other hand, the detection of either T or B cells speaks against a major stem cell cause. B cells of substantial capability are found in CID. Recent studies by Gelfand (1981) showed T cell precursors which could be "matured" under the influence of thymus, theophylline or thymic factors in a majority of 12 patients with CID. These results are at variance with data obtained by Pahwa and his coworkers (1979), but even the latter group find some CID patients with thymic precursor cells. All workers would agree that many CID patients do not have a stem cell defect. The disagreement is over the percentage.

On the basis of published data and my own experience, I would propose that only those patients who present with reticular dysgenesis, demonstrating both severe hematologic and immunologic deficiency, can be readily defined as having a stem cell defect (De Vaal and Seynhaeve, 1959). In those without significant hematologic abnormalities, only those patients in whom there is a profound deficiency of B cells and in vitro B cell responses as well as T cell defects should be accepted as having a stem cell origin for their disease. I believe that this group will turn out to be very small in number.

The Thymus Defect

Most of the consequences of an in utero thymic defect have been considered in the previous section. As mentioned, I believe that in all cases significant in utero dysplasia presents clinically as combined immunodeficiency.

Less effect upon the B cell system would be expected in less profound malfunctions of the thymus gland. Obvious examples of these defects could be caused by thymic hormone deficiencies. There are probably 10 or 20 different hormones produced by the thymus; many are presumed to be important in promoting T cell maturation. One can easily imagine a series of different maturation arrests and/or a series of T cell subset deficiencies as a result of single enzyme lesions. Unfortunately, the ability to quantitate specific hormones is not refined to the point where this postulate can be tested. However, we should soon have that capability.

An important consequence of the requirement for a defined site for maturation of T cell precursors is that the stem cells must recognize and be attracted to this site and ingress of cells must be allowed. It is therefore possible that the thymus might not elaborate a chemotactic influence or, alternatively, that a T cell precursor might not bear a receptor which can respond to such a stimulus. No examples of the former have been observed, but ''bare'' lymphocytes lacking histocompatibility markers have been seen in combined immunodeficiency. Although it is unlikely that HLA antigens are the receptors which respond to thymic chemoattractants, the actual receptor may be a product of the major histocompatibility locus and absent as an associated defect in the bare lymphocytes (Touraine et al., 1978). Cells enter the substance of the lymph nodes via high endothelial venules whose walls are uniquely adapted to promote the lymphocyte ingress. Similar vessels occur also in the thymus, so one can reason by analogy that T cell precursors enter the thymus through the high endothelial venules. A defect in this structure could hinder thymocyte traffic.

A defect akin to those just discussed was suggested by findings of Pyke et al. (1975). They observed that supernates of a cultured thymic monolayer, derived from a patient with combined immunodeficiency, were able to increase E rosette numbers when incubated with fractionated bone marrow cells of normal patients. Also, this patient's thymus monolayer showed the same growth characteristics in vitro as normal thymus tissue. Pyke et al. (1975) postulated that the patient's immunodeficiency might be caused by an intrathymic defect, in which the thymus in situ was unable to differentiate precursors but was competent when cultured in vitro. However, the increase of rosette number, although an interesting phenomenon, can hardly be equated with normal capability. A direct test of their hypothesis would be accomplished by orthotopic autotransplantation of the thymus in a combined immunodeficiency patient.

The Bursa Defect

The bursa of Fabricius in chickens serves as a site for induction of plasma cell differentiation. It seems clear that differentiation of the B cells occurs in an extrathymic site in all species examined to date, but, in those which do not have a bursa, the anatomical counterpart has been difficult to define. The most likely candidate in man is the fetal liver, which is the original repository of bone marrow cells (Owen et al., 1974). An absence of the liver is incompatible with life, there is no human counterpart of thymic dysplasia and one can only hypothesize deficiency of bursal function but an otherwise normal liver. Under such circumstances, one should find B stem cells. Counts of pre-B cells which are at a very early stage of B cell lineage are now possible. Studies by Pearl et al. (1978) show normal numbers of pre-B cells in X-linked congenital agammaglobulinemia. Further differentiation appears to be blocked, as the more mature surface immunoglobulin-positive Ig cells are lacking. This observation supports the notion that an inability to differentiate a precursor B is the fundamental fault in X-linked congenital hypogammaglobulinemia.

Although no bursal hormones are known, it seems attractive to hypothesize that a series of humoral factors, similar to thymic factors, could play important roles in maturation and differentiation of the B cells and could account for various types of Ig deficiency states. Demonstration of this disorder must await definition of agents appropriately classified as bursal hormones.

Selective immunoglobulin deficiency is known; the most common involves IgA. The cells committed to production of a single immunoglobulin isotype ultimately derive from a precursor B cell which carries IgM molecules on its surface (Cooper et al., 1972). Acquisition of the ability to synthesize other isotypes is accomplished by deletion of various segments of what might be termed a master gene which then undergoes rearrangement. Successive deletions and rearrangements allow production of, in turn, IgM, IgG and IgA. which is a phenomenon known as switching (reviewed by Molgaard, 1980). Failure of this switching mechanism could account for Ig class deficiencies. The order of the H chain genes seems to be, as indicated above, mu, gamma, alpha. From this, one can infer that failure of switching of IgM to IgG should also be associated with IgA deficiency, accounting for combined IgG and IgA deficiency with normal or even elevated IgM. Such a disorder has been described as dysgammaglobulinemia type I. Selective IgA deficiency could occur with normal production of IgM and IgG and is commonly seen. The precise position of IgD and IgE constant region genes is not defined as yet, but they apparently come after IgA. If one continues reasoning in the above manner, IgA deficiency would also be constantly associated with IgD and IgE deficiencies. Combined IgA and IgE deficiencies are known; they are mostly seen in ataxia telangiectasia (Polmar et al., 1972). However, IgD values in ataxia telangiectasia are normal (Buckley and Fiscus, 1975). The failure to regularly observe immunoglobulin deficiencies according to predictions based upon constant region heavy chain gene position suggests to me that a failure of switching is not a common mechanism for antibody deficiency which does not involve all immunoglobulins. Numerous studies suggest that the switching process is predetermined and not dependent upon external signals (e.g., antigen) delivered to early B cells [reviewed by Seligmann (1979)]. It is also conceivable that a gene controlling switching and serving as an initiator occupies a position prior to the constant region genes or could occur on a different chromosome. Failure of this gene to initiate switching would result in either panhypogammaglobulinemia or only IgM synthesis, depending upon the normal site of action of the switching gene.

In view of the relative infrequency of the pattern of selective deficiencies which would be predicted by failure of gene switching, the selective deficiencies might be more adequately explained on extrabursal defects involving T helper or suppressor imbalance or terminal differentiation processes of the isotype-committed B cell.

Extrathymic and Extrabursal Defects

If the bursa is viewed as the site where the pre-B cell must undergo maturation and differentiation to acquire the ability to synthesize all isotypes (and perhaps also to respond to antigen and T cell signals), bursa failure should be denoted by presence of pre-B cells or SIgM+ B cells only.

Surface Ig+ cells of other classes should be absent. Whether the pre-B cells or SIgM+ cells of such patients could be further differentiated in vitro is unknown. It would seem most likely that they could not, except perhaps under the influence of a bursal hormone. A major difficulty in testing this hypothesis lies in the paucity of available cells for study. However, a number of years ago Lawton et al. (1973) showed that all patients with selective IgA deficiency possessed SIgA+ cells in the peripheral blood. They further showed that pokeweed mitogen increased the number of cytoplasmic IgA-containing cells in these patients to the same degress as in normal patients. They also found that these cells secreted IgA, but this observation was not subsequently confirmed (Waldmann et al., 1976; Atwater and Tomasi, 1978). Waldmann et al. (1976) showed that patients with IgA deficiency also possessed SIgA+ cells in the peripheral blood, but secretion of IgA was possible only in some patients and required the addition of normal T helper cells. Atwater and Tomasi (1978) showed that selective IgA deficiency was due either to deficiency of T helper or excess of T suppressor. These studies of selective IgA deficiency suggest plausible extrabursal mechanisms which could readily explain a number of Ig deficiencies involving one or a few isotypes. The serologic marker of these defects should be the presence of surface Ig+ cells of the relevant isotype in the absence of secreted immunoglobIulin.

In common variable hypogammaglobulinemia, usually observed in adults and some agammaglobulinemic female children, SIg+ cells are regularly seen. This could represent a partial bursal failure or failure of an extrabursal mechanism.

Some final maturation of T cells may occur after migration from the thymus. As an illustration of this fact, we know that thymocytes are less effective than peripheral blood or lymph node T cells in graft versus host killing and in proliferative responses to mitogens. One could assume that such maturational events occur in the peripheral lymphoid tissue of the gut. Again, hormones could be essential for these processes; alternatively, they could be antigen-induced. Faulty mechanisms of this type could result in inadequate helper and suppressor cells, but a more likely result would be the inadequate secretion of lymphocyte products such as migration inhibitory factor and macrophage activation factor, which augment the T cell immune processes.

Autoimmune processes can lead to gradual destruction of tissues or cells. The immune system itself is not spared from this type of attack. Loss of suppressor T cells as a manifestation of systemic lupus erythematosus and rheumatoid arthritis is now well documented (Strelkauskas et al., 1978; Sakane et al., 1979). These processes do not generally lead to immunodeficiency; however, antibodies against lymphocytes in general (August et al., 1969) or T or B lymphocytes have also been described (Brouet et al., 1980; Rubinstein et al., 1981). The consequences of these aberrations are as yet not fully defined, but they could produce any variety of clinical syndromes depending upon the target of the immune attack.

Nutrition is important in maintaining a healthy environment for cell replication and some elements are particularly important in maintaining the immune system. Protein-calorie malnutrition tends to disrupt the T cells more than the B cells [reviewed by Chandra (1972) and Good (1981)]. Zinc deficiency has been shown to result in profound thymic atrophy, T cell deficiency and increased risk of cancer (Good, 1981). In transcobalamin II deficiency, Ig deficiency in the face of normal T cell function was observed (Hitzig et al., 1974).
Viral infections in utero can cause immunodeficiency, ostensibly by altering the differentiation potential of lymphocyte precursors. Immunodeficiency has been observed as part of the rubella syndrome [reviewed in Horowitz and Hong (1976)]. Another mechanism of viral immunosuppression is seen as a result of E-B virus infection in a genetically susceptible host (Purtilo et al., 1977).

Thus, there are any number of mechanisms which can cause immunodeficiency. A characteristic of these extrabursal and extrathymic disorders is that a more selective deficiency (predominantly T or B) is usually seen.

Enzyme Deficiencies

Enzymes important in the catabolic pathways of pyrimidines and purines would be expected to play important roles in all cellular replication processes. One might guess that a deficiency of adenosine deaminase which catalyzes the catabolism of adenosine to inosine would result in a condition incompatible with life. However, the major consequence of this deficiency is in the lymphoid system (Meuwissen et al., 1975). Apparently the T cells are most sensitive to the disorder. With time, there is loss of B cell function as well and recent studies in our laboratory suggest detrimental effect upon thymic epithelial tissue as well. The cellular deficiency is attributed to the buildup of toxic metabolites which accumulate as a result of the failure of adenosine conversion (Cohen et al., 1978). These metabolites act in a manner similar to a powerful lymphocyte poison leading to progressive dropout of the relevant cell population.

An even more striking example of the selectivity of this process is seen in nucleoside phosphorylase deficiency, in which a true isolated T cell loss occurs (Ammann and Wara, 1979). Loss of B cell function has not been described in this defect, which involves the next metabolic step along the adenosine pathway.

It seems likely that more examples of this type of biochemical disorder will be found with time. Except for the presence of bony defects in adenosine deaminase deficiency, there is no obvious clinical difference in the presentation of these cases. Pure red cell aplasia was seen in the index case of NP deficiency. On the basis of previous clinical experience, perhaps one should think of an enzyme defect when there appears to be a selective loss of only T cell function.

The absence of enzymes results in immunodeficiency because of the unique susceptibility of a particular cell line to the metabolic consequences. At the moment, one can only assume a fortuitous association of the two. I would assume that there exist enzymes required for specific immune processes and that their malfunction could cause deficiency states. Diseases of these types might present with lacunar defects (i.e., most of this immune system is intact, but a particular function is lost). This might lead to unique susceptibility for only a few organisms. In cartilage hair hypoplasia, for example, unusual susceptibility to overwhelming varicella is seen, but other infections usually do not occur with inordinate frequency or unexpected severity.

Summary

The above discussion is presented to correlate possible mechanisms of generating immunodeficiency with clinical experience. It is intended to be a starting point for future discussion and not to close debate. It is presented to encourage continuing testing of the hypotheses tendered in an effort to come to a useful understanding of the mechanisms involved in the development of a fully competent immune system. Hopefully, these exercises can ultimately lead to correction of the myriad of deficiencies which presently frustrate the clinician and devastate the patient.

Acknowledgments

This work was supported by National Institutes of Health grants HD-07778 and AI 14354.

References

Ammann, A.J., and Wara, D. 1979. Clinical and laboratory features of purine nucleoside phosphorylase deficiency and immunodeficiency. In: Inborn Errors of Specific Immunity, eds. B. Pollara, R.J. Pickering, H.J. Meuwissen, and I.H. Porter, pp. 17–29. Academic Press; New York.

Atwater, J.S., and Tomasi, T.B., Jr. 1978. Suppressor cells and IgA deficiency. Clin Immunol Immunopathol 9:379–384.

August, C.S., Rosen, F.S., Filler, R.M., Janeway, C.A., Markowski, A., and Kay, H.E.M. 1968. Implantation of a foetal thymus restoring immunological competence in a patient with thymic aplasia (DiGeorge syndrome). Lancet ii: 1210–1212.

August, C.S., Rosen, F.S., Janeway, C.A., and Kretschmer, R. 1969. Recurrent infections, episodic lymphopenia and impaired cellular immunity. N Engl J Med 281:285–290.

Brouet, J.C., Grillot-Courvalin, C., and Seligmann, M. 1980. Human antibody reacts with a B cell subset in man to induce B cell differentiation. Nature 283:668–669.

Buckley, R.H., and Fiscus, S.A. 1975. Serum IgD and IgE concentrations in immunodeficiency diseases. J Clin Invest 55:157–165.

Chandra, R.K. 1972. Immunocompetence in undernutrition. J Pediatr 81:1194–1200.

Claman, H.N., Chaperon, E.A., and Triplett, R.F. 1966. Thymus-marrow cell combinations. Synergism in antibody production. Proc Soc Exp Biol (NY) 122:1167–1171.

Cohen, A., Hirschhorn, R., Horowitz, S.D., Rubenstein, A., Polmar, S.H., Hong, R., and Martin, D.W., Jr. 1978. Deoxyadenosine triphosphate as a toxic metabolite in adenosine deaminase deficiency. Proc Natl Acad Sci 75:472–476.

Cooper, M.D., Lawton, A.R., and Kincade, P.W. 1972. A developmental approach to the biological basis for antibody diversity. In: Contemporary Topics in Immunobiology, vol. 1, ed. M.G. Hanna, Jr., pp. 33–47. Plenum Press; New York.

De Vaal, O.M., and Seynhaeve, V. 1959. Reticular dysgenesia. Lancet ii:1123–1125.

DiGeorge, A.M. 1967. Congenital absence of the thymus and its immunologic consequences: Concurrence with congenital hypoparathyroidism. In: Immunologic Deficiency Diseases in Man, eds. D. Bergsma and R.A. Good, pp. 116–123. The National Foundation; New York.

Fudenberg, H., Good, R.A., Goodman, H.C., Hitzig, W., Kunkel, H.G., Roitt, I.M., Rosen, F.S., Rowe, D.S., Seligmann, M., and Soothill, J.R. 1971. Primary immunodeficiencies. Report of a World Health Organization Committee. Pediatr 47:927–946.

Gatti, R.A., Meuwissen, H.J., Allen, H.D., Hong, R., and Good, R.A. 1968. Immunological reconstitution of sex-linked lymphopenic immunological deficiency. Lancet ii:1366–1369.

Gelfand, E.W., and Dosch, H.M. 1981. Severe combined immune deficiency disease. A T cell disorder. Ped Res 15:595.

Good, R.A. 1981. Nutrition and immunity. J Clin Immunol 1:3–11.

Good, R.A., and Bach, F.H. 1974. Bone marrow and thymus transplants. Clin Immunobiol 2:63–114.

Good, R.A., Dalmasso, A.P., Martinez, C., Archer, O.K., Pierce, J.C., and Papermaster, B.W. 1962. The role of the thymus in development of immunologic capacity in rabbits and mice. J Exp Med 116:773–796.

Hitzig, W.H., Dohmann, V., Pluss, H.J., and Vischer, D. 1974. Hereditary transcobalamin II deficiency: Clinical findings in a new family. J Pediatr 85:622–628.

Horowitz, S.D., and Hong, R. 1977a. The Pathogenesis and Treatment of Immunodeficiency, pp. 97–99. S. Karger; Basel.

Horowitz, S.D., and Hong, R. 1977b. The Pathogenesis and Treatment of Immunodeficiency, pp. 74–77. S. Karger; Basel.

Lawton, A.R., Bockman, D.E., and Cooper, M.D. 1973. Treatment of autosomal recessive lymphopenic agammaglobulinemia by transplantation of matched allogeneic bone marrow. Am J Med 54:98–110.

Lawton, A.R., Royal, S.A., Self, K.S., and Cooper, M.D. 1972. IgA determinants on B lymphocytes in patients with deficiency of circulating IgA. J Lab Clin Med 80:26–33.

Meuwissen, H.J., Pickering, R.J., Moore, E.C., and Pollara, B. 1975. Impairment of adenosine deaminase deficiency in combined immunological deficiency disease. In: Combined Immunodeficiency Disease and Adenosine Deaminase Deficiency: A Molecular Defect. eds. H.J. Meuwissen, B. Pollara, R.J. Pickering, and I. Pater, pp. 73–87. Academic Press; New York.

Miller, J.F.A.P. 1961. Immunological function of the thymus. Lancet ii:748–749.

Molgaard, H.V. 1980. Assembly of immunoglobulin heavy chain genes. Nature 286:657–659.

Owen, J.J.T., Cooper, M.D., and Raff, M.D. 1974. In vitro generation of B lymphocytes in mouse foetal liver. A mammalian "bursa equivalent." Nature 249:361–363.

Pahwa, R.N., Pahwa, S.G., and Good, R.A. 1979. T-lymphocyte differentiation in vitro in severe combined immunodeficiency. J Clin Invest 64: 1632–1641.

Pearl, E.R., Lawton, A.R., and Cooper, M.D. 1979. Informative defects of B lymphocyte differentiation in human antibody deficiency disorders. In: B Lymphocytes in the Immune Response, eds. M. Cooper, D.E. Mosier, I. Scher, and E.S. Vitetta, pp. 341. Elsevier/North Holland; New York.

Pearl, E.R., Vogler, L.B., Okos, A.J., Cust, W.M.,

Lawton, A.R. and Cooper, M.D. 1978. B lymphocyte precursors in human bone marrow: An analysis of normal individuals and patients with antibody-deficiency states. J Immunol 120: 1169–1175.

Peterson, R.D.A., Cooper, M.D., and Good, R.A. 1965. The pathogenesis of immunologic deficiency diseases. Amer J Med 38:579–604.

Polmar, S.H., Waldman, T.A., Balestra, J.T., Jost, M.C., and Terry, W.D. 1972. Immunoglobulin E in immunologic deficiency diseases I. Relation of IgE and IgA to respiratory tract disease in isolated IgE deficiency, IgA deficiency and ataxia telangiectasia. J Clin Invest 51:326–330.

Purtilo, D.T., DeFloria, D., Jutt, M., Jr., Bhawan, J., Yang, J.P.S., Oho, R., and Edwards, W. 1977. Variable phenotype expression of an X-linked recessive lymphoproliferative syndrome. N Engl J Med 297:1077–1081.

Pyke, K.W., Dosch, H-M, Ipp, M.M., and Gelfand, E.W. 1975. Demonstration of an intrathymic defect in a case of severe combined immunodeficiency. N Engl J Med 293:424–428.

Rubinstein, A., Sicklick, M., Mehra, V., Rosen, R.S., and Levy, R.H. 1981. Anti-helper T cell autoantibody in acquired agammaglobulinemia. J Clin Invest 67:42–50.

Sakane, T., Steinberg, A.D., Reeves, J.P., and Green, I. 1979. Studies of immune functions of patients with systemic lupus erythematosus. J Clin Invest 64:1260–1269.

Seligmann, M. 1979. Neoplasias and B-cell precursors. Nature 279:578.

Seligmann, M., Griscelli, C., Preud'homme, J.L., Sasportes, M., Herzog, C., and Brouet, J.C. 1974. A variant of severe combined immunodeficiency with normal in vitro response to allogeneic cells and an increase in circulating B lymphocytes persisting several months after successful bone marrow graft. Clin Exp Immunol 17:245–252.

Strelkauskas, A.J., Callery, R.T., McDowell, J., Borel, Y., and Schlossman, S.F. 1978. Direct evidence for loss of human suppressor cells during active autoimmune disease. Proc Natl Acad Sci 75:5150–5154.

Touraine, J-L., Betuel, H., Souillet, G., and Jeune, M. 1978. Immunodeficiency diseases II. The "bare lymphocyte syndrome," a partial combined immunodeficency with absence of cell surface HLA antigens. J Pediatr 93:47–51.

Wagner, H., Hardt, C., Heeg, K., Rollinghoff, M., and Pfizenmaier, K. 1980. T cell derived helper factor allows in vivo induction of cytotoxic T cells in nu/nu mice. Nature 284:278–279.

Waksman, B.H., Arnason, B.G., and Jankovic, B.D. 1962. Role of the thymus in immune reactions in rats. III. Changes in the lymphoid organs of thymectomized rats. J Exp Med 116:187–206.

Waldmann, T.A., Broder, S., Krakauer, R., McDermott, R.P., Durm, M., Goldmann, C., and Meade, B. 1976. The role of suppressor cells in the pathogenesis of common variable hypogammaglobulinemia and the immunodeficiency associated with myeloma. Fed Proc 35:2067–2072.

Chapter 7

Secondary Immunodeficiencies

Gabriel Virella and H. Hugh Fudenberg

Introduction

The importance of the study of primary immunodeficiencies for our understanding of the biology of the human immune system is well documented in Chapter 6 of this book. Each patient with congenital immune deficiency is an experiment of nature from which priceless information can be obtained. In terms of clinical impact, however, secondary immune deficiencies far outweigh primary immune deficiencies. Nonetheless, immunologists have been considerably slower in grasping the importance of secondary immune deficiency. Often insidious in onset and of complicated pathogenesis, secondary immune deficiency is frequently regarded as only one more complication in the difficult treatment of a patient. This is reflected in the way in which the subject is approached in most immunology texts, either by total omission or by some short sentences coupled with a table listing a variety of diseases associated with secondary immune deficiency.

To present a concise and clear picture of the secondary immune deficiencies is no easy task. The number of factors suspected of leading to secondary immune deficiency has grown exponentially and the data supporting these suspicions are often fragmentary and controversial. It is often difficult to determine whether the infection is the consequence of immune depression or whether the state of immune depression is a result of the infection. Longitudinal studies showing the precise timing of the several factors involved in a specific type of secondary immune deficiency are scarce. Despite these difficulties, considerable progress has been made in our understanding of secondary immune deficiencies. We have attempted to summarize recent progress in this chapter.

Immunodeficiencies of Nutritional Basis

Malnutrition and Immune Deficiency

The association between malnutrition and predisposition to infectious disease has too often been thought to be merely coincidental. Increased incidence or severity of tuberculosis, measles, chickenpox, rubella, mumps and infection by *Pneumocystis carinii* has been noted by several authors (Edelman, 1977). Striking abnormalities of the lymphoid organs, including thymic atrophy and to a lesser degree atrophy of all lymphoid tissues, have attracted the attention of many investigators (Smythe et al., 1971; Douglas and Schopfer, 1976; Edelman, 1977). However, this has been an area plagued by controversy due to the lack (or impossibility) of controlled studies, the discrepancies between human data and data obtained in experimental models and, above all, the impossibility of dissociating the effects of malnutrition from those of infection when both are present simultaneously, as is often the case.

Such discrepancies, as well as observations contrary to the accepted dogma (e.g., higher mortality from the influenza pandemic in 1914–18 among the well fed, low incidence of typhus and measles among the underfed in concentration camps during the 1934–1945 war, lack of significant increase of infection among patients with anorexia nervosa, poor susceptibility to viral infections by hibernating animals) and observations suggesting that gram negative sepsis, malaria, brucellosis and tuberculosis show sharp outbreaks in starved populations as soon as feeding is begun, led Murray and Murray (1977) to develop an alternative perspective. According to these authors, malnutrition may be associated with resistance to infection, perhaps due to lack of metabolic conditions favorable to the replication of micro-organisms. As soon as feeding starts and metabolism begins to be restored, with ample supply of nutrients in an overcrowded and hygenically deficient setting, ideal conditions for the outbreak of infections are created.

Indeed, the interplay of malnutrition, poor sanitation and infection is difficult to separate into simple, experimentally testable components. In any event, there is ample evidence both from in vitro studies and from studies in animal models to justify as real the belief that protein-calorie malnutrition and a deficiency of elements such as iron, zinc and certain vitamins are often associated with abnormalities of the immune functions.

Cell-mediated Immunity in Protein-Calorie Malnutrition

Most reports agree on the finding of cutaneous anergy to both natural and artificial antigens in children with protein-calorie malnutrition (Smythe et al., 1971; Chandra, 1972; Neumann et al., 1977: Schlesinger et al., 1977). The most striking defects are seen in children with severe kwashiorkor, who usually are more affected than those with marasmus (Smythe et al., 1971; Douglas and Schopfer, 1976). Schlesinger et al. (1977) in a study of marasmic children from Chile noted that the frequency of negative PPD reactions was not significantly different among the malnourished group from that in a group of infected children with normal nutritional status. The authors pointed out that their population did not suffer from vitamin and iron deficiencies, which may explain some differences with relation to kwashiorkor and marasmus in African and Asian children.

In vitro correlates of cell-mediated immunity, such as the T cell count, the reactivity of peripheral blood lymphocytes to mitogens such as PHA and the release of macrophage inhibitory factor (MIF) by stimulated lymphocytes, have been reported to be depressed in malnourished children (Smythe et al., 1971; Chandra, 1972; 1977a; Neumann et al., 1977; Schlessinger et al., 1977; Kulapongs et al., 1977; Smith et al., 1977; McFarlane, 1977). Several authors have found correlations between the degree of malnutrition and the degree of depression of these parameters (Chandra, 1979a; Neumann et al., 1977; McFarlane, 1977). Several studies (e.g., Fig. 7.1) showed that with improved nutrition most in vitro parameters would normalize (Chandra, 1979a; Neumann et al., 1977; Kulapongs et al., 1977). However, some controversy exists about the degree or nature of the apparent T cell depletion, since depending on the way T cells are counted normal numbers can be obtained (Douglas, 1977).

It is also noteworthy that a depression of cell-mediated immunity very similar to that reported in malnutrition is often observed in children born with low weight for age, sometimes even when studied at 5 years of age (Chandra et al., 1977). Prolonged immunological deficits are particularly frequent among children who fail to show normal-for-age growth (Chandra et al., 1977a), which suggests that fetal malnutrition may lead to irreversible changes. In animals, both F_1 and F_2 offspring of starved females show deficiencies in immune responses, suggesting that the damage which occurred in fetal life is not only irreversible but even transmittable to the following generation. This is perhaps a result of a general deficiency in metabolic functions in the F_1 offspring that may result in intrauterine malnutrition of the F_2 offspring even when food is made freely available to the F_1 animals (Chandra, 1975a).

The nature of the cell-mediated immune deficiency in protein-calorie malnutrition is not fully understood. There is some evidence for a general metabolic depression affecting not only phagocytic cells (Selvaraj and Bhat, 1972) but also the lymphocyte. A lowering of the levels of thymic hormone (Chandra, 1979b), perhaps secondary to thymic aplasia, could also play an important role. Finally, some studies have suggested that in protein-calorie malnutrition there is a relative increase of null cells with suppressive effects on the (reduced) T cell population (Chandra, 1977a). These studies are obviously difficult to reproduce, and their significance has to be judged in the perspective of the above-mentioned controversy concerning whether there is really a decrease in T cells or just a reduction in the expression of the sheep red blood cell (SRBC) receptor in malnourished children (Douglas, 1977).

It is most interesting that chronic calorie malnutrition in experimental animals fails to depress cell-mediated immunity. If anything, starved animals showed enhanced function (increased resistance to viral infections, for example). It is therefore tempting to speculate that most of the abnormalities seen in human protein-calorie malnutrition are secondary perhaps to associated deficiency of vitamins or minerals (such as iron or zinc) or to the suppressive effect of infecting agents, since the overwhelming majority of malnourished children studied for their immune reactivity had more or less overt evidence of infection.

Humoral Immune Deficiency in Malnutrition

Humoral immune deficiency is the major consequence of protein-calorie malnutrition in experimental animals (Good et al., 1979; Chandra, 1975a). However, depending on whether acute or chronic starvation is induced and whether only protein or both proteins and calories are restricted, different effects are seen. For example, the humoral immune response appears to increase during acute starvation, whereas chronic protein and/or protein-calorie malnutrition affects humoral immunity very adversely (Good et al., 1977). On the other hand, chronic moderate protein deficiency can maintain the humoral immune response to T-dependent antigens and delay the appearance of autoantibodies in NZB mice, although the lifespan of the animals is prolonged only when the animals are deprived of both protein and calories or of calories alone (Good et al., 1977).

In humans, humoral immunity appears to be less affected by malnutrition than cell-mediated immunity and can be described as normal, increased or decreased in different studies (Chandra, 1972; Douglas and Schopfer, 1976). In general, however, most reports agree that numbers of B cells and levels of serum immunoglobulins remain normal (Chandra, 1977b; Kulapongs et al., 1977; Suskind et al., 1977a), although it has been observed that malnutrition in the first months of life can result in a marked delay of the maturation of serum immunoglobulin levels (Neumann et al., 1977b). On the other hand, some humoral responses, such as that to *Salmonella typhi*, have been reported to be decreased in malnutrition (Chandra, 1972; Suskind et al., 1977a), whereas others, such as the response to tetanus toxoid, were normal (Chandra, 1972; Kielman, 1977). Secretory immunoglobulins have been found to be decreased (Chandra, 1975b, 1977b, 1979a; Sirisinha et al., 1977) and the mucosal antibody response to attenuated polio vaccine has been found to be deficient (Chandra, 1975b). This apparent deficiency of the secretory IgA system may be related to the increased incidence of food antibodies in malnourished children (Chandra, 1975c, 1977b), but such antibodies are of unknown pathogenic significance (Chandra, 1977b); furthermore, there is no apparent relationship between the decreased levels of secretory IgA and any increase in the frequency of intestinal infection (Sirisinha et al., 1977a).

The apparent contradiction between the effects of protein-calorie malnutrition in man and experimental animals is most interesting. To date, it is unexplained. Another unanswered question is whether or not immunization is of protective value for malnourished children. In

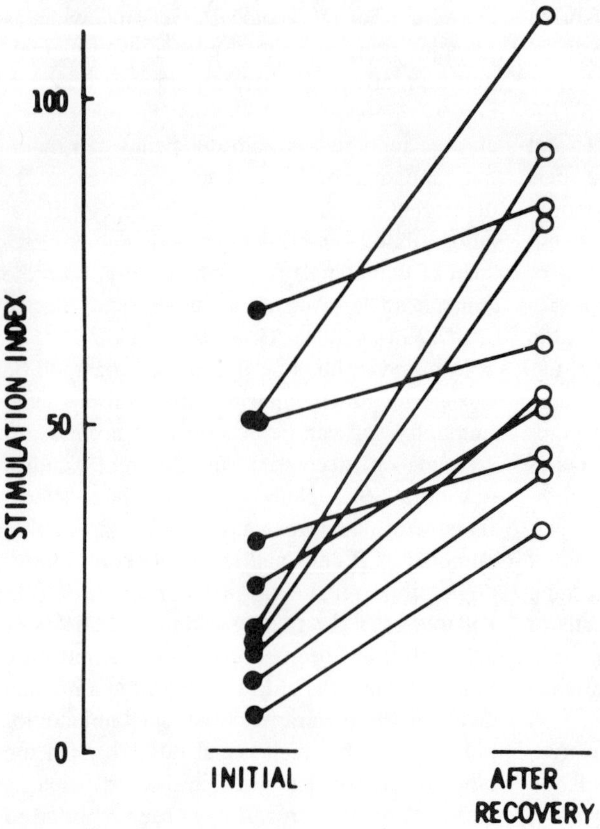

Fig. 7.1 Lymphocyte stimulation response in 10 children with energy-protein undernutrition, before and after nutritional recovery. Lymphocytes isolated from the peripheral blood were cultured in the presence of phytohemagglutin. Stimulation index represents the ratio of counts per minute in PHA-containing culture to counts in buffer-containing culture. Reproduced with permission from Chandra, R.K., 1979a, Acta Pediat Scand 68:137–144.

view of the evidence supporting a deficiency of cell-mediated immunity it appears that live-attenuated vaccines are contraindicated in malnourished children. Also, whether food intake is adequate to support an active immune response must be considered; if not, vaccination may have a negative effect on the nutritional status. Furthermore, since secretory IgA production is also impaired in malnourished children (Chandra, 1977b; Sirisinha et al., 1977a), it would appear that attempts at mucosal immunization are not likely to succeed. On the other hand, malnourished children have been shown to be able to produce adequate antibody responses to tetanus toxoid (Chandra, 1972; Kielmann, 1977) and children undergoing nutritional rehabilitation may show adequate responsiveness to typhoid vaccine (Pretorius and de Villiers, 1962). These observations suggest that perhaps active immunization with those vaccines that do not contain live viruses should be carried out simultaneously with nutritional rehabilitation.

Complement Levels in Protein-Calorie Malnutrition

Several authors have reported direct and indirect evidence of complement deficiency in malnutrition. Indirect evidence includes decreased opsonizing and bactericidal activity of whole serum, deficient development of inflammatory responses and increased susceptibility to gram negative infection and sepsis (Sirisinha et al., 1977b). Direct evidence includes decreased hemolytic activity of the serum of malnourished children and quantitative deficiencies of all complement components with the exception of C4 (Sirisinha et al., 1973, 1977b; Chandra, 1975c).

The levels of complement appear to be lower in children with kwashiorkor (Sirisinha et al., 1973; Neumann et al., 1977c), suggesting impaired synthesis as seen in animal models (McGhee et al., 1974). Levels are also lower in infected children, suggesting excessive consumption (Sirisinha et al., 1973, 1977b; Chandra, 1975c). The role of infection in determining low complement levels is suggested by findings of circulating fragments of C3 (Chandra, 1975c, 1977c), anticomplementary activity (Sirisinha et al., 1977b) and the presence of circulating endotoxin (Klein et al., 1977) in the serum of malnourished children. It appears likely that complement deficiency reflects the effects of infection in a debilitated organism rather than being the cause of the predisposition to infection seen in protein-calorie malnutrition.

Phagocytic Dysfunction in Malnutrition

Children with severe protein-calorie malnutrition, particularly those with kwashiorkor, have been found to have delayed chemotaxis and deficient intracellular killing of phagocytized bacteria (Selvaraj and Bhat, 1972; Seth and Chandra, 1972; Douglas and Schopfer, 1977; Chandra et al., 1977b). There is also evidence of a differential capacity of monocytes and PMN to be mobilized. Studies performed with Rebuck skin windows have shown that in kwashiorkor most of the cells that become adherent to the coverslip are polymorphonuclear leukocytes (PMN), with very few monocytes (Edelman et al., 1977b; Freyre et al., 1973); this can be correlated with apparently normal PMN chemotaxis reported by other authors in children with severe malnutrition (Rich et al., 1977). Indeed, there is less unanimity in the results concerning defective chemotaxis than in those concerning defective intracellular killing; perhaps, as noted by Chandra et al. (1977b), the presence of infection has a particular impact on chemotaxis. Theoreticaly infection could lead to reduced chemotaxis by decreasing complement levels and hence the generation of chemotactic factors C3a and C5a would be deficient in the serum of malnourished individuals. This mechanism appears to be the main one responsible for defective phagocytosis in experimental protein-calorie malnutrition induced in rats (Keusch et al., 1977a, 1978). In human malnutrition, however, the opsonic activity of serum is normal or even increased (Seth and Chandra, 1972); addition of normal serum to PMN of malnourished children does not correct their defective function (Leitzman et al. 1977). One must then dissociate two possible defects of the phagocytic cells in malnutrition. These are defects in chemotaxis, probably related to infection-induced complement deficiency, and defects in intracellular killing, probably related to a general metabolic slowdown of the leukocytes (Selvaraj and Bhat, 1972) or to an associated lack of some specific nutrient such as iron (Chandra et al., 1977b). However, the degree of metabolic and functional deficiencies in the phagocytic cells of malnourished children appears mild; it is much less striking than the abnormalities seen in chronic granulomatous disease and it seems unlikely that they are an important factor predisposing to infection (Keusch et al., 1977b).

In summary, our current knowledge concerning immune deficiency associated with protein-calorie malnutrition is that the most striking defects occur in cell-mediated immunity and the complement system and that humoral immunity and phagocytic function are only mildly and inconsistently affected. However, this is a particularly difficult subject for two major reasons. First, the effects of co-existing infection at the time of immunological studies are extremely hard to separate from the effects of primary malnutrition; secondly, human malnutrition is the complicated sum of many deficiencies, not only in protein and calories but also in vitamins, iron and other important nutrients. The degree of deficiency of each important nutrient varies among geographical regions and possibly even among individuals of the same geographical origin. This variability may explain some of the discrepancies observed in studies by different authors; more importantly, since there is little knowledge of what nutrients should be assessed and what the precise effects of their lack in humans are, progress beyond the descriptive point has been extremely slow. The complexity of human malnutrition, in addition to interspecies variation, probably accounts for the marked differences observed between human malnutrition and experimental malnutrition in animals. However, it seems obvious that at this point the most valuable information will originate from animal models; only after proper understanding of the consequences of experimental malnutrition will we be able to reexamine the human situation in a more scientific fashion.

Immune Deficiency Associated with Single Nutrient Deficiencies

Zinc Deficiency and Immune Function

The association of zinc deficiency and hypoplasia of the lymphoid tissue was first recognized in cattle with genetically determined malabsorption (Luecke, 1966). Soon a human counterpart was recognized in acrodermatitis enteropathica, which is a congenital disease characterized by diarrhea (with malabsorption of zinc, among other substances), epidermolysis bullosa and other dermatoses and, in some cases, generalized moniliasis. Most features of the disease can be corrected by dietary supplementation with zinc (Moynahan and Barnes, 1976). Good et al. (1979) studied the immunological function of some of these patients and found a form of combined immunodeficiency that could be corrected entirely through zinc supplementation.

These early observations resulted in great interest in studies of the effects of zinc deprivation in experimental animals and in humans. In experimental animals, zinc deprivation results in dysfunction of the immune system. The lymphoid system, particularly the T-dependent areas of the lymph nodes and the thymus itself, suffers marked involution (Fraker et al., 1977; Fernandes et al., 1979). Such animals show impairment of many parameters of cell-mediated immunity, such as depressed delayed hypersensitivity, defective cytotoxicity, low natural killer cell activity and progressive loss of circulating T cells. Antibody formation against T-dependent antigens is also impaired (Schloen et al., 1979; Fernandes et al., 1979). Some compartments of the immune system appear less affected than others. Antibody-dependent cell-mediated cytotoxicity appears enhanced (Schloen et al., 1979) and B cell function appears to be normal, since the transfer of T lymphocytes from normal syngeneic donors can restore the ability of zinc-deprived animals to produce antibodies (Fraker et al., 1977). A deficiency of thymosin and of the "serum thymic factor" of J.F. Bach has been reported in zinc-deprived experimental animals (Fig. 7.2) (Iwata et al., 1979; Chandra et al., 1980) and in humans (Cunningham-Rundles et al., 1979). It has been speculated that the impairment of thymic function underlies the deficiency of cellular immunity.

However, zinc is essential to the proper function of at least 70 enzymes, and to initiation of the action of at least 35 (Kirchessner et al., 1976); it would therefore seem likely that its effects on the immune system are rather complex. This has been substantiated by many experimental studies carried out in recent years. On one hand, zinc appears to be an absolute requirement for lymphocyte transformation after PHA stimulation (Alford, 1970); on the other hand, zinc by itself is able to stimulate T cells (Berger and Skinner, 1974) and B cells (Cunningham-Rundles et al., 1980). Although at the present time it is not clear whether this is a T-cell dependent function, the mitogenic effect of zinc, as a whole, seems to require the presence of monocytes (Ruhl and Kirchner, 1978). The mechanism of action of zinc has not been elucidated, but it has been found that zinc-transferrin can potentiate the mitogenic effect of PHA (Phillips and Azari, 1974) and that under these circumstances the cellular uptake of zinc-transferrin is increased (Phillips, 1978). It appears likely that zinc can operate at the intracellular level by stimulating nucleic acid metabolism (Hsu and Anthony, 1975), but a direct effect on the lymphocyte membrane is suggested by the fact that unsaturated Zn:8-hydroxyquinoline complexes, unable to permeate the cell membrane, are also able to enhance lymphocyte mitosis (Chapil et al., 1972). Such membrane modulatory effects of zinc could be the basis for the reported in vitro enhancement of the proportion of E rosette-forming cells on peripheral blood lymphocytes from cancer patients (McMahon et al., 1976).

The question of the importance of zinc deficiency in humans as a cause of immune deficiency then arises. Acrodermatitis enteropathica is a very rare disease, even when compared with the primary immune deficiencies. The intriguing question as to whether some of the presumed congenital combined immune deficiencies are clinical expressions of zinc deficiency is being cautiously examined (Good et al., 1979). It is possible that much larger segments of the population may be affected by chronic subclinical zinc deficiency, due to poor dietary habits and/or low meat consumption (Sandstead, 1973), which can have a significant impact in periods of rapid growth and during pregnancy (Hambridge and Walravens, 1976; Henkin et al., 1971). Diets rich in phytic acid and fiber may decrease the biological availablity of zinc, reducing its intestinal absorption (Rheinhold, 1971). Pathological conditions that lead to failure of absorption of dietary zinc (malabsorption syndromes) and loss of zinc through urine (chronic renal disease), gut (chronic diarrhea) or skin (burns, psoriasis) can also lead to secondary zinc deficiencies (Prasad, 1978). Parenteral alimentation deficient in zinc may cause a syndrome similar to acrodermatitis enteropathica and/or impaired parameters of T-cell function that show a total normalization after zinc supplementation (Obske et al., 1979; Schloen et al., 1979; Fudenberg, Galbraith, and Goust, unpublished observations). Obese patients have also been shown to have variable compromises of cell-mediated immune responses apparently correlated with subclinical deficiencies of zinc and iron (Chandra and Kutty, 1980). Thus it appears likely that zinc deficiency may become recognized as a more common cause of secondary immune deficiency than is apparent at present.

Iron Deficiency and Immune Function

Although iron deficiency is certainly widespread and relatively easy to diagnose, its precise effect on immune function remains controversial. Chandra and Saraya (1975) reported a defect in

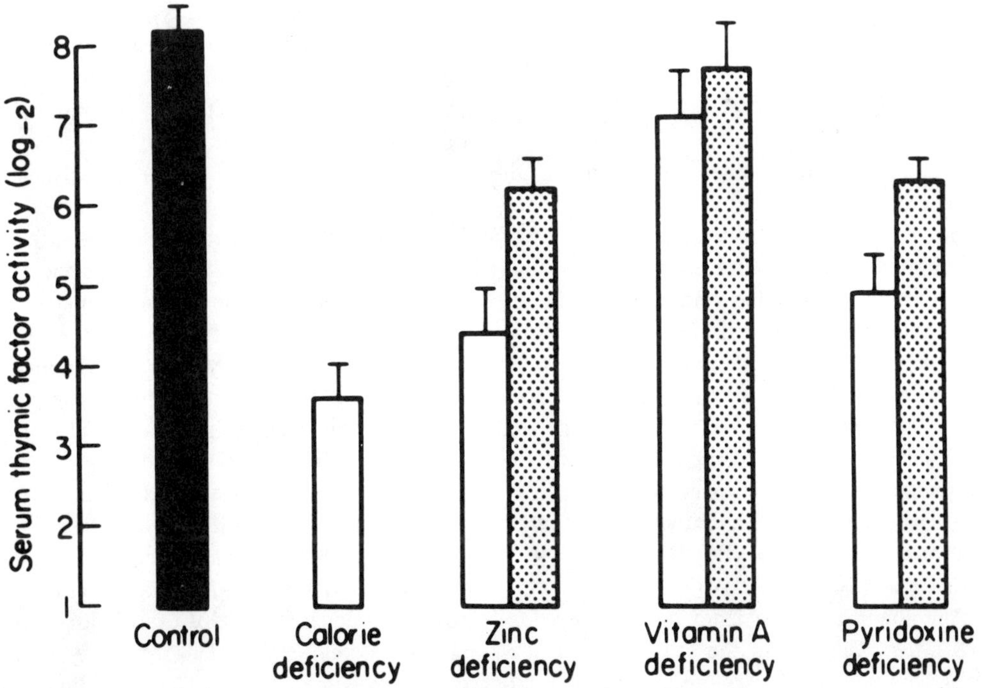

Fig. 7.2 Serum thymic factor activity in controls fed standard laboratory diet (■), deprived rats given a diet deficient in a single nutrient (□) and pair-fed controls (□). Data are based on 7 to 10 animals and are shown as mean ± standard error. Reproduced with permission from Chandra, R.K., Heresi, G., and Au, B., 1980, Clin Exp Immunol 42:332–335.

delayed hypersensitivity, reduced mitogenic responses to phytohemagglutinin (PHA), slight reduction of E rosette-forming cells and a defect of intracellular killing by PMN in iron-deficient children, which was reversible upon iron administration. Other reported abnormalities include reduction of MIF production by peripheral blood leukocytes (PBL) stimulated with purified protein derivative (PPD) and *Candida* antigens, which returned to normal after iron supplementation (Suskind et al., 1977b).

As in other forms of malnutrition, the concomitant existence of infectious disease and other deficiencies complicates the analysis of data. Not much has been published concerning experimental models of iron deficiency, except for some data (Chandra, 1976) suggesting a poor immune response to *S. typhimurium*. However, given the high frequency of iron deficiency all over the world and the repeated hints of its possible deleterious effects in the immune system not only in malnutrition but also in obesity (Chandra and Kutty, 1980), a serious effort to further investigate the consequences of iron deficiency in the immune response appears warranted.

Vitamin Deficiencies

Deficiencies of pyridoxine, pantothenic acid, folic acid, vitamin A and vitamin E have been reported to be associated with abnormalities of the immune response (Beisel et al., 1981). A deficiency of pyridoxine (vitamin B6) causes atrophy of the lymphoid tissues, cutaneous anergy, delayed rejection of skin transplants, poor responses of PBL to mitogens and decreased humoral immune responses, both primary and secondary. There is a decreased thymic hormones level, but the primary consequence of pyridoxine deficiency is an impairment of DNA and protein synthesis (Beisel et al., 1981; Chandra and Newberne, 1977).

Pantothenic acid deficiency has a more selective effect, depressing the primary and secondary immune responses in experimental animals and in human volunteers submitted to brief pantothenic acid deprivation (Axelrod, 1971; Hodges et al., 1962).

Folic acid deficiency is a relatively common condition and is associated with deficiency of cell-mediated immunity in man and experimental animals (Newberne, 1977; Chandra and Newberne, 1977). In guinea pigs and rats folic acid deficiency can also be associated with reduced humoral immune responses (Beisel et al., 1981).

Vitamin A deficiency in experimental animals results in increased frequency and severity of infections of all types; the study of immune functions reveals a depression of T lymphocyte numbers and of PBL responses to mitogens. Humans deficient in vitamin A are also reported to be affected by increased incidence of infections and the production of secretory IgA appears impaired. It has been postulated that the effects of this vitamin deficiency are related to its role in maintaining the composition of external cell membranes and surface glycopropteins and promoting cell differentiation (Chandra and Newberne, 1977; Beisel et al., 1981).

Of the fat-soluble vitamins, vitamin E is the only other one the deficiency of which appears to be reflected by impaired immune responses, both cellular and humoral. A stimulatory effect on immune functions in experimental animals, on the other hand, can be obtained by doses exceeding two to ten times the minimal requirements (Biesel et al., 1981).

Although most of the data concerning the effects of isolated vitamin deficiencies have been obtained in experimental animals, the significance is obvious. Vitamin deficiencies are always present in populations with protein-calorie malnutrition and, depending on the severity of the deficiency and the vitamins involved, the clinical expression of immune deficiency varies. The significance of vitamin deficiencies, like that of deficiencies of iron and zinc, goes beyond the overt cases of malnutrition. Folic acid deficiency, for example, is not uncommon in developed countries and can be associated with a multitude of conditions, such as pregnancy, use of oral contraceptives, chronic alcoholism, malabsorption syndromes, etc. (Newberne, 1977). The full clinical significance of the depression of the immune response that may take place in such patients remains to be clarified.

Parenteral Nutrition and Predisposition to Infections

Given the striking association between malnutrition, infection and poor immunological response, it would appear logical that vigorous refeeding would be the best approach. This appears to be true in animals undergoing experimental malnutrition, in which parenteral nutrition induces a rapid recovery of immune function which is faster than oral feeding (Diogni et al., 1976). In humans, however, parenteral feeding with concentrated solutions of amino acids or monosaccharides is often associated with secondary septicemia, either fungal or bacterial. The frequency of complicating infections appears to be rather high. In a series of 15 infants and children fed parenterally for periods ranging from 7 to 461 days, 12 developed infections. Eight episodes of bacerial sepsis with *Klebsiella, Escherichia coli* and *Staphylococcus aureus* and six with *Candida albicans* were documented. Five patients died from infections; they were documented as fungal in three and probably bacterial in two (Boeckman and Krill, 1970). In another study, it was found that, out of 33 patients with fungal sepsis, 22 had received parenteral hyperalimentation; septicermia appeared as a complication in 13 out of 49 patients treated with parenteral hyperalimentation (Curry and Quie, 1971). A correlation of the length of hyperalimentation and the presence of intravenous catheters with the development of septicemia has been noted (Boeckman and Krill, 1970). The co-existence of infections with parenteral alimentation also appeared to favor the development of sepsis (Boeckman and Krill, 1970).

No specific immunologic abnormality has been suggested as associated with the tendency to infection. It appears that supplying large amounts of simple nutrients for prolonged periods of time, involving intravenous catheterization and other sources of infection, creates ideal conditions for the systemic dissemination of infectious agents (Kettlewell et al., 1979).

Immunodeficiency Secondary to Infectious Diseases

In 1908, von Pirquet published the first observations of cutaneous anergy, as reflected by a loss of tuberculin reactivity, during measles. Subsequent authors published similar observations sporadically (Westwater, 1935; Coovadia et al., 1977a); this was for many years the paradigmatic example of immunosuppression apparently caused by an infectious agent. In recent years interest in the immunology of infectious diseases has increased, due in part to the recognition of its epidemiological and biological significance and in part to the availability of sophisticated new methodology developed during the past two decades. These have been applied to problems such as the study of immunosuppression induced by infectious agents. Soon it became obvious that measles virus was not an isolated agent capable of inducing immune suppression; bacteria, other viruses, and parasites can also induce immunosuppression by a variety of mechanisms.

Immunodeficiency Associated with Bacterial Infection or Induced by Bacterial Products

The bacterial infections most often referred to as being associated with secondary immune suppression are syphilis and lepromatous leprosy.

Syphilis

The peripheral blood lymphocytes of patients with primary and secondary syphilis have been reported to have impaired ability to respond to PHA stimulation (Levene et al., 1969; Kantor, 1975). In the case of patients with secondary syphilis, an inhibitory factor can be demonstrated; when added to the PBL of normal donors, it reduces the mitogenic responses (Levene et al., 1969; Kantor, 1975). This inhibitor is either not present or only very sporadically pre-

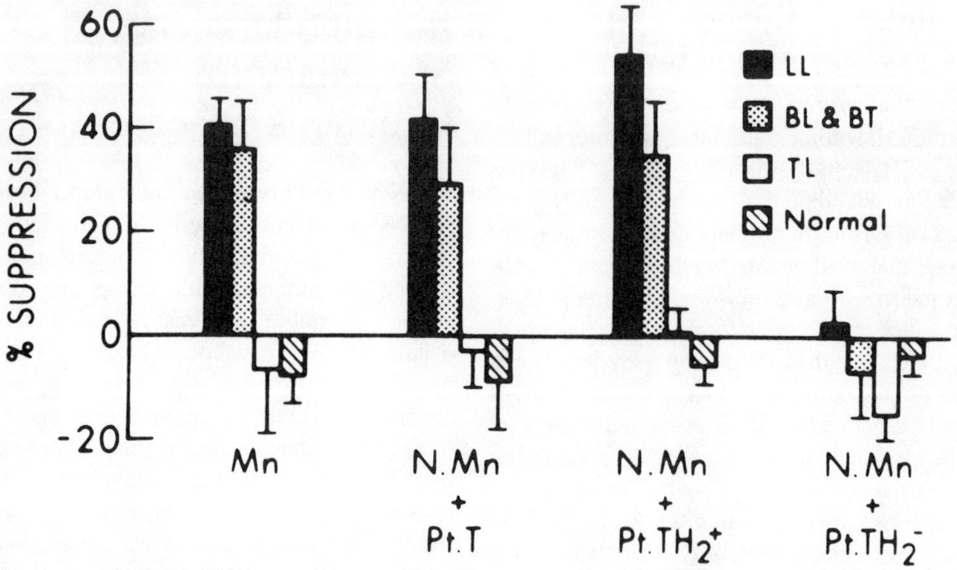

Fig. 7.3 Effect of TH_2^+ and TH_2^- subsets of T cells from 10 patients with lepromatous leprosy, 5 with borderline leprosy, 5 with tuberculoid leprosy and 7 normal subjects on the mitogenic response of normal mononuclear cells to Con A in the presence of lepromin. The statistical significance of lepromin-induced suppression of Con A response of normal mononuclear cells in the presence of T cells and TH_2^+ and TH_2^- subsets of T cells from leprosy patients was determined by analysis of variance and Duncan's multiple range test. Suppression obtained in the presence of T cells and the TH_2^+ subset of T cells from lepromatous and borderline leprosy patients was highly significant ($p < 0.005$). No significant suppression was obtained in the presence of T cells and the TH_2^+ subset of T cells from tuberculoid leprosy patients and normals ($p > 0.3$). The TH_2^- subset failed to induce any appreciable suppression in any group ($p > 0.05$). Reproduced with permission from Mehra, V., Mason, L.H., Rothman, W., Reinhers, E., Schlossman, S.F., and Bloom, B.R., 1980, with permission from Mehra, J Immunol 125:1183–1188. Copyright 1980 by The Williams & Wilkins Co., Baltimore.

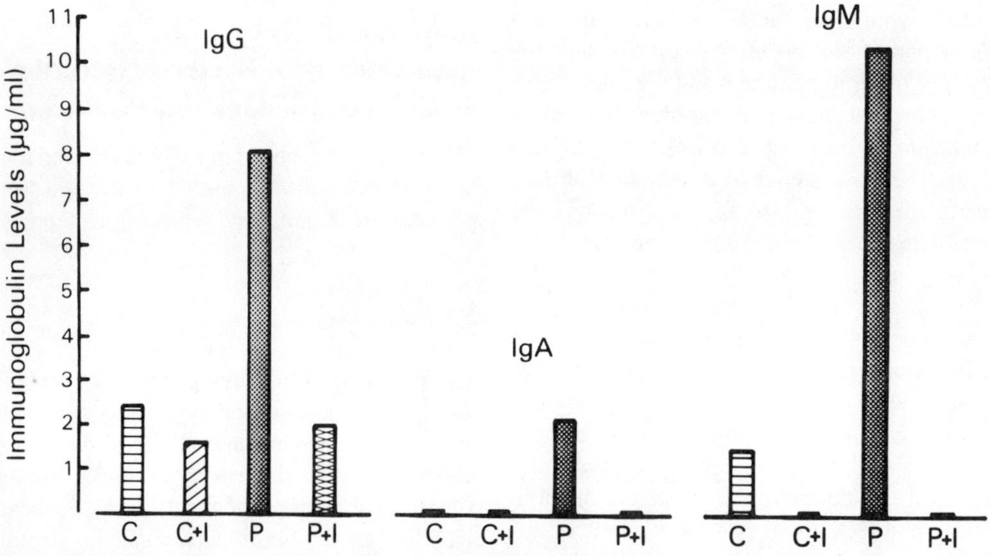

Fig. 7.4 Immunoglobulin levels in the supernatants of lymphocyte cultures to which an extracellular immunosuppressive substance released by *Streptococcus intermedius* was added. C, control culture; C + I, cells cultivated in the presence of 10% FCS and the inhibitory substance; P, PWM-stimulated culture; P + I, PWM-stimulated culture to which the immunosuppressive substance was added. Reproduced with permission from Munoz, J., Virella, G., Arala-Chaves, M.P., and Fudenberg, H.H., 1980, Haematologia 13:213–223.

sent in the plasma of patients with primary syphilis. Very little has been learned about the nature of this factor. Studies with an experimental animal model, using rabbits, have shown that in the phase of disseminated infection equivalent to human secondary syphilis the response of the infected rabbit's PBL to SRBC is nearly obliterated. Cells obtained from the spleen or lymph nodes at that time suppress the response of normal PBL to SRBC. The suppressive activity is present in cell-free washings of cells from infected animals and can be correlated with the presence of soluble immune complexes (IC). Sera containing soluble IC added to cultures of lymphocytes from uninfected SRBC-sensitized rabbits cause dose-related suppression of the antibody response (Baughn et al., 1980). Since IC can also be demonstrated in syphilitic patients (Gamble and Reardan, 1975), it appears that the investigation of IC as the responsible factors for the suppression induced by plasma from patients with secondary syphilis would be highly rewarding. However, other alternatives also appear to merit consideration. A tryptic fragment of C3, similar to C3a, has been shown recently to inhibit mitogen and antigen-induced lymphocyte proliferation in a dose-related manner (Needleman et al., 1981) and the presence of circulating C3a would appear to be likely in patients with disseminated bacterial infection. Interferon (immune interferon), produced in response to the bacterial infection, could also be responsible for the inhibition of mitogenic responses (Blalock et al., 1980). Finally, the possibility that *Treponema pallidium* can induce the production of antilymphocyte antibodies, similar to what happens after infections with rubella, measles and other viruses (Mottironi and Terasaki, 1970), should be considered.

Lepromatous Leprosy

Patients with this type of leprosy show anergy when stimulated with lepromin and a lack of cutaneous sensitization when simple substances such as 1-chloro-2,4-dinitrobenzene (DNCB) are used; they also show delayed rejection of allogeneic skin grafts, correlated to the concentration of *M. leprae* in the skin at the site of the transplantation. In vitro parameters of CMI are also impaired, including lack of lymphocyte reactivity to *M. leprae* and depressed mitogenic response to PHA. Mediator production in response to *M. leprae* is also depressed in PBL isolated from patients with lepromatous leprosy. The serum of these patients does not show any suppressor activity on normal lymphocytes and culture in normal serum fails to improve the reactivity of the patient's lymphocytes. Therefore, it appears that in lepromatous leprosy lymphocytes have an intrinsic defect, being unable to proliferate and release lymphokines in response to adequate specific and nonspecific stimuli (Abe et al., 1973; Bullock, 1978).

One obvious mechanism to explain the depressed CMI seen in lepromatous leprosy would be an increase in the number and/or activity of suppressor cells. Evidence in favor of such a mechanism was first reported by Bullock (1978) and Bullock and Carlson (1978) based on experimental work in mice infected with *Mycobacterium lepramurium*. They found that two suppressor cell populations are involved; these are a monocytic suppressor cell in the early stages and a T suppressor cell in later stages. Evidence suggesting the involvement of suppressor T cells in human patients was reported by Mehra et al. (1979). The same group later demonstrated that the TH^+ subset of patients with tuberculoid leprosy or normal individuals failed to induce such activity (Mehra et al., 1980).

Immunosuppression in Other Bacterial Infections

A general depression of the immune response during the acute phase of bacterial infection is suggested by several observations. Heiss and Palmer (1974) reported that patients with leukocytosis, many of whom had associated acute infections ranging from pneumonia to urinary tract infections, showed cutaneous anergy to microbial antigens, DNCB and croton oil, and had lowered mitogenic responses to PHA. In vitro lymphocyte transformation to bacterial antigens is more depressed than the responses to PHA in patients with acute bacterial meningitis; this depression is both nonspecific (affecting the response to antigen of the causative organism and to antigens of other micro-organisms) and transient (Andersen et al., 1976). Lymph node or splenic cells from mice innoculated with *Pseudomonas aeruginosa* have been shown to be able to induce cutaneous anergy when transferred to normal recipients (Garzelli et al., 1978).

In recent years, considerable effort has been expended on studies of the in vitro and in vivo effects of bacterial products or extracts on the immune response. Although the precise biological meaning of the observed effects is not clear, the published data clearly demonstrate that many bacterial products have the capacity to depress either the immune response in vivo or the in vitro activation of immunocompetent cells. Some enzymes released by bacteria, including ribonuclease (Carpenter et al., 1972), *L*-glutamine (Hersh, 1971) and asparaginase (Hersh, 1973), have been shown to have immunosuppressive properties while being noncytotoxic. Other bacterial substances have also been shown to have similar properties. Streptococcal species appear particularly abundant in suppressive substances. Whole cellular extracts from group A streptococci, group A streptococcal membranes, streptococcal teichoic acid, group A streptococcal and staphylococcal pyrogenic exotoxins and noncytotoxic extracellular substances released by several mutant strains of streptococci (particularly, from *S. intermedius*) have been shown to have immunosuppressive activity in vivo or in vitro (Malakian and Schwab, 1968, 1971; Gaumer and Schwab, 1972; Toffaletti and Schwab, 1979; Schlievert, 1980; Higerd et al., 1978; Arala-Chaves et al., 1979). All these substances and extracts appear to act directly on the lymphocyte. The extracellular substances released by *S. intermedius* induce a general depression of cell proliferation affecting both T and B lymphocytes (Fig. 7.4) as well as other cell types (Higerd et al., 1978; Munoz et al., 1980; Arala-Chaves et al., 1979). The streptococcal and staphylococcal pyrogenic toxins appear to activate a suppressor cell population (Schlievert, 1980), whereas the streptococcal membrane appears to depress selectively the proliferation of immature B cells, without enhancing suppressor cells (Toffaletti and Schwab, 1979).

Tetanus toxoid and cholera toxoid have been shown to have suppressor activity (Fevrier et al., 1977; Pierce and Koster, 1980). Tetanus toxoid appears to stimulate two types of suppressor cells; one is specific for tetanus toxoid and the other is nonspecific and able to abrogate the one-way mixed lymphocyte reaction. Cholera toxoid, when given parenterally, can induce antigen-specific immunodepression reflected at the mucosal level through a mechanism as yet unexplained.

It is interesting that some bacteria and bacterial products classically considered as immunostimulants can also induce immunosuppression. *Corynebacterium parvum*, for example, when injected 1 to 16 days prior to SRBC, can suppress the primary immune response. Two mechanisms have been proposed to explain this immunosuppression; they are rapid elimination of the antigen by a hyperstimulated reticuloendothelial system and generation of suppressor cells of monocytic nature (Ghaffar and Sigel, 1978). Lipopolysaccharide, classically considered as an immunostimulant (Anderson et al., 1972; Gery et al., 1972), can have an immunosuppressant effect when added to unseparated mononuclear cells, reducing by 36 to 84% the responses to PHA and streptokinase-streptodornase over a wide range of concentrations. Apparently, this suppression is dependent on adherent cells. LPS has been shown to activate monocytes and the supernatants of LPS-activated monocytes have been shown to suppress T lymphocyte function (Ellner and Spagnuolo, 1979).

Whether or not these bacterial immunosuppressants play a role in preventing the activation of host defense mechanisms, allowing the infection to persist, is not clear. It could be that in vivo these substances either are not released or are very quickly inactivated by host enzymes. But even if their biological significance is limited, some of these substances appear to have great potential as immunomodulators. The most attractive substances are those able to depress cell division without inducing cytotoxicity, such as the extracellular substance produced by *S. intermedius* (Arala-Chaves et al., 1979). Large scale production systems are being tested and, if a reliable method for the bulk preparation of a substance with consistent properties is developed, we may see a revolution in the area of immunomodulation similar to that which resulted from the introduction of penicillin as an anti-infectious agent.

Immunodeficiency Associated with Viral Infections

As described above, an early observation of infection-associated immunodeficiency was the cutaneous anergy that develops during the acute phase of measles. Laboratory studies in recent years have shown that measles patients develop lymphopenia, but the precise degree of involvement of T and B cells has been the subject of contradictory results. According to Coovadia et al. (1977a, b), B cells and null cells are predominantly affected, whereas Whittle et al. (1978) showed a predominant depression of T lymphocyte counts. Whether the discrepancies were due to methodological or population differences is not clear. Mitogenic stimulation with PHA also reveals a depression in patients with acute measles (Coovadia et al., 1977a, b; Whittle et al., 1978). Some contradictory observations also exist in this area, since Coovadia et al. (1977a, b) observed a depression of PHA stimulation in the presence of AB serum, whereas Whittle et al. (1978) found depressed responses only in the presence of autologous serum and not when the cells were activated in the presence of fetal calf serum. The response of PBL to microbial antigens such as *Candida* has also been found to be depressed in the presence of 10% autologous serum in the acute phase, with normalization during convalescence. Similarly, the production of MIF after stimulation with host-killed *Candida* cells was also found to be reduced in the acute phase and to increase during convalescence (Whittle et al., 1978). Patients with lymphopenia who fail to produce antimeasles antibodies during the disease (Coovadia et al., 1977a, b) appear to have a poorer prognosis and higher death rate.

The nature of the immunodepression in measles has not been totally clarified. Evidence showing that both T and B lymphocytes (particularly the former) harbor measles virus has been obtained by Whittle et al. (1978). A direct cytopathic effect could account for the depression of lymphocyte functions and, if the cytopathic effect were severe enough, cytotoxicity could ensue, resulting in lymphopenia. However, the fact that some of the parameters of depressed function could only be demonstrated when the cells were cultivated in autologous serum led Whittle et al. (1978) to postulate the presence of a serum inhibitor of lymphocyte function. One could speculate on the nature of such a factor; either C3a (Needleman et al., 1981) or interferon (De Maeyer et al., 1975) are likely candidates. However this is an aspect that requires clarification due to the contradictory observations of Coovadia et al. (1977a, b).

In measles, the immunological defect appears rather nonspecific. In children congenitally infected with cytomegalovirus (CMV) and in their mothers, cell-mediated immunity has also been found to be impaired, but in this case the defect seems to be specific, affecting the response of PBL to CMV but not to PHA. Interferon production in response to CMV is also depressed (Starr et al., 1979). It appears that the depression of lymphocyte function can be correlated with active infection, since it is most obvious in viruric infants and since lymphocyte function tends to improve in aviruric children and in their mothers after the ninth month post partum. Some cases of dual infection with CMV and other agents (bacterial or viral) (Bale et al., 1980) in infants suggest that the immunodepression caused by CMV can in some instances affect the capacity to respond against unrelated agents, although all parameters of nonspecific immunity studied in these patients were normal.

Children with congenital rubella also show transient immunological deficits that induce impairment of the cellular immune response to rubella-specific antigens with normal PHA responses, depression of PHA responses, depression of immunoglobulin levels (particularly IgA) and loss of antibody to rubella (South et al., 1975). It has been proven that the addition of rubella viruses to normal lymphocytes depresses their proliferation to all types of stimuli, perhaps in relation to the capacity of this virus to suppress cell proliferation in general. It has yet to be proven that the abnormalities in lymphocyte function observed in infected children can be correlated with the presence of circulating viruses (South et al., 1975). In adults infected with rubella, responses to PHA have been reported to be depressed during convalescence; this depression was obvious only when the PBL were activated in autologous sera, with normal responses being observed when the cultures were carried out in homologous sera (Maller et al., 1978). This suggests the existence of a suppressor factor in the serum.

Sporadic cases of immunodepression apparently associated with viral infections have been reported in the literature. Provisor et al. (1975) reported three males in one family who were affected by a severe acute febrile disease with lymphadenopathy and hepatosplenomegaly. Two patients surviving the disease developed acquired agammaglobulinemia and Epstein-Barr virus was implicated as a possible causative agent by the finding of positive heterophile antibody titers and positive fluorescent antibody titers. The authors postulated that perhaps an abnormal T cell response to virus-transformed B lymphocytes, leading to massive cytotoxicitiy of the infected B cells, could be the origin of the acquired agammaglobulinemia; however, they did not produce any data in support of this hypothesis.

Experimental studies using dogs and canine distemper virus as the infecting agent showed that this infection induced a decrease in the absolute lymphocyte count, which did not return to normal in animals that died from the disease. In those animals, the thymuses were atrophic, the lymph nodes were depleted of lymphocytes, and viral nucleoprotein was demonstrated in thymic and lymph node cells. Dogs in which the disease ran a benign course showed normalization of lymphocyte count, no lymphoid lesions and, in some cases, hypertrophy of the thymus (McCullough et al., 1974). This could be a very useful model for future studies on the effects of viral infection on different immunocompetent cell populations.

Basically, four mechanisms could lead to immunosuppression during viral infection. These are a direct cytopathic effect of the virus on immunocompetent cells, a selective effect of the virus on suppressor cell populations, the production of substances able to suppress nonspecifically the proliferation of immunocompetent cells and the production of lymphocytotoxic antibodies. Evidence for the first mechanism can be found in the severe lymphocytopenia that accompanies both human and experimental viral infections, but this is an area in which hard data are practically nonexistent.

In contrast, there is some solid evidence suggesting that viral infections can induce alterations in the distribution and function of immunocompetent cells. Adults vaccinated with rubella develop a depression of the response to PHA 7 to 10 days after vaccination (Arneborn et al., 1980). This suppression is obvious when the cells are cultured in AB serum and is associated with an increase in the T_γ subpopulation (with Fc receptors for IgG), which has been postulated to have suppressor function. An increase in the number of suppressor cells also present during the acute phase of infectious mononucleosis; T cells with the phenotype $T5^+$, Ia^+ are increased in number and activity; these cells can suppress autologous T cell proliferation to antigens and the response of B cells to pokeweed mitogen (Reinherz et al., 1980). On the other hand, Wybran and Fudenberg (1972) reported that patients in the acute phase of viral upper respiratory tract infections had low levels of "active" T cells which is a subpopulation of T cells that appears to include, among other types of cells, the effector T lymphocytes involved in cytotoxicity (Robbins et al., 1981).

Evidence for the activation of suppressor cells has also been obtained from in vivo studies with experimental animals. Liew and Russell (1980) showed that animals infected with a given strain of influenza virus had depressed delayed hypersensitivity to a crossreactive strain. This suppressive activity could be transferred to cytoxan-treated recipients. Treatment of the PBL population from the immune donors with antisera to Thy-1.2 or Lyt-1.1 plus complement abrogated the transfer of the suppressive activity. In contrast, treatment with anti-Lyt-2.1 or anti-Ia^k did not, suggesting that T cells with the phenotype Thy1 + ,Lyt1 + 2 − , Ia − are responsible for the suppression of CMI mice infected with influenza virus. Interestingly, the same animals showed enhanced antibody production to influenza virus, suggesting that the virus acti-

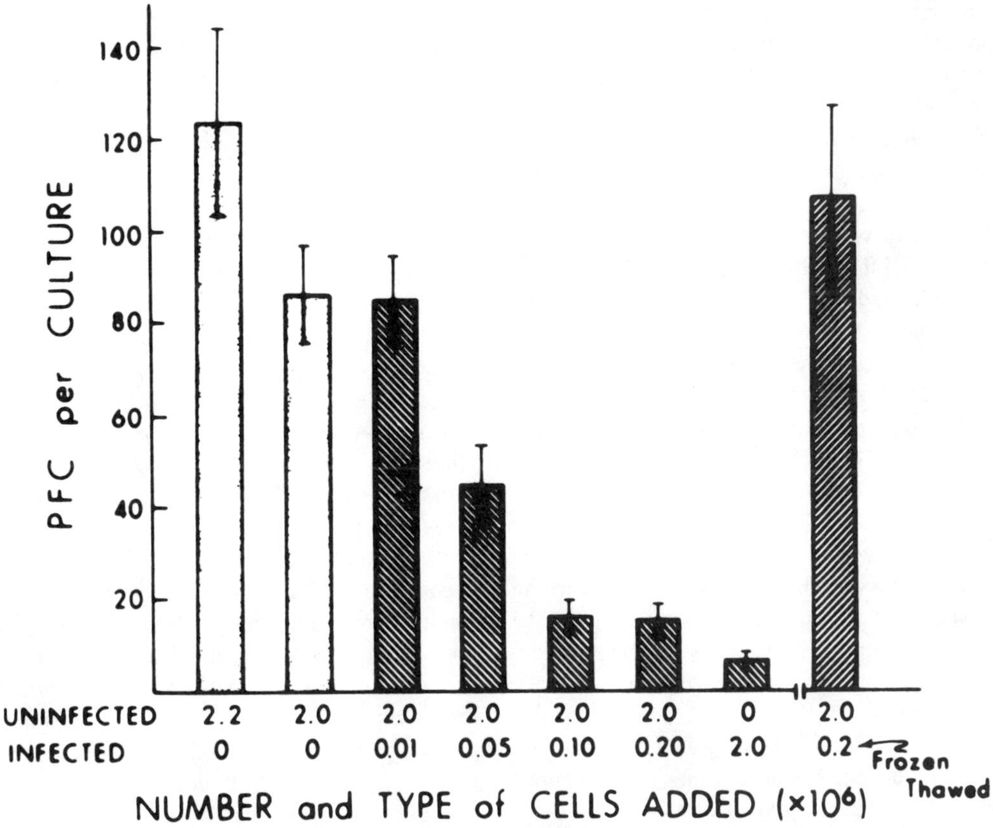

Fig. 7.5 Effect of influenza-infected cells on the antibody-forming response of uninfected CBA spleen cells. Suspensions of either 2.2 or 2.0 × 10^6 uninfected splenocytes were placed in microculture. To designated wells were added various concentrations of either viable or frozen-thawed influenza-infected ($10^{3.0}$ HAU/cell) spleen cells. Each culture then received 3 × 10^5 sheep red blood cells and was incubated for 4 days. Values represent the mean of octuplicate determinations ± SEM. Reproduced with permission from Daniels, C.A., and Marbrook, J., 1981, J Immunol 126:1737–1741. Copyright 1981 by The Williams & Wilkens Co., Baltimore.

vates two different T cell subsets; one has helper effects on the B cells producing antibody and the other has suppressor effects on the cell-mediated immune response.

Reovirus type 3 has been shown to inhibit the in vitro proliferative response of PBL to ConA by generating suppressor T cells. This inhibition is apparently mediated by the viral hemagglutinin of this virus; other viruses of the same family, such as reovirus type 1, are not able to induce suppressor cells. The existence of a receptor on murine lymphocytes for the type 3 hemagglutinin has been demonstrated. It appears logical to conclude that the differentiation of suppressor T cells is a direct result of the interaction between this hemagglutinin and its corresponding lymphocyte receptor (Fontana and Weiner, 1980). Influenza A_2 virus can also inhibit the in vitro antibody-forming cell response of mouse spleen cells to SRBC; this effect can be transferred by adding viable, infected cells to normal, uninfected spleen cell cultures (Fig. 7.5). The precise nature of the cell(s) involved in this suppression has not been clarified (Daniels and Marbrook, 1981).

Using avian retroviruses, Wainberg and Israel (1980) demonstrated similar abrogation of mitogen- and alloantigen-driven cell proliferation when murine lymphocytes were incubated with the virus. Apparently, in this particular case the induction of suppressor cells does not require live viruses; similar effects can be induced when plasma membrane vesicles derived from normal cells and of the approximate size of a virus are used. These results appear to favor a nonspecific activation of suppressor lymphocytes, but this is strongly contradicted by the results on Fontana and Weiner (1980) with reoviruses. At this point, although there is good evidence for the activation of suppressor cells in experimental animals both in vivo and in vitro, we are still far from understanding all the mechanisms involved.

Beneke and Pearson (1980) showed that the supernatant fluids of two herpes virus-transformed cell lines produced factors able to inhibit DNA snythesis by B cells, T cells and even nonlymphoid cells. Antibody-dependent cell-mediated cytotoxicity, which apparently requires cells able to produce protein but not necessarily to replicate, was not affected, but PHA blastogenesis was strongly inhibited when these suppressor substances were added early in the culture. Preliminary investigations have shown this suppressor substance to be a protein of molecular weight 60,000 to 70,000 (Beneke et al., 1980).

Another factor that could play a role in inducing immunosuppression during viral infections is interferon. Depressive effects on delayed hypersensitivity (De Maeyer et al., 1975), primary antibody response to T-dependent (Johnson et al., 1975a) and T-independent (Johnson et al., 1975b) antigens primary and secondary immune responses to SRBC, and DNA synthesis induced by ConA, PHA and LPS (Brodeur and Merigan, 1974) have been demonstrated. A recent publication has shown that cultivation of human mononuclear cells in the presence of interferon changes the ratio of T_γ to T_μ cells with depression of T_μ and enhancement of the T_γ cells, which are assumed to have suppressor functions (Itoh et al., 1980). This is similar to effects seen in children vaccinated with live attenuated rubella vaccine (Arneborne et al., 1980) and in individuals with infectious mononucleosis (Reinherz et al., 1980). Johnson and Blalock (1980) showed that interferon can induce suppressor cell activity in cultures of mouse splenocytes and that a soluble factor produced by these suppressor cells can in turn affect the B cell response, without inhibiting viral replication.

Finally, the relatively old observation that some viral infections (rubella, measles, infectious mononucleosis) apparently trigger the production of antibodies cytotoxic to normal lymphocytes (Mottironi and Terasaki, 1970) should be recalled and perhaps reinvestigated in terms of its mechanisms and biological implications.

The effects of viruses on the immune response are extremely complex. Detailed studies by Bixler and Booss (1980) using a murine model of cytomegalovirus infection showed that, although virus suppressed primary immune responses, the capacity to elicit a secondary immune response was intact and immunological memory could be generated in the absence of an obvious immune response. Whether these puzzling observations are an indication of general events is unclear; the nonspecific depression of delayed hypersensitivity in humans during the acute phase of measles and the results of several experimental models discussed above would suggest that the capacity to express secondary responses involving cell-mediated immunity can also be impaired. The data concerning humoral responses both in humans and in animal models are compatible with this selective effect on primary responses, which deserves to be more exhaustively investigated in different viral infections with different approaches.

In closing the discussion of the immunosuppressive effects of viral infection it should be recalled that other cells and systems can be affected, perhaps with relevance to the final effect. Ruutu et al. (1977), for example, showed that incubation of human neutrophils with both infective and noninfective viruses, even in the presence of inhibitors of viral replication, resulted in a reduction of neutrophil mobility affecting random locomotion, chemokinesis and chemotaxis. Such depression could obviously be of importance in determining increased susceptibility to bacterial infections.

Immunodepression Associated with Fungal Infections

Fungal infections are frequent complications of immunodeficiency states, but very little is known about the capacity of fungi or products elaborated by fungi to suppress the immune response. Rogers and Balish (1978) published the results of a study in which mice were systemically challenged with *Candida albicans* and the mitogenic responses of spleen cells harvested 7 and 14 days after challenge to PHA, concanavalin A (ConA) and PPD (in mice previously vaccinated with bacille de Calmet-Guerin (BCG) were studied. A general suppression of lymphocyte blastogenesis was observed at day 7 in cultures with heterologous (fetal calf) serum. At day 14 the lymphocyte responses had normalized. Given the isolated nature of this work its significance is hard to assess, but it represents a promising point of departure for future investigations.

Immunosuppression Associated with Parasitic Infections

In recent years there has been an outburst of interest in the study of the mechanisms by which parasites evade the immune response of the host. It soon became obvious that several parasites were able to suppress the immune response of the host.

It has been observed that peripheral blood mononuclear cells from patients with schistosomiasis are unable to generate strong in vitro proliferative responses to parasite antigens, while responses to mitogens and nonschistosomal antigens are normal (Ottensen, 1979). Fractionation of the mononuclear cells on nylon wool columns, to remove adherent cells, resulted in enhancement of the proliferative responses to parasitic antigens (Fig. 7.6) while the response to nonspecific antigens was inconsistently affected and the response to mitogens was depressed. These observations suggest that adherent suppressor cells (probably monocytes) play a key role in inducing the immunosuppression associated with chronic schistosomiasis. This, however, does not appear to be the only mechanism to explain the immunosuppression in human schistosomiasis. According to Rocklin et al. (1980), there was a significant difference in the response of PBL from some infected children to schistosomal antigens when the culture was carried out in autologous serum or in normal AB-positive serum. Sera containing immune complexes appeared to affect PBL proliferation adversely; this inhibition of proliferation was selective to schistosomal antigens. Antigen-specific suppressor cells affecting antigen-driven immune responses were also demonstrated by this group for some antigens. Finally, it has been shown that this parasiste can elaborate a substance that inhibits mast cell degranulation in vitro and anaphylactic reactions in vivo. The inhibition of mast cell degranulation can be correlated with a significant decrease in the in vitro IgG2a-dependent cytotoxicity mediated by eosinophils (Capron et al., 1980).

Experimental trypanosomiasis is one of the models more extensively used from the point of view of defining parasite-dependent suppressor mechanisms. Earlier work suggested that parasitic infection generated a suppressor T cell population (Jayawardena and Waksman, 1977; Jayawardena et al., 1978). A population of adherent cells with suppressor activity was later identified by Cunningham et al. (1980). It soon became obvious, however, that other mechanisms could also account for an immunosuppressive effect in experimental trypanosomiasis. Cunningham and Kuhn (1980) characterized a suppressor substance in the serum of infected animals which could inhibit antibody responses when added to normal spleen or lymph node cell cultures. It had a molecular weight of 196,000 to 210,000 and was proteic in nature but apparently unrelated to any known immunoglobulin. This inhibition was nonspecific and required the presence of T cells, B cells, and macrophages in the culture. Absorption experiments suggested that its main targets were B cells. The type(s) of suppressor cell stimulated by this substance has not yet been defined. Another possible mechanism of suppression, apparently not involving suppressor cells of any type, was identified by Albright and Albright (1980), who showed that the reactivity of T-depleted spleen cell culture to TNP-LPS (a T-independent antigen) was abolished when *Trypanosoma musculi* was added to the cultures. The possibility that this parasite could stimulate a B suppressor cell population was excluded by showing that enriched B cells from infected animals failed to display suppressor activity on normal spleen cell responses to both T-dependent and T-independent antigens. To complicate further the picture of altered immunoregulation in trypanosomiasis, evidence was obtained showing that infected animals appear to have an increase population of specific helper cells, the activity of which, however, is overridden by that of adherent suppressor cells (Cunningham et al., 1980).

The activation of adherent suppressor cells also seems to be involved in the immunosuppression that occurs in human or experimental malaria (Greenwood et al., 1972; Jayawardena et al., 1975; Warren and Weidanz, 1976; Finerty and Krehl, 1976). Spleen cells from infected animals can suppress responses to SRBC and mitogens by spleen cells obtained from normal donors. The population responsible for this suppressive activity is adherent to plastic and resistant to irradiation and to anti-Thy-1 plus complement treatment (Correa et al., 1980). Lelchuck and Playfair (1980), comparing the extent and nature of immunosuppression in mice infected with *Plasmodium yoelii* and *P. berghei*, with or without prior vaccination, and using lethal and nonlethal strains of *P. yoelii*, showed that suppression of the response to mitogens was greater in sublethally infected animals. The suppression of the response to SRBC was equal in all infections, with maximum at the peak of parasitemia; the suppression of contact sensitivity to oxazolone was stronger in mice with fatal infections. On the basis of these observations, Lelchuck and Playfair (1980) postulated that more than one suppressor mechanism is operative and that, while the suppression of mitogen stimulation and antibody production does not seem to have serious consequences, the suppression of delayed hypersensitivity is associated with lack of recovery.

At present it seems clear that more human studies are needed to clarify the importance of the mechanisms for immunosuppression identi-

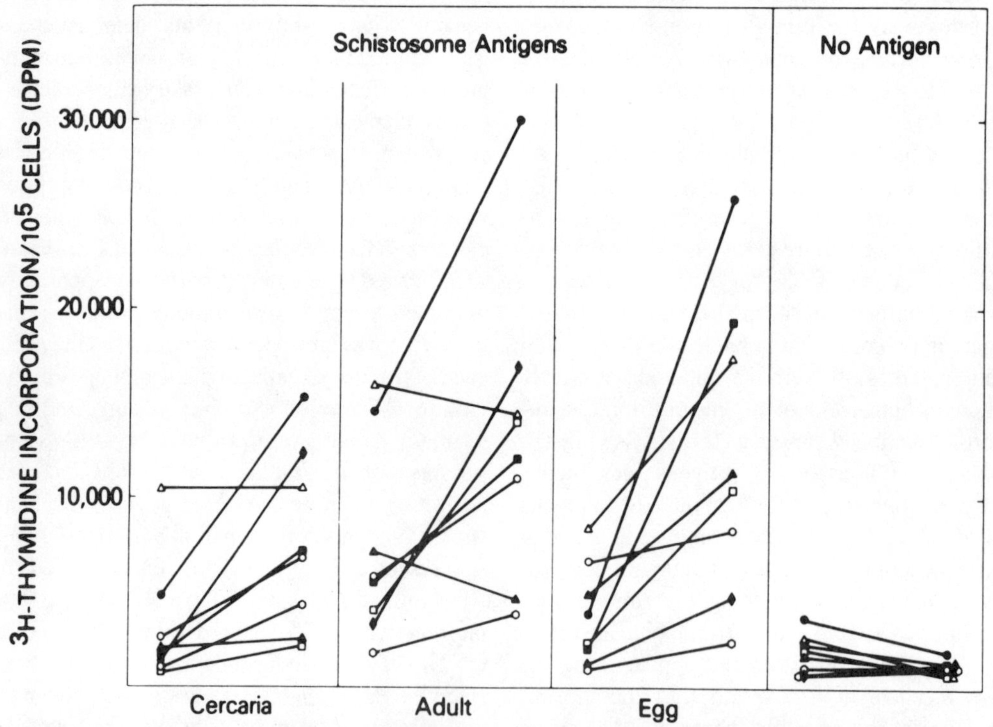

Fig. 7.6 Effects of removing adherent cells on lymphocyte proliferative responses of patients with chronic schistosomiasis. Responses of eight patients are depicted for three different schistosome antigens and for unstimulated cell cultures. The left end of each line marks the proliferative response of the unfractionated peripheral blood mononuclear cell (PBMC) culture. The right end works the response of nonadherent cells obtained after passage of PBMC over nylon-wool columns. Each symbol designates a different patient. Cells were cultured in autologous plasma. Reproduced with permission from Ottesen, E.A., 1979, J Immunol 123:1639–1649. Copyright 1979 by The Williams & Wilkens Co., Baltimore.

fied through experimental models and in vitro experiments in human disease. The physiological importance of those mechanisms in the evolution of experimental infections also must be better addressed. Finally, experiments designed to test whether immunodulating agents can influence the immunosuppression induced in vivo and whether this can be correlated with increased recovery from infection would be of the greatest significance.

Immunodeficiency Secondary to Protein Loss

Protein-losing Enteropathy

The association between protein-losing enteropathy and immunodeficiency has been cited as a classic example of secondary immunodeficiency for many years. Intestinal lymphangiectasia is perhaps the best known cause of protein-losing enteropathy. In this situation a combined immune deficiency state develops, with depression of all immunoglobulin levels, lymphocytopenia and depressed cell-mediated immunity, as reflected by cutaneous anergy, prolonged graft survival and depressed mitogenic responses to several stimuli (Strober et al., 1968; Weiden et al., 1972). Both immunoglobulins and lymphocytes are lost into the gastrointestinal tract (Strober et al., 1968; Weiden et al., 1972). Intestinal lymphangiectasia can be a primary or a secondary disorder, e.g., secondary to constrictive pericarditis. Nelson et al. (1975) reported a cure of intestinal lymphangiectasia developing as a complication of constrictive pericarditis. After pericardectomy the patient progressively recovered with normalization not only of his severe protein imbalance but also of his immune functions, which by 18 months after surgery were totally normal. This observation corroborates the concept that the intestinal loss of antibodies and immunocompetent cells is the primary cause of immune deficiency in intestinal lymphangiectasia.

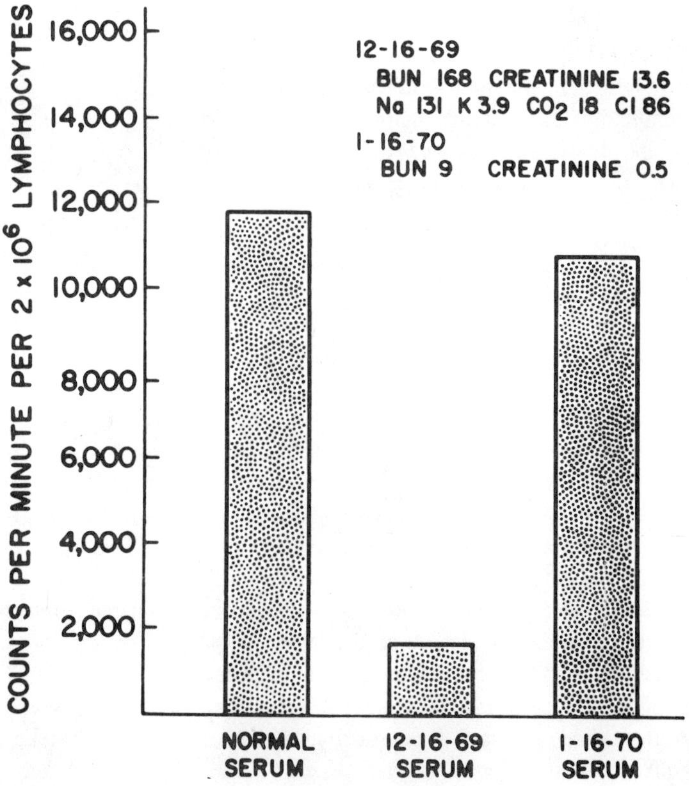

Fig. 7.7 The response of PHA-stimulated normal lymphocytes cultured in normal, acute renal falure and postrecovery phase sera. Reproduced with permission from Newberry, W.M., and Sanford, J.P., 1971, J Clin Invest 50:1262–1271.

Nephrotic Syndrome

The nephrotic syndrome is among the more frequent causes of secondary hypogammaglobulinemia. It primarily affects IgG due to its relatively low molecular weight, but several authors have pointed out that the magnitude of the urinary loss of IgG is not sufficient to explain the reduction in its serum levels (Hobbs, 1968; Shakib et al., 1977). A loss of the feedback mechanism that would usually lead to a compensatory increase of IgG synthesis has been postulated by Shakib et al. (1977), who advanced two possibilities. These are exhaustion of the feedback mechanism due to continuous stimulation and lack of stimulation of the feedback mechanism normally triggered by catabolic peptides, which would not be present in patients leaking intact IgG molecules directly into the urine.

Another possibility is in the triggering of suppressor cells or lack of helper cells; a dysfunction of immunoregulatory mechanisms has been proposed as the cause of the persistently low IgG concentration in children with minimal-change nephrotic syndrome, persisting even during long-term remission, when the loss of IgG has practically ceased. These children fail to switch from IgM to IgG synthesis after antigenic stimulation. This is a further argument in support of an abnormality of the immunoregulatory mechanisms (Giangiacomo et al., 1975).

Immunodeficiency Associated with Uremia

Patients with renal failure and uremia are known to be predisposed to infection (Montgomerie et al., 1968). The suggestion that cell-mediated immunity is affected in uremia was made early in the transplantation era, when it was found that uremic patients had depressed delayed hypersensitivity (Kirkpatrick et al., 1964) and delayed graft rejection (Hume et al., 1955; Dammin et al., 1957). Experimentally induced renal insufficiency in dogs also results in prolonged graft survival compared to the survival of similar grafts in normal dogs (Mannick et al., 1960). Wilson et al. (1965), in their classic systematic study of immune function in uremia, found evidence for a combined defect of cellular and humoral immunity. The uremic patient had lymphopenia, low incidence of positive skin test reactions to a battery of common antigens and low antibody response to the flagellar and somatic antigens of *Salmonella typhi*. These authors also observed that graft rejection was delayed in uremic patients with cutaneous anergy.

The depression of humoral immunity in uremia does not appear to be complete. Severe depression of all immunoglobulins can be observed in patients treated with hemodialysis and immunosuppressants (Riches and Hobbs, 1979; Virella, unpublished observations), but it is impossible to ascribe this effect to uremia. In patients with uremic renal failure not under cytotoxic therapy, humoral immune responses appear to be variably affected. Depressed immune responses to *S. typhi* and *S. paratyphi* antigens have been reported (Wilson et al., 1965), but other investigators have found normal responses to toxoids (Balch, 1955; Stoloff et al., 1958). In experimental animals, uremia seems to result in impairment of the primary immune response, with conservation of secondary immune responses (Gowland and Smiddy, 1962).

The depression of cellular immunity, on the other hand, appears to be more consistent and has been more thoroughly studied. Patients with chronic renal failure have been shown to have reduced PBL mitogenesis in response to PHA and PPD. Interestingly, the depression was more pronounced in patients with urea levels below 200 mg/dl than in those with levels exceeding this value, showing that urea is not responsible for this suppression (Nakhla and Goggin, 1973). A suppressor cell population apparently consisting of adherent cells (monocytes/macrophages) has been demonstrated in uremic animals in a graft-versus-host model (Raskova and Morrison, 1976) and by comparison of the reactivity of spleen cells from uremic animals and normal controls (Alvey et al., 1981). In both cases the removal of adherent cells restored the immunological competence of the remaining cells from uremic animals. Some differences in antigen make-up and sensitivity to pharmacological agents have been demonstrated between uremic suppressor cells and normal splenic adherent cells (Alevy and Slavin, 1981). Whether two entirely different cell populations or a modified monocyte/macrophage cell is in question is not clear.

In humans, most evidence has been obtained with regard to the presence of soluble suppressor factors. Plasma or serum from uremic patients was found to have a suppressor effect on the mitogenic responses of normal lymphocytes in vitro (Fig. 7.7) (Silk, 1967; Newberry and Sanford, 1971). The nature of the suppressive factor, however, has not been determined. Newberry and Sanford (1971) showed that the suppressive activity was found in uremic serum dialysates of molecular weight less than 20,000. Traeger et al. (1976) showed that methylguanidine and "middle molecules" (molecular weight approximately 1,200) isolated from uremic sera could suppress the in vitro mitogenesis of normal lymphocytes. However, they failed to induce immunosuppression in mice by injecting sublethal doses of methylguanidine, perhaps due to the fact that the animals had normal renal function. The in vitro effect of methylguanidine and "middle molecules" is not toxic in nature, nor does it alter the expression of E receptors.

Recently, Musatti et al. (1979), using an approach similar to that of Newberry and Sanford (1971), found that the immunosuppressive activity of uremic serum dialysates could be removed by absorption with sheep erythrocytes and concluded that accumulation of soluble E receptors in uremic serum is the main cause of its immunosuppressive properties. However, more solid evidence is needed to prove that the suppressor substance is indeed an E receptor.

If the suppressor substance is dialyzable, it should be expected that hemodialysis would improve lymphocyte function. This has been suggested in several studies (Webel et al., 1976; Holdsworth et al., 1978) and contradicted by others (Nelson and Penrose, 1975). On the other hand, one would expect to find the suppressive activity in the dialysate and less suppressive activity in the plasma of the patient. The first point was demonstrated by Hanicki et al. (1976), but the plasma of the patient appears, if anything, to have more suppressive activity after dialysis (Holdsworth et al., 1978).

In conclusion, immunodepression in uremia appears to be complex. A suppressive factor(s), still not properly characterized, appears to exist in the sera of uremic patients. Experimental studies, not corroborated in humans, suggest that a population of adherent suppressor cells is increased in uremia. Both areas deserve more detailed studies for a proper characterization of the effects of chronic renal failure on the immune response.

Burn-associated Immunodeficiency

Bacterial infections are a frequent and severe complication in burn patients; they often lead to death. There are several factors that may contribute to the incidence of infections in burn patients, ranging from the presence of open and infected wounds to a general metabolic disequilibrium.

Burn patients present a wide spectrum of immunological abnormalities. Neutrophil function has been reported to be abnormal, with defective chemotaxis (Warden et al., 1974) and depressed oxidative metabolism (Canonico et al., 1979). Monocyte chemotaxis is also depressed (Altman et al., 1977) and circulatory fragments reflect intense complement consumption (Bjornson et al., 1976). Alexander and Moncrief (1966) reported one of the first studies carried out to investigate a possible alteration of the immune response in burn patients, including studies of both humoral and cell-mediated immune responses. They found an inability to produce a primary humoral response to heterologous erythrocytes (very likely a T-dependent antigen in humans), but normal to enhanced secondary immune responses to tetanus toxoid. An impairment of cell-mediated immunity was suggested by a prolongation of the survival of skin homographs. The same authors (Alexander and Moncrief, 1966) complemented their human investigations with studies in experimental animals. They found a correlation between the magnitude of the burned body surface and the effects on the humoral immune response; apparently a burn of 30% of the body surface was required for any inhibition of the humoral immune response to become evident, with the inhibition being more pronounced when the antigen was given between 24 hours and 4 days after the burn. The prolongation of skin graft survival, later confirmed by many groups, would immediately suggest that cell-mediated immunity was affected in these patients. This impairment was also suggested by the fact that many of the secondary infections involved gram-negative bacteria, virus and fungi (Liedberg et al., 1954; Liljedahlal, 1963). Confirmatory evidence of a depression of cell-mediated immunity was obtained by in vitro studies showing a depressed response to mitogenic stimuli (Mahler and Batchelor, 1971) and a depressed mixed lymphocyte culture reaction (Sakai et al., 1974) in patients with burns. This lack of reactivity was associated wth severe lymphopenia, apparently due to a decrease in the number of T lymphocytes, probably associated with a decrease in their function (Sakai et al., 1974).

A controversy soon arose with regard to the nature of the putative T-cell defect in burned patients. Some authors reported findings of nonspecific immunosuppressive activity in the serum of infected patients (MacLean et al., 1975; Constantian et al., 1977) and others claimed that lymphocytes from burn patients may react normally to in vitro mitogenic stimulation if previously washed and tested in AB homologous serum (Munster et al., 1973). This last observation is contradicted in part by the findings of Sakai et al. (1974) since their studies on the mixed lymphocyte culture reaction were carried out in homologous AB serum, although the lymphocytes were not previously washed.

The nature of the immunosuppressive factor in the serum of burn patients is also somewhat controversial. According to Constantian (1978), this factor is noncytotoxic, has a molecular weight below 10,000 and is polypeptidic in composition. However, Ninnemann et al. (1979) have found that patients recovering their immune function after burns have an increased gamma globulin fraction, the IgG component of which forms precipitates with sera containing the post-burn suppressor factor in double immunodiffusion studies and can neutralize its in vitro suppressive effect on normal lymphocytes. These findings have been interpreted as proving that the suppressive factor is immunogenic and, as such, likely to have a molecular weight greater than 10,000. Actually, Ninnemann et al. (1979) suggested that the immunosuppressive activity could reside within a lipid-protein complex released by damaged epithelial cells of molecular weight 10^6, previously described by Schoenenberg et al. (1975). How to reconcile these two drastically different estimates of the molecular size of the post-burn serum immunosuppressive factor is not clear with the evidence at hand. In any case, this factor appears to be relevant to the clinical course of the patient. On one hand, the levels of this factor are greater in patients with more severe, more extense or more complicated burns (Ninnemann et al., 1979). The levels of the suppressive factor also correlate roughly with the clinical course, with spikes immediately preceding or concomitant with septic episodes, although it is not quite clear whether infections are the consequences of immunosuppression or vice versa (Constantian, 1978; Ninnemann et al., 1979). On the other hand, patients with higher levels of suppressive factor seem to retain skin homografts for longer periods of time (Ninnemann et al., 1979).

An alternative mechanism to explain the depression of cell-mediated immune response in burns would be an increase in suppressor cell activity. Evidence suggesting that suppressor T cells are increased in burn patients (Miller and Baker, 1979) and thermally injured experimental animals (Miller and Claudy, 1979) has been published. Both in humans and in animals, increased suppressor T cells can be demonstrated 4 to 8 days after thermal injury, preceding severe sepis by 4 to 5 days (Miller and Claudy, 1979; Baker et al., 1979, 1980). The increased suppressor cell activity, similar to the serum suppressive reactivity, was associated with very poor prognosis (66% mortality versus 0% mortality in those patients with no evidence of suppressor activity). In humans, suppressor activity was reflected by depressed mitogenic responses to PHA of unfractionated leukocytes; when lymphocytes from patients showing depressed mitogenic responses were added to mixtures of lymphocytes showing strong mixed lymphocyte reaction, a depression of the MLC was observed (Fig. 7.8) (Miller and Baker, 1979). In experimental animals, a reduction in the humoral response to SRBC has been observed and T lymphocytes from animals showing this depression suppressed the responsiveness of normal syngeneic cells (Miller and Claudy, 1979).

It appears logical to conclude that in burn patients there are three possible mechanisms by which the cellular arm of the immune response may become defective and lead to a defect in humoral immunity by failing to provide adequate help. Two of the mechanisms involve suppressor substances; one appears to be macromolecular and the other is a small polypeptide. The third mechanism involves an increased population of suppressor T cells. Two areas of research which appear to be of immediate interest are the study of the interrelationships between these three mechanisms and the study of possible ways to counteract them. In the first area, it would be interesting to know whether the same patient can present all three types of immunosuppression and, if so, whether they appear simultaneously or in given order. In vitro experiments aimed at determining whether the humoral factor(s) can induce the differentiation of suppressor T cells or if suppressor T cells release suppressor factor(s) would be welcome. Another interesting line of research would be to attempt the purification of the postulated antisuppressor antibodies for better characterization of their nature. A better understanding of this phenomenon could lead to attempts to reverse the immunosuppressed state using antisuppressor immunoglobulins in the hope that this reversion could have a positive impact on the outcome of therapy for the burn patient.

Iatrogenically Induced Immune Deficiencies

X-Ray- and Drug-induced Immune Deficiencies

The use of potentially immunosuppressive drugs in several types of clinical situations (mainly homografted patients and patients with malignancies, immune diseases or hypersensitivity diseases) has been associated with a progressive increase of infectious complications apparently related to excessive suppression of the normal immune response.

In most cases, immunosuppression is induced by a combination of drugs, either "immunosuppressive" or "cytotoxic," combinations of drugs with antilymphocyte or antithymocyte globulin or combinations of drugs with x-ray therapy. It becomes practically impossible to determine whether any single drug is responsible for the excessive depression of the normal immune response or for any specific characteristic of the infectious complications in the patient.

Two main features characterize the infections that appear in immunodepressed patients. First, they usually involve low-grade pathogens, bacteria or other micro-organisms not usually associated with clinical disease; second, the extent of and areas affected by the infection are unusual in noncompromised hosts.

Several nonpathogenic micro-organisms are frequently involved in the immunosuppression associated with drug therapy; these are *Pneumocystis carinii*, cytomegalovirus, *Candida albicans* and other fungi. Systemic infection with *Candida* species (Rifkind et al., 1967; Williams et al., 1971; Zazgornick et al., 1975) and deep tissue infections with other fungi have been reported frequently in immunosuppressed patients (Burton et al., 1972; Rifkind et al., 1967). Both localized and disseminated infections with herpes zoster varicella virus are also more frequent and severe in immunosuppressed hosts (Dolin et al., 1978). In this case there is some degree of association with x-ray therapy. Whether the irradiation of the skin is associated with local activation of the virus or whether it creates better local conditions for viral proliferation has not been elucidated.

Involvement of the eye and central nervous system by viral infections is a frequent event in immunosuppressed patients. Measles encephalopathy and/or retinopathy have been reported repeatedly (Breitfeld et al., 1973; Mellor, 1976; Pullan et al., 1976; Haltia et al., 1978a, b; Agamanolis et al., 1979) and, although its occurrence is more frequent in children treated with cytotoxic drugs for leukemia or other malig-

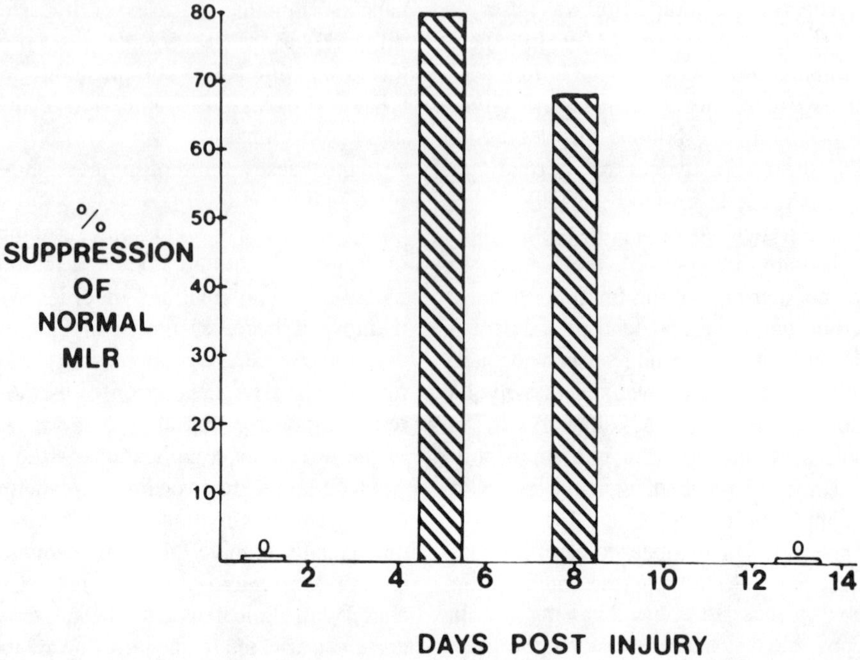

Fig. 7.8 Development of suppressive activity in the mononuclear cells of burn patients. The effect of adding 1×10^5 mononuclear cells from severely burned patients to triplicate cultures containing 2×10^5 cells from a highly responsive normal responder and 1×10^5 mitomycin treated normal stimulator cells was assessed. The bars represent percentage disease of the normal mixed leukocyte reaction (MLR) when cells from burn patients were studied at various times after injury. Reproduced with permission from Miller, C.L., and Baker, C.C., 1979, J Clin Invest 66:202–210.

nancies, it can also complicate immunosuppressive treatment (Haltia et al., 1978a, b). Other organisms, such as cytomegalovirus, toxoplasma and *Candida*, can also be responsible for eye infections in immunosuppressed patients (Egbert et al., 1980; Nicholson and Wolchock, 1976; Edward et al., 1974). Subacute sclerosing panencephalitis has been reported in immunosuppressed patients with a history of infection with measles virus 2 to 8 years prior to its onset (Loirat et al., 1971; Wolinski et al., 1977; Coulter et al., 1979). Finally, it has been suggested that infection with adenovirus type II may be involved in causing hemorrhagic cystitis in patients treated with cyclophosphamide or other immunosuppressant drugs (Fiala et al., 1974). This hypothesis is based on the recovery of the virus from serum and urine and increase in antibody titers during the disease and also on several other observations, such as the occurrence of hemorrhagic cystitis in patients treated with cytosine arabinoside, the lack of remission with discontinuation of cyclophosphamide in some patients, the lack of relapse of hemorrhagic cystitis in patients restarted on cyclophosphamide after remission of the cystitis (Fiala et al., 1974) and the observation of inclusions suggestive of cytomegalovirus infection in the bladder mucosa of a cyclophosphamide-treated patient with hemorrhagic cystitis (Goldman and Warner, 1970). However, all this evidence can be considered circumstantial and, at this point, it is not possible to consider this interesting hypothesis as proven.

The mechanisms of action of most immunosuppressive agents have been characterized in clinical and experimenal studies. Corticosteroids have been shown to induce lympholysis in corticosteroid-sensitive species (mouse, rat and rabbit), while in humans the effects on some leukocytes (including lymphocytes) appear more related to changes in distribution than to actual lysis. The main effects of corticosteroids in humans seem to be related to depressed function of neutrophils and monocytes, as well as depressed effector function of lymphocytes, such as release of lymphokines and cytotoxicity (Webb and Winkelstein, 1980). It seems likely that this inability of lymphocytes and monocytes to participate in an adequate immune response may be the best explanation for the development of cutaneous anergy in corticosteroid-treated patients. Corticosteroid therapy has variable effects on humoral immunity. Decreased gammaglobulin levels were reported in patients with rheumatoid arthritis treated with ACTH (Ragan et al., 1949); decreased IgG levels were observed in patients receiving short courses of high dosage corticosteroids (Butler and Rossen, 1973) and in asthmatic patients treated for an average of 15 days (Settipane et al., 1978). This reduction of serum IgG appears to be related to a decrease in immunoglobulin synthesis, particularly in the bone marrow. Decreased immunoglobulin concentrations were also shown in patients with autoimmune thrombocytopenia 3 weeks after beginning therapy (McMillan et al., 1976). The decrease could reflect either a primary effect of corticosteroids on B cells, lack of help by T cells or excessive suppression by T cells. An effect over regulatory cells is suggested by the fact that both in experimental animals and humans the production of IgG and IgA is predominantly affected, while levels of IgM do not show any changes (Berglund, 1962; McMillan et al., 1976; Settipane et al., 1978).

Most cytotoxic drugs destroy cells more or less nonspecifically and their effects on immunocompetent cells depend on the proliferative state of the cell and the cell cycle specificity. In general, they are effective in suppressing primary immune responses and ineffective in suppressing immunological memory (Webb and Winkelstein, 1980). The same difference in sensitivity between primary and secondary responses can be observed with irradiation, although an interesting difference is observed in the radiosensitivity of the primary immune response when soluble or aggregated protein antigens are used; the response to the latter is not affected by x-ray exposure (Stoner et al., 1974). This would suggest that the impairment of the afferent limb of the immune response is only partial and that, somehow, the participation of macrophages (processing the aggregated antigen) may short circuit the depressed stages of the immune response. Additional studies of the precise mechanism by which aggregated antigen induces an adequate immune response in x-irradiated animals should be undertaken.

Surgically Induced Immunodeficiences

In general, surgical intervention and general anesthesia are associated with immunodeficiency, affecting the mitogenic responses of PBL, cutaneous hypersensitivity and humoral immune responses. A transient severe lymphopenia can be seen in the immediate postoperative period and complete normalization of immune function may take 10 days (for mitogenic responses) to a month (for delayed hypersensitivity reactions and the humoral immune response) (WHO Report, 1978).

Some surgical interventions can have a more long-lasting effect on the immune response. Splenectomy is a particularly important cause of immune depression. Splenectomized patients have normal humoral immune responses following injection of soluble antigen, but are weakly responsive to particulate antigens. As such, these patients are prone to severe septicemia and the offending organisms are common pyogenic bateria, including *Streptococcus pneumoniae* (50% of the cases), *Haemophilus influenzae, Staphylococcus aureus,* group A *Steptococcus* and *Neisseria meningitidis*. The rate of mortality is high (Likhite, 1976).

These findings can be correlated with the role of the spleen in trapping and clearing cellular antigens and in recruiting immunocytes in the initial phases of the immune response. Splenectomized patients have been shown to have depressed serum IgM levels (depressed primary immune response), delayed macrophage mobilization and suboptimal levels of opsonins and cytophilic antibodies. The levels of tuftsin also appear to be decreased (Schumacher, 1970; Likhite, 1976).

Opportunistic infections with ''nonpathogenic'' organisms such as *Staphylococcus epidermidis* and *Candida albicans* are a definite risk after surgery, both in immunosuppressed and in apparently immunocompetent individuals. Cardiac surgery is particularly associated with a significant risk of infective endocarditis and/or speticemia, involving bacteria and fungi. The combination of sources of contamination (catheters, transducers, blood products) with local conditions favorable to bacterial proliferation (grafts, artificial valves, etc) and the immunodepression induced by surgery itself leads to a high risk of infection (Feigin and Shearer, 1975). Other types of invasive procedure, such as intravenous fluid therapy, parenteral alimentation and urethal catheterization, involve a high risk of opportunistic infections, particularly if other predisposing factors, such as malnutrition, are present (Feigin and Shearer, 1975). Some specific surgical interventions, such as jejunoileal bypass, can also lead to a depressed immunocompetence that can be reflected by increased incidence of histoplasmosis and tuberculosis. It is likely that malnutrition secondary to malabsorption due to the bypass is the primary cause of immunoincompetence in these patients (Dons, 1979).

The success of any therapeutic intervention is often based on a very delicate balance between positive and negative effects. This is particularly true for immunosuppressive and cytotoxic therapies and radiotherapy, which should always be reserved for those cases in where there is no other therapeutic option. It is also important that physicians and surgeons realize that there is no invasive procedure or surgical intervention without immunological risk. The immunological consequences of general surgery and general anesthesia, and of specific types of surgical interventions such as splenectomy and intestinal or gastrointestinal bypass, have to be taken into consideration, together with all other risk factors, when a decision is made with regard to the advisability of surgery.

Acknowledgments

This work was supported in part by U.S. Public Health Service grant CA-25746. We thank Charles L. Smith for editorial assistance.

References

Abe, M., et al., 1973. Immunological problems in leprosy research (A WHO Memorandum). Bull WHO 48:345–354.

Agamanolis, D.P., Tan, J.S., and Parker, D.L. 1979. Immunosuppressive measles encephalitis in a patient with renal transplant. Arch Neurol 36:686–690.

Albright, J.W., and Albright, J.F. 1980. Trypanosome-mediated suppression of murine humcral immunity independent of typical suppressor cells. J Immunol 124:2481–2484.

Alevy, Y.G., and Slavin, R.G. 1981. Immune response in experimentally induced uremia. II. Suppression of PHA response in uremia is mediated by an adherent Ia-negative and indomethacin-insensitive suppressor cell. J Immunol 126: 2007–2010.

Alevy, Y.G., Slavin, R.G., and Hutcheson, D. 1981. Immune response in experimentally induced uremia. I. Suppression of mitogen responses by adherent cells in chronic uremia. Clin Immunol Immunopathd 19:8–18.

Alexander, J.W., and Moncrief, J.A. 1966. Alteration of the immune response following severe thermal injury. Arch Surg 93:75–83.

Alford, R.M. 1970. Metal cation requirements for phytohenagglutinin-induced transformation of human peripheral blood lymphocytes. J Immunol 109:698–703.

Atlman, L.C., Furukawa, C.T., and Kelbanoff, S.J. 1977. Depressed mononuclear leukocyte chemotaxis in thermally injured patients. J Immunol 119:199–205.

Andersen, V., Hansen, N.E., Karle, H., Lind, I., Hoiby, N., and Weeke, B. 1976. Sequential studies of lymphocyte responsiveness and antibody formation in acute bacterial meningitis. Clin Exp Immunol 26:469–477.

Anderson, J., Moller, G., and Sjoberg, O. 1972. Selective induction of DNA synthesis in T and B lymphocytes. Cell Immunol 4:381–393.

Arala-Chaves, M.P., Higerd, T.B., Porto, M.T., Munoz, H., Goust, J.M., Fudenberg, H.H., and Loadholt, C.B. 1979. Evidence for the synthesis and release of strongly immunosuppressive, noncytotoxic substances by *Streptococcus intermedius*. J Clin Invest 64:871–883.

Arneborn, P., Biberfeld, G., and Wasserman, J. 1980. Immunosuppression and alterations of T-lymphocyte subpopulations after rubella vaccination. Infect Immun 29:265–271.

Axelrod, A.E. 1971. Immune process in vitamin deficiency states. Amer J Clin Nutr 24:265–271.

Baker, C.C., Miller, C.L., Trunkey, D.D., and Lim, R.C. 1979. Identity of mononuclear cells which compromise the resistance of trauma patients. J Surg Res 26:4787–487.

Baker, C.C., Trunkey, D.D., and Baker, W.J. 1980. A simple method of predicting severe sepsis in burn patients. Amer J Surg 139:513–517.

Balch, H.H. 1955. The effect of severe battle injury and of post-traumatic renal failure on resistance to infection. Ann Surg 142:145–163.

Bale, J.F., Reilly, T.T., Bray, P.F., and Kelsey, D.K., 1980. Cytmegalovirus and dual infection in infants. Arch Neurol 37:236–238.

Baughn, R.E., Turg, K.S.K., and Musher, D.M. 1980. Detection of circulatory immune complexes in the sera of rabbits with experimental syphilis: Possible role in immunoregulation. Infect Immun 29:575–582.

Beisel, W.R., Edelman, R., Nauss, K., and Suskind, R.M. 1981. Single-nutrient effects on immunologic functions. Report of a workshop sponsored by The Department of Food and Nutrition and Its Nutrition Advisory Group of The American Medical Association. J Amer Med Ass 245:53–58.

Beneke, J., and Pearson, G.R. 1980. Inhibitors of DNA snythesis produced by herpes virus transformed cell lines. J Immunol 124:2944–2949.

Beneke, J.S., Qualtiere, L.F., Nesheim, M.C., and Pearson, G.R. 1980. Purification and biochemical characterization of an inhibitor of DNA synthesis produced by an Epstein-Barr virus-transformed B cell line. J Immunol 124:2950–2955.

Berger, N.A., and Skinner, A.M. 1974. Characterization of lymphocyte transformation induced by zinc ions. J Cell Biol 61:45–55.

Berglund, K. 1962. Inhibition of antibody formation by predinisone: Location of a short sensitive period. Acta Path Microbiol Scand 55:187–202.

Bixler, G.S., and Booss, J. 1980. Establishment of immunological memory concurrent with suppression of the primary immune response during acute cytomegalovirus infection of mice. J Immunol 125:893–896.

Bjornson, A.B., Altemeier, W.A., and Bjornson, H.S. 1976. Reduction in C3 conversion in patients with severe thermal injury. J Trauma 16:905–911.

Blalock, J.E., Georgiades, J.A., Langford, M.P., and Jonson, H.M. 1980. Purified human immune interferon has more potent anticellular activity than fibroblast or leukocyte interferon. Cell Immunol 49:390–394.

Boeckman, C.R., and Krill, C.E. 1970. Bacterial and fungal infectious complicating parenteral alimentation in infants and children. J Pediat Surg 5: 117–126.

Breitfeld, V., Hashida, Y., Sherman, F.E., Odagiri, K., and Vunis, E.J. 1973. Fatal measles in children with leukemia. Lab Invest 28:279–291.

Brodeur, B.R., and Merigan, T.C. 1974. Suppressive effect of interferon on the humoral immune response to sheep red blood cells in mice. J Immunol 113:1319–1325.

Bullock, W.E. 1978. Leprosy: A model of immunological perturbation in chronic infection. J Infect Dis 137:341–354.

Bullock, W.E., and Carlson, E.M. 1978. The evolution of immunosuppressive cell populations in experimental mycobacterial infection. J Immunol 120:1709–1716.

Burton, J.R., Zachery, J.B., Bessin, R., Rathbun, H.F., Grennough, W.B., Sterioff, S., Wright, J.R., Slavin, R.E., and Williams, G.M. 1972. Aspergillosis in four renal transplant patients. Diagnosis and effective treatment with amphotericin B. Ann Int Med 77:383–388.

Butler, W.T., and Rossen, R.D. 1973. Effects of corticosteroid on immunity in man. I. Decreased serum IgG concentration caused by 3 or 5 days of high doses of methylprednisolone. J Clin Invest 52:2629–2640.

Canonico, P.G., McManus, A.T., and Powanda, M.C. 1979. Bichemistry and function of the neutrophil in infected, burned and traumatized hosts. Front Biol 48:287–326.

Capron, A., Dessaint, J.P., and Capron, M. 1980. Immunoregulation of parasite infections. J Allergy Clin Immunol 66:91–96.

Carpenter, C.B., Milton, J.D., Mowbray, J.F., and Butterworth, A.E. 1972. Immunosuppressive properties of a ribonuclease-containing fraction from bacterial cultures. Immunol 23:171–182.

Chandra, R.K. 1972. Immunocompetence in undernutrition. Pediat 81:1194–1200.

Chandra, R.K. 1975a. Antibody formation in first and second generation offspring of nutritionally deprived rats. Science 190:289–290.

Chandra, R.K. 1975b. Reduced secretory antibody response to live attennated measles and poliovirus vaccines in malnourished children. Brit Med J 2:583–585.

Chandra, R.K. 1975c. Food antibodies in malnutrition. Arch Dis Child 50:532–534.

Chandra, R.K. 1975d. Serum complement and immunoconglutinin in malnutrition. Arch Dis Child 50:225–229.

Chandra, R.K. 1976. Iron and immunocompetence. Nutr Rev 34:129–144.

Chandra, R.K. 1977a. Lymphocyte subpopulations in human malnutrition: Cytotoxic and suppressor cells. Pediatrics 59:423–427.

Chandra, R.K. 1977b. Immunoglobulins and antibody response in protein-calorie malnutrition—A review. In: Malnutrition and the Immune Response, Kroc Fdtn. Series, vol. 7, ed. R.M. Suskind, pp. 155–168. Raven Press; New York.

Chandra, R.K. 1977c. Serum complement components in malnourished Indian children. In: Malnutrition and the Immune Response, Kroc Fdtn. Series, vol. 7, ed. R.M. Suskind, pp. 329–332. Raven Press; New York.

Chandra, R.K. 1979a. Interactions of nutrition, infection and immune response. Acta Pediat Scand 68: 137–144.

Chandra, R.K. 1979b. Serum thymic hormone activity in protein-energy malnutrition. Clin Exp Immunol 38:228–230.

Chandra, R.K., Ali, S.K., Kutty, K.M., and Chandra, S. 1977a. Thymus-dependent lymphocytes and delayed hypersensitivity in low birth weight infants. Biol Neonate 31:15–18.

Chandra, R.K., Heresi, G., and Au., B. 1980. Serum thymic factor activity in deficiencies of calories, zinc, vitamin A and pyndoxine. Clin Exp Immunol 42:332–335.

Chandra, R.K., and Kutty, K.M. 1980. Immunocompetence in obesity. Acta Paediatr scand 69:25–30.

Chandra, R.K., and Newberne, R.M. 1977. Nutrition, immunity and infection. In: Mechanisms of Interactions, pp. 152–171.

Chandra, R.K. and Saraya, A.K. 1975. Impaired immunocompetence associated with iron deficiency. J Pediat 86:899–902.

Chandra, R.K., Seth, V., Chandra, A., Bhujwala, R.A., and Ghai, O.P. 1977b. Polymorphonuclear leukocyte function in malnourished Indian children. In: Malnutrition and the Immune Response, Kroc Fdtn. Series, vol. 7, ed. R.M. Suskind, pp. 259–264. Raven Press; New York.

Chapil, M., Ryan, J.N., and Zukoski, C.F. 1972. The effect of zinc and other metals on the stability of lysosomes. Proc Soc Exp Biol Med 140:642–646.

Constantian, M.B. 1978. Association of sepsis with an immunosuppressive polypeptide in the serum of burn patients. Ann Surg 188:209–215.

Constantian, M.B., Menzoian, J.D., and Nimberg, R.B. 1977. Association of circulatng immunosuppressive polypeptide with operative and accidental trauma. Ann Surg 185:73–79.

Coovadia, H.M., Wesley, A., Brain, P., Henderson, L.G., Hallet, A.F., and Vos, G.H. 1977a. Immunoparesis and outcome in measles Lancet i:619–621.

Coovadia, H.M.N., Wesley, A., and Brain, P. 1977b. Immunological events in acute measles influencing outcome. Arch Dis Child 53:861–867.

Correa, M., Narayanan, P.R., and Miller, H.C. 1980. Suppressive activity of splenic adherent cells from *Plasmodium chabandi*-infected mice. J Immunol 125:749–754.

Coulter, J.B.S., Balch, N., and Best, P.V. 1979. Subacute sclerosing panencephalitis after drug-induced immunosuppression. Arch Dis Child 54:640–642.

Cunningham, D.S., Benarides, G.R., and Kuhn, R.E. 1980. Differences in the regulation of humoral responses between mice infected with *Trypanosoma cruzi* and mice administered *T. cruzi*-induced suppressor substance. J Immunol 125:2317–2321.

Cunningham, D.S., and Kuhn, R.E. 1980. *Trypanosoma cruzi*-induced suppressor substance. I. Cellular involvement and partial characterization. J Immunol 124:2122–2129.

Cunningham-Rundles, C., Cunningham-Rundles, S., Garofalo, J., Iwata, T., Incefy, G., Twomey, J., and Good, R.A. 1979. Increased lymphocyte function and thymopoietin following zinc repletion in man. Fed Proc 38:1222.

Cummingham-Rundles, S., Cunningham-Rundles, C. Dupont, B., and Good, R.A. 1980. Zinc-induced activation of human B lymphocytes. Clin Immunol Immunopath 16: 115–122.

Curry, C.R., and Quie, P.G. 1971. Fungal septicemia in patients receiving parenteral hyreralimentation. New Engl J Med 285:1221–1225.

Dammin, G., Couch, J., and Murray, J.E. 1957. Prolonged survival of skin homografts in uremic patients. Ann NY Acad Sci 64:967–976.

Daniels, C.A., and Marbrook, J. 1981. Influenza Az inhibits murine *in vitro* antibody synthesis. J Immunol 126:1737–1741.

DeMaeyer, E., Demaeyer-Guignard, J., and Vandepuite, M. 1975. Inhibition by interferon of delayed-type hypersensitivity in the mouse. Proc Nat Acad Sci USA 72:1753–1757.

Diogni, R., Zonta, M., Dominioni, L., and Gres, C. 1976. Malnutrition, immunocompetence and total parenteral nutrition: experimental studies. In: Total Parenteral Alimentation, ed. C. Manni, S.I. Magalini, and E. Scrascia, p. 86. Excerpta Media; Amsterdam.

Dolin, R., Reichman, R.C., Mazur, M.H., and Whitley, R.J. 1978. Herpes zoster-varicella infections in immunosuppressed patients. Ann Int Med 89:375–388.

Dons, R.F. 1979. Opportunistic pulmonary infections, malnutrition, and immunocompetence after jejunoileal bypass. Amer Rev Resp Dis 120:961.

Douglas, S.D. 1977. Discussion: The cell-mediated immune system. In: Malnutrition and the Immune Response, Kroc Fdtn. Series, vol. 7, ed. R.M. Suskind, pp. 135. Raven Press; New York.

Douglas, S.D., and Schopfer, K. 1976. Analytical review: Host defense mechanisms in protein-energy malnutrition. Clin Immunol Immunopathol 5:1–5.

Douglas, S.D., and Schopfer, K. 1977. The phagocyte in protein-calorie malnutrition. A review. In: Malnutrition and the Immune Response, Kroc. Fdnt. Series, vol. 7, ed. R.M. Suskind, pp. 230–244. Raven Press; New York.

Edelman, R. 1977. Cell-mediated immune response in protein-calorie malnutrition. A review. In: Malnutrition and the Immune Response, Kroc Fdtn.

Series, vol. 7, ed. R.M. Suskind, pp. 47–76. Raven Press; New York.

Edelman, R., Kulapongs, P., Suskind, R.M., and Olson, R.E. 1977. Leukocyte mobilizaton in Thai children with Kwashiorkor. In: Malnutrition and the Immune Response, Kroc Fdtn. Series, vol. 7, ed. R.M. Suskind, pp. 265–270. Raven Press; New York.

Edwards, J.E., Jr., Foos, R.Y., Montgomerie, J.Z., and Guze, L.B. 1974. Ocular manifestations of *Candida* septicemia; Review of seventy-six cases of hematogenous *Candida* endophtalmitis. Medicine 53:47–75.

Egbert, P.R., Pollard, R.B., Gallhager, J.G., and Merigan, T.C. 1980. Cytomegalo virus retinitis in immunosuppressed hosts. II. Ocular manifestations. Ann Intern Med 93: 664–670.

Ellner, J.J., and Spagnuolo, P.J. 1979. Suppression of antigen and mitogen induced human T lymphocyte DNA synthesis by bacterial lipopolysaccharide: Mediation by monocyte activation and production of prostaglandins. J Immunol 123:2689–2695.

Feigin, R.D., and Shearer, W.T., 1975. Opportunistic infection in children. I. In the compromised host. J Pediat 87:507–514.

Fernandes, G., Nair, M., Onoe, K., Tanaka, T., Floyd, R., and Good, R.A. 1979. Impairment of cell-mediated immunity functions by dietary zinc deficiency in mice. Proc Natl Acad Sci USA 76:457–461.

Fevrier, M., Bona, C., Eyqueim, A., and Licecopoulos, P. 1977. Inhibition of mixed lymphocyte reactions in humans after immunization with tetanus toxoid. Transplantation 23:199–209.

Fiala, M., Payne, J.E., Berne, T.V., Poolsawat, S., Schieble, J., and Guze, L.B. 1974. Role of adenovirus Type II in hemorrhagic cystitis secondary to immunosuppression. J Urol 112:595–597.

Finerty, J.F., and Krehl, E.P. 1976. Cyclophosphamide pretreatment and protection against malaria. Infect Immun 14:1103–1105.

Fontana, A., and Weiner, H.L. 1980. Interaction of reovirus with cell surface receptors. II. Generation of suppressor T cells by the hemagglutinin of reovirus type 3. J Immunol 125:2660–2664.

Fraker, P.J., Haas, S.M., and Luecke, R.W. 1977. Effect of zinc deficiency on the immune response of the young adult A/J mouse. J Nutr 107:1889–1895.

Freyre, E.A., Chabes, A., Poemape, O., and Chabes, A. 1973. Abnormal rebuck skin window response in Kwashiorkor. J Pediat 82:523–526.

Gamble, C.N., and Reardan, J.B. 1975. Immunopathogenesis of syphilitic glomerulonephritis. Elution of antitreponemal antibody from glomerular immune-complex deposits. New Engl J Med 292: 449–454.

Garzelli, C., Colizzi, V., and Falcone, G. 1978. Attivazione di linfociti con funzione soppressora sulla sensibilita da contatto da parte di *Pseudomonas aeruginosa*. Folia Allerg Immunol Clin 25:418–420.

Gaumer, H.R., and Scwab, J.H. 1972. Differential susceptibility of mouse lymphocytes to an immunosuppressant from group A streptococci. Cell Immunol 4:394–406.

Gery, I., Krueger, K., and Spiesel, S.Z. 1972. Stimulation of B-lymphocytes by endotoxin. J Immunol 108:1088–1091.

Ghaftar, A., and Sigel, M. 1978. Immunomodulation by Corynebacterium parvum. I. Variable effects on anti-sheep erythrocyte responses. Immunology 35:685–693.

Giangiacomo, J., Cleary, T.G., Cole, B.R., Hoffsten, P., and Robson, A.M. 1975. Serum immunoglobulins in the nephrotic syndrome. N. Engl J Med 293:8–12.

Goldman, R.L., and Warner, N.E. 1970. Hemorrhagic cystitis and cytomegalic inclusions in the bladder associated with cyclophosphamide therapy. Cancer 25:7–11.

Good, R.A., Fernandes, G., and West, A. 1979. Nutrition, immunity, and cancer. I. Influence of protein or protein-calorie malnutrition and zinc deficiency on immunity. Clin Bull 9:3–12.

Good, R.A., Jose, D., Cooper, W.G., Fernandes, G., Kramer, T., and Junis, E. 1977. Influence of nutrition on antibody production and cellular immune responses in man, rats, mice, and guinea pigs. In: Malnutrition and the Immune Response, Kroc Fdtn. Series, vol. 7, ed. R.M. Suskind, pp. 169–184. Raven Press; New York.

Gowland, G., and Smiddy, F.G. 1962. The effect of acute experimental uremia on the immunological responses of the rabbit to bovine serum albumin. Brit J Urol 34:274–279.

Greenwood, B.M., Playfair, J.H.L., and Torrigiani, G. 1971. Immunosuppression in murine malaria. Clin Exp Immunol 8:467–478.

Haltia, M., Paetau, A., Vaheri, A., and Salmi, A. 1978a. Measles encephalopathy during immunosuppression. Scand J Infect Dis 10:159.

Haltia, M., Tarkkanen, A., Vaheri, A., Paetau, A., Kaakinen, K., and Erkkila, H. 1978b. Measles retinopathy during immunosuppression. Brit J Ophtalmol 62:356–360.

Hambridge, K.M., and Walravens, P.A. 1976. Zinc deficiency in infants and preadolescent children. In: Trace elements in human health and disease, vol. I: Zinc and Copper, ed. A. Prasad, pp. 21–32. Academic Press; New York.

Hanicki, Z., Cichocki, T., Sarnecka-Keller, M., Klein, A., and Komorowska, Z. 1976. Influence of middle-sized molecule aggregates from dialysate of uremic patients on lymphocytes transformation *in vitro*. Nephron 17:73–80.

Heiss, L.I., and Palmer, D.L. 1974. Allergy in patients with leukocytosis. Amer J Med 56: 323–332.

Henkin, R.I., Marshal, J.R., and Meret, S. 1971. Maternal fetal metabolism of copper and zinc at term. Amer J Obstet Gynecol 110:131–134.

Hersh, E.M. 1971. L-glutamine: Suppression of lymphocyte blastogenic reponses *in vitro*. Science 172:736–738.

Hersh, E.M., 1973. Immunosuppressive enzymes. Transplant Proc 5:1211–1214.

Higerd, T.B., Vesole, D.H., and Goust, J.M. 1978. Inhibitory effects of extracellular products from oral bacteria of human fibroblasts and stimulated lymphocytes. Infect Immun 21:567–574.

Hobbs, J.R., 1968. Secondary antibody deficiency. Proc Roy Soc Med 61:883–887.

Hodges, R.E., Bean, W.B., Ohlson, M.A., and Bleiler, R.E. 1962. Factors affecting human antibody response. V. Combined deficiencies of pathotenic acid and pyridoxine. Am J Clin Nutr 11:187–199.

Holdsworth, S.R., Fitzgerald, M.G., Hosking, C.S., and Atkins, R.C. 1978. The effect of maintenance dialysis on lymphocyte function. I. Hemodialysis. Clin Exp Immunol 33:95–101.

Hsu, J.M., and Anthony, W.L. 1975. Effect of zinc deficiency and repletion on thymidine metabolism. Clin Chem 21:544–550.

Hume, D.M., Merrill, J.P., Miller, B.F., and Thorn, G.W. 1955. Experiences with renal homotransplantation in the human: Report of nine cases. J Clin Invest 34:327–382.

Itok, K., Inone, M., Kataoka, S., and Kumaji, K. 1980. Differential effect of interferon in the expression of IgG- and IgM-Fc receptors on human lymphocytes. J Immunol 124:2589–2595.

Iwata, T., Incefy, G.S., and Tanaka, T. 1979. Circulatory thymic hormone levels in zinc deficiency. Cell Immunol 47:100–105.

Jayawardena, A.N., Targett, G.A.T., Leuchars, E., Carter, R.L., Doenhoff, M.J., and Davies, A.J.S. 1975. T-cell activation in murine malaria. Nature 258:149–151.

Jayawardena, A.N., and Waksman, B.H. 1977. Suppressor cells in experimental trypanosomiasis. Nature 265:539–541.

Jayawardena, A.N., Waksman, B.H., and Eardley, D.D. 1978. Activation of distinct helper and suppressor T cells in experimental trypanosomiasis. J Immunol 121:622–628.

Johnson, H.M., and Blalock, J.E. 1980. Interferon immunosuppression: Mediation by a suppressor factor. Infect Immun 29:301–305.

Johnson, H.M., Bukovic, J.A., and Baron, S. 1975a. Interferon inhibition of the primary in vitro antibody response to a thymus-independent antigen. Cell Immunol 20:104–109.

Johnson, H.M., Smith, B.G., and Baron, S. 1975b Inhibition of the primary in vitro antibody response by interferon preparations. J Immunol 114:403–409.

Kantor, F.S. 1975. Infection, allergy and cell-mediated immunity. New Engl J Med 292: 629–634.

Keusch, G.T., Douglas, S.D., Hammer, G., and Braden, K. 1978. Antibacterial functions of macrophages in experimental protein-calorie malnutrition. II. Cellular and humoral factors for chemotaxis, phagocytosis, and intracellular bactericidal activity. J Infect Dis 138:134–142.

Keusch, G.T., Douglas, S.D., Hammer, G., and Ugurbil, K. 1977a. Macrophage function in experimental protein-calorie malnutrition. In: Malnutrition and the Immune Response, Kroc Fdtn. Series, vol 7, ed. R.M. Suskind, pp. 245–252. Raven Press; New York.

Keusch, G.T., Umitia, J.J., Fernandez, R., Guerrero, O., and Casteneda, G. 1977b. Humoral and cellular aspects of intracellular bacterial killing in Guatemalan children with protein-calorie malnutrition. In: Malnutrition and the Immune Response, Kroc Fdtn. Series, vol 7, ed. R.M. Suskind, pp. 245–252. Raven Press; New York.

Kielman, A.A. 1977. Nutritional status and immune responses of subclinically malnourished Indian children. In: Malnutrition and the Immune Response, Kroc Fdtn. Series, vol. 7, ed. R.M. Suskind, pp. 195–200. Raven Press; New York.

Kirchgessner, M., Roth, H.P., and Weigland, E. 1976. Biochemical changes in zinc deficiency. In: Trace Element in Human Health and Disease, vol. 1, Zinc and Copper, ed. A. Prasad, pp. 189–225. Academic Press; New York.

Kirkpatrick, C.H., Wilson, W.E.C., and Talmage, D.W. 1964. Immunologic studies in human organ transplantation. I. Observation and characterization of suppressed cutaneous reactivity in uremia. J Exp Med 119:727–742.

Klein, K., Suskind, R.M., Kupalongs, P., Mertz, G., and Olson, R.E. 1977. Endotoxemia, a possible cause of decrease complement activity in malnourished Thai children. In: Malnutrition and the Immune Response, Kroc Fdtn. Series, vol 7, ed. R.M. Suskind, pp. 321–328. Raven Press; New York.

Kupalongs, P., Suskind, R.M., Vilhayasai, V., and Olson, R.E. 1977. *In vitro* cell-mediated immune response in Thai children with protein-calorie malnutrition. In: Malnutrition and the Immune Response, Kroc Fdtn. Series, vol 7, ed. R.M. Suskind, pp. 99–104. Raven Press; New York.

Leitzmann, C., Vithayasai, V., Windecker, P., Suskind, R.M., and Olson, R.E. 1977. Phagocytosis and killing function of polymorphonuclear leukocytes in Thai children with protein-calorie malnutrition. In: Malnutrition and the Immune Response, Kroc Fdtn. Series, vol. 7, ed. R.M. Suskind, pp. 253–258. Raven Press; New York.

Lelchuck, R., and Playfair, J.H.L. 1980. Two distinct types of non-specific immunosuppression in murine malaria. Clin Exp Immunol 42:428–435.

Levene, G.M., Turk, J.L., Wright, D.J.M., and Grimble, A.G.S. 1969. Reduced lymphocyte transformation due to a plasma factor in patients with active syphilis. Lancet ii: 246–247.

Liedberg, N.C.F., Reiss, E., and Artz, C.P. 1954. Infection in burns. III. Septicemia, a common cause of death. Surg Gynec Obst 99:15158.

Liew, F.Y., and Russell, S.M. 1980. Delayed-type hypersensitivity to influenza virus. Induction of antigen-specific suppressor T cells for delayed-type hypersensitivity to hemagglutinin during influenza virus infection in mice. J Exp Med 151:799–814.

Likhite, V.V. 1976. Immunological impairment and susceptibility infection after splenectomy. J Amer Med Ann 236:1376–1377.

Liljedahl, S.O., Olhagen, B., and Plantin, L.D. (1963) Studies on burns. VII. The problem of infection, with special reference to gammaglobulin. Acta Chirurg Scand Suppl 309:1–25.

Loirat, C., Danon, F., and Broyer, M. 1971. Panencephalite subaigue sclerosante suvenant au cours d'un syndrome rephrotique traite par les immunosuppresseurs. Arch Franc Ped 29:641–654.

Luecke, R.W. 1966. The role of zinc in animal nutrition. In: Zinc Metabolism, ed. A.S. Prasad, pp. 202–214. Charles C Thomas; Springfield, Ill.

MacLean, L.D. 1975. Host resistance in surgical patients. J Trauma 19:297–304.

Mahler, D., and Batchelor, J.R. 1971. Phytohemagglutinin transformation of lymphocytes in burned patients. Transplantation 12:409–411.

Malakian, A.H., and Schwab, J.H. 1968. Immunosuppressant from group A streptococci. Science 159:880–881.

Malakian, A.H., and Schwab, J.H. 1971. Biological characterization of an immunosuppressant from group A streptococci. J Exp Med 139:1253–1265.

Maller, R., Fryden, A., and Soren, L. 1978. Mitogen stimulation and distribution of T- and B-lymphocytes during natural rubella infection. Arch Path Microbiol Scand 85C:93–98.

Mannick, J.A., Powers, J.H., Mithoefer, J., and Ferrebee, J.W. 1960. Renal transplantation in azotemic dogs. Surgery 47:340–345.

McCullough, B., Krakowka, S., and Koestner, A. 1974. Experimental canine distemper virus-induced lymphoid depletion. Amer J Pathol 74:155–170.

McFarlane, H. 1977. Cell-mediated immunology in clinical and experimental protein-calorie malnutrition. In: Malnutrition and the Immune Response, Kroc Fdtn. Series, vol. 7, ed. R.M. Suskind, pp. 127–134. Raven Press; New York.

McGhee, J.R., Michalek, S.M., Ghania, V.K., and Stewart, G. 1974. Complement levels in malnourished animals: Quantification of serum complement in rats and their offspring. J Reticuloendothel Soc 16:204–212.

McMahon, L.J., Montgomery, D.W., Guschewsky, A., Woods, A.H., and Zukoski, C.F. 1976. In vitro effects of $ZnCl_2$ on spontaneous sheep red blood cells (E) rosette formation by lymphocytes from cancer patients and normal subjects. Immunol Commun 5:53–67.

McMillan, R., Longmire, R., and Yelenosky, R. 1976. The effect of corticosteroids on human IgG synthesis. J Immunol 116:1592–1595.

Mehra, V., Mason, L.H., Fields, J.P., and Bloom, B.R. 1979. Lepromin-induced suppressor cells in patients with leprosy. J Immunol 123:1813.

Mehra, V., Mason, L.H., Rothman, W., Reinherz, E., Schlossman, S.F., and Bloom, B.R. 1980. Delineation of a human T cell subset responsible for lepromin-induced suppression in leprosy patients. J Immunol 125-1183–1188.

Mellor, D. 1976. Encephalitis and encephalopathy in childhood leukemia. Dev Med Child Neur 18: 90–98.

Miller, C.L., and Baker, C.C. 1979. Changes in lymphocyte activity after thermal injury. The role of suppressor cells. J Clin Invest 63:202–210.

Miller, C.L., and Claudy, B.J. 1979. Suppressor T-cell activity induced as a result of thermal injury. Cell Immunol 44:201–208.

Montgomerie, J.Z., Kalmanson, G.M., and Giuze, L.B. 1968. Renal failure and infection. Medicine 47:1–32.

Mottironi, V.D., and Terasaki, P.I. 1970. Lymphocytotoxins in disease. I. Infectious mononucleosis, rubella and measles. In: Histocompatibility Testing 1970, ed. P.I. Terasaki, pp. 301–307. Munksgaard; Copenhagen.

Moynahan, E.J., and Barnes, P.M. 1973. Zinc deficiency and a synthetic diet for lactose tolerance. Lancet i:676.

Munoz, J., Virella, G., Arala-Chaves, M.P., and Fudenberg, H.H. 1980. Measurement of extracellular immunoglobulins as an index of B cell function. Haematologia 13:213–223.

Munster, A.N., Eurenius, K., and Katz, R.M. 1973. Cell-mediated immunity after thermal injury. Ann Surg 177:139–143.

Murray, M.T., and Murray, A.B. 1977. Starvation suppression and refeeding activation of infection. An ecological necessity? Lancet i:123–125.

Musatti, C.C., Soares, V.A., Santos, L.M.B., De-Lima, J.J.G., and Mendes, N.F. 1979. Immunosuppressive effect of soluble E receptors in uremic serum. Clin Immunol Immunopathol 14:403–410.

Nakhla, L.S., and Goggin, M.J. 1973. Lymphocyte transformation in chronic renal failure. Immunology 24:229–235.

Needleman, B.W., Weiler, J.M., and Feldbush, T.L. 1981. The third component of complement inhibits human lymphocyte blastogenesis. J Immunol 126:1586–1591.

Nelson, D.L., Blaese, R.M., Strober, W., Bruce, R.M., and Waldmann, T.A. 1975. Constrictive pericarditis. J Pediat 86:548–554.

Nelson, D.S., and Penrose, J.M. 1975. Effects of hemodialysis and transplantation on inhibition of lymphocyte transformation by sera from uremic patients. Clin Immunol Immunopathol 4:143–146.

Neumann, C.G., Stiehm, E.R., Swenseid, M., Fergerson, A.C., and Lawton, G 1977a. Cell-mediated immune response in Ghanian children with protein-calorie malnutrition. In Malnutrition and the Immune Response, Kroc Fdtn. Series, vol. 7, ed. R.M. Suskind, pp. 77–90. Raven Press; New York.

Neumann, C.G., Stiehm, E.R., and Swenseid, M. 1977b. Immunoglobulin levels in Ghanian children with protein-calorie malnutrition. In: Malnutrition and the Immune Response, Kroc Fdtn. Series, vol 7, ed. R.M. Suskind, pp. 191–194. Raven Press; New York.

Neumann, C.G., Stiehm, E.R., and Swenseid, M. 1977c. Complement levels in Ghanian children with protein-calorie malnutrition. In: Malnutrition and the Immune Response, Kroc Fdtn. Series, vol 7, ed. R.M. Suskind, pp. 333–336. Raven Press; New York.

Newberne, P.M. 1977. Effect of folic acid B, choline and methionine on immunocompetence and cell-mediated immunity. In: Malnutrition and the Immune Response, Kroc Fdtn. Series, vol. 7, ed. R.M. Suskind, pp. 375–386. Raven Press; New York.

Newberry, W.M., and Sanford, J.P. 1971. Defective cellular immunity in renal failure: Depression of reactivity of lymphocytes to phytohemagglutinin by renal failure serum. J Clin Invest 50:1262–1271.

Nicholson, D.H., and Wolchock, E.B. 1976. Ocular toxoplasmosis in an adult receiving long-term articosteroid therapy. Arch Ophtalm 94:248–254.

Ninnemann, J.L., Fisher, J.C., and Wachtel, T.L 1979. Thermal injury-associated immunosuppression occurrence and *in vitro* blocking effect of post recovery serum. J Immunol 122:1736–1741.

Obske, J.M., Westphal, M.L., Stan, S.E., Shore, S., Gorden, O., Bogden, J., Coplen, D.B., and Nahmias, A. 1979. Correction with zinc therapy of depressed cellular immunity in acrodermatitis enteropathica. Amer J Dis Child 133:915–918.

Ottensen, E.A. 1979. Modulation of the host response in human schisomiasis. I. Adherent suppressor cells that inhibit lymphoproliferative response to parasite antigens. J Immunol 123:1639–1644.

Phillips, J.L. 1978. Uptake of transferrin-bound zinc by human lymphocytes. Cell Immunol 35:318–329.

Phillips, J.L., and Azari, P. 1974. Zinc transferrin enhancement of nucleic acid synthesis in phytohemagglutinin-stimulated human lymphocytes. Cell Immunol 15:94–99.

Pierce, N.F., and Koster, F.T. 1980. Priming and suppression of the intestinal immune response to cholera toxoid/toxin by parenteral toxoid in rats. J Immunol 124:307–311.

Prasad, A.S. 1978. Trace Elements and Iron in Human Metabolism, pp. 312–328. Plenum; New York.

Pretorius, P.J., and deVilliers, L.S. 1962. Antibody response in children with protein malnutrition. Amer J Clin Nutr 10:379–383.

Provisor, A.J., Iacuone, J.J., Chilcote, R.R., Neiburger, R.G., Crussi, F.G., and Bahener, R.L. 1975. Acquired agammaglobulinemia after a life-threatening illness with clinical and laboratory features of infectious mononucleosis in three related male children. N Engl J Med 293:62–65.

Pullan, C.R., Noble, T.C., Scott, D.J., Wisniewski, K., and Gardner, P.S. 1976. Atypical measles infections on leukaemic children on immunosuppressive treatment. Brit Med J 1:1562–1565.

Ragan, C., Grokoest, A.W., and Boots, R.H. 1949. Effects of adrenocorticotrophic hormone (ACTH) on rheumatoid arthritis. Am J Med 7:741–750.

Raskova, J., and Morrison, A.B. 1976. A decrease in cell-mediated immunity in uremia associated with an increase on activity of suppressor cells. Amer J Path 84:1–10.

Reinherz, E.L., O'Brien, C., Rosenthal, P., and Schlossman, S.F. 1980. The cellular basis for viral-induced immunodeficiency: Analysis by monoclonal antibodies. J Immunol 125:1269–1274.

Rheinhold, J.G. 1971. High phytate content of rural Indian bread: A possible cause of human zinc deficiency. Am J Clin Ntr 24:1204–1206.

Rich, K.C., Neumann, C.G., and Stiehm, E.R. 1977. Neutrophil chemotaxis in malnourished Ghanian children. In: Malnutrition and the Immune Response, Kroc Fdtn. Series, vol. 7, ed. R.M. Suskind, pp. 271–276. Raven Press; New York.

Riches, P.G., and Hobbs, J.R. 1979. Mechanisms in secondary hypogammaglobulinemia. J Clin Path 32(suppl 13):15–22.

Rifkind, D., Marchioro, T.L., Achneck, S.A., and Hill, R.B. 1967. Systemic fungal infections complicating renal transplantation and immunosuppressive therapy. Amer J Med 43:28–38.

Robbins, D.S., Donnan, G.G., Fudenberg, H.H., and Strelkauskas, A.J. 1981. Functional subsets of human T cells defined by ''active'' rosette formation. Cell Immunol 59:205–218.

Rocklin, R.E., Brown, A.P., Warren, K.S., Pelley, R.P., Houba, V., Siongok, T.K.A., Ouma, J., Sturrock, R.F., and Butterworth, A.E. 1980. Factors that modify the cellular immune response in patients infected by *Schistosoma mausoni*. J Immunol 125:1916–1923.

Rogers, T.J., and Balish, E. 1978. Suppression of lymphocyte blastogenesis by *Candida albicans*. Clin Immunol Immunopathol 10:298–305.

Ruhl, H., and Kirchner, H. 1978. Monocyte-dependent stimulation of human T cell by zinc. Clin Exp Immunol 32:484–488.

Ruuti, P., Vaheri, A., and Kosuren, T.V. 1977. Depression of human neutrophil mobility by influenza virus in vitro. Scand J Immunol 6:897–906.

Sakai, H., Daniels, J.C., Beathard, G.A., Lewis, S.R., Lynch, J.B., and Ritzman, S.E. 1974. Mixed lymphocyte culture reaction in patients with acure thermal burns. J Trauma 14:53–57.

Sandstead, H.H. 1973. Zinc nutrition in the United States. Am J Clin Ntr 26:1251:1260.

Schleisinger, L., Ohlbaum, A., Grez, L., and Stekel, A. 1977. Cell-mediated immune studies in marasmic children from Chile: delayed hypersensitivity, lymphocyte transformation, and interferon production. In: Malnutrition and the Immune Response, Kroc Fdtn. Series, vol. 7, ed. R.M. Suskind, pp. 91–98. Raven Press; New York.

Schlievert, P.M. 1980. Activation of murine T-suppressor lymphocytes by group A streptococcal pyrogenic exotoxins. Infect Immune 28:876–880.

Schloen, L.H., Fernandes, G., Garofalo, J.A., and Good, R.A. 1979. Nutrition, immunity and cancer—A review. Part II. Zinc, immune function and cancer. Clin Bull 9:63–75.

Schoenenberger, G.A. 1975. Burn toxins isolated from mouse and human skin. Monog Allergy 9:72–139.

Schoenenberger, G.A., Burckhardt, F., Kalberer, F., Muller, W., Stadtler, K., Vogt, P., and Allgower, M. 1975. Experimental evidence for a significant impairment of host defense for gram-negative organisms by a specific cutaneous toxin produced by severe burn injuries. Surg Gyn Obstet 141:555–561.

Schumacher, M.J. 1970. Serum immunoglobulin and transferrin levels after childhood splenectomy. Arch Dis Child 45:114–117.

Selvaraj, R.J., and Bhat, K.S. 1972. Metabolic and bactericidal activities of leukocytes in protein-calorie malnutrition. Amer J Clin Nutr 25: 166–174.

Seth, V., and Chandra, R.K. 1972. Opsonic activity, phagocytosis, and bactericidal capacity of polymorphs in undernutrition. Arch Dis Child 47:282-284.

Settipane, G.A., Pudupakkam, R.K., and McGowan, J.H. 1978. Corticosteroid effect on immunoglobulins. J Allergy Clin Immunol 62:162–166.

Shakib, F., Hardwicke, J., Stanworth, D.R., and White, R.H.R. 1977. Asymmetric depression in the serum level of IgG subclasses in patients with nephrotic syndrome. Clin Exp Immunol 28:506–511.

Silk, M.R. 1967. The effect of uremic plasma on lymphocyte transformation. Invest Urol 5:195–199.

Sirisinha, S., Suskind, R., Edelman, R., Charupatana, C., and Olson, R.E. 1973. Complement and C_3-proactivator levels in children with protein-calorie malnutrition and effect of dietary treatment. Lancet i:1016–1024.

Sirisinha, S., Suskind, R.M., Edelman, R., Asvapaka, C., and Olson, R.E. 1977a. Secretory IgA in Thai children with protein-calorie malnutrition. In: Malnutrition and the Immune Response, Kroc Fdtn. Series, vol. 7, ed. R.M. Suskind, pp. 195–200. Raven Press; New York.

Sirisinha, S., Suskind, R.M., Edelman, R., Kulapongs, P., and Olson, R.E. 1977b. The complement system in protein-calorie malnutrition—A review. In: Malnutrition and the Immune Response, Kroc Fdtn. Series, vol. 7, ed. R.M. Suskind, pp. 105–110. Raven Press; New York.

Smythe, P.M., Schonland, M., Brereton-Stiles, G.G., Coovadia, H.M., Grace, J.H., Loening, W.E.K., Mafoyane, A., Parent, M.A., and Vos, G.H. 1971. Thymolymphatic deficiency and depression of cell-mediated immunity in protein-calorie malnutrition. Lancet ii:939–944.

South, M.A., Montgomery, J.R., and Rawls, W.E. 1975. Immune deficiency in congenital rubella and other viral infections. Birth Defects: Original Article Series 11:234–238.

Starr, S.E., Toloin, M.D., Friedman, H.M., Paucker, K., and Plotkin, S.A. 1979. Impaired cellular immunity to cytomegalovirus in congenitally infected children and their mothers. J Infect Dis 140:500–505.

Stoloff, I.L., Stout, R., Myerson, R.M., and Havens, W.P. 1958. Production of antibody in patients with uremia. N Engl J Med 259:320–323.

Stoner, R.D., Hess, M.W., and Terres, G. 1974. Primary and secondary antibody responses related to radiation exposures. In: Interaction of Radiation and Host Immune Defense Mechanisms in Malignancy, Conference Proceedings, pp. 152–166. Greenbrier; West Virginia.

Strober, W., Wochner, R.D., and Carbone, P.P. 1968. Intestinal lymphangiectasia, lymphocytopenia and impaired homograft rejection. J Clin Invest 46:1643–1656.

Suskind, R.M., Kulapongs, P., Vitahaysai, V., and Olson, R.E. 1977b. Iron deficiency anemia and the immune response. In: Malnutrition and the Immune Response, Kroc Fdtn. Series, vol. 7, ed. R.M. Suskind, pp. 387–394. Raven Press; New York.

Suskind, R.M., Sirisinha, S., Edelman, R., Vitahayasai, V., Damrongsak, D., Charupatana, C., and Olson, R.E. 1977a. Immunoglobulins and antibody response in Thai children with protein-calorie malnutrition. In: Malnutrition and the Immune Response, Kroc Fdtn. Series, vol. 7, ed. R.M. Suskind, pp. 185–190. Raven Press; New York.

Toffaletti, D.L., and Schwab, J.H. 1979. Modulation of lymphocyte functions by group A streptococcal membrane. Cell Immunol 42:3–17.

Traeger, J., Touraine, J.L., Revillard, J.P., Brochier, J., and Navano, J. 1976. Role of methylguanidine and middle molecules in the immunodeficiency secondary to uremia. In: Proc. 6th Int. Cong. Nephrol., Florence 1975, pp. 584–589. Karger; Basel.

von Pirquet, C. 1908. Das Verhalten der kutanen Tuberkulinreaktion whröend der Masern. Dtsch Med Wochenschr 34:1297–1300.

Wainberg, M.A., and Israel, E. 1980. Viral inhibition of lymphocyte mitogenesis. J. Immunol 124: 64–70.

Warden, G.D., Mason, A.D., and Pritt, B.A. 1974.

Evaluation of leukocyte chemotaxis *in vitro* in thermally injured patients. J Clin Invest 54: 1001–1004.

Warren, H.S., and Weindanz, W.P. 1976. Malarial immunodepression in vitro: Adherent spleen cells are functionally defective as accessory cells in the response to horse erythrocytes. Eur J Immunol 6:816–819.

Webb, D.R., Jr., and Winkelstein, A. 1980. Immunosuppression and immunopotentiation. In: Basic and Clinical Immunology, eds. H.H. Fudenberg, D.P. Stites, J.L. Caldwell, and J.V. Wells, pp. 313–326. Lange; Los Altos, Calif.

Webel, M.L., Ritts, R.E., Briggs, W.A., and Light, J.A. 1976. Lymphocyte blastogenesis in patients receiving hemodialysis. Arch Intern Med 136:682–687.

Weiden, P.L., Blaese, R.M., and Strober, W. 1972. Impaired lymphocyte transformation in intestinal lymphangiectasia. Evidence for at least two functionally distinct lymphocyte populations in man. J Clin Invest 51:1319–1325.

Westwater. 1935. Tuberculin allergy in acute infectious diseases. Quart J Med 4:203–225.

Whittle, H.C., Dossetor, J., Oduloju, A., and Bryceson, A.D.M. 1978. Cell-mediated immunity during natural measles infection. J Clin Invest 62:678–684.

WHO Scientific Report. 1978. Immune deficiency diseases. WHO Technical Reports No. 630. WHO; Geneva.

Williams, R.J., Chandler, J.G., and Orloff, M.J. 1971. Candida septicaemia. Arch Surg 103:8–11.

Wilson, W.E.C., Kirkpatrick, C.H., and Talmage, D.W. 1965. Suppression of immunologic responsiveness in uremia. Ann Intern Med 62:1–14.

Wolinski, J., Sweveland, P., Johnson, K.P., and Baringer, J.R. 1977. Subacute measles encephalitis complicating Hodgkin's disease in an adult. Ann Neurol 1:452–457.

Wybran, J., and Fudenberg, H.H. 1972. Thymus-derived rosette-forming cells in various human disease states: Cancer, lymphoma, bacterial and viral infections, and other diseases. J Clin Invest 52:1026–1032.

Zazgornik, J., Schmidt, P., Kopsa, H., Fill, W., and Deutsch, E. 1974. Septic candidiasis with intrahepatic cholestasis and immunoglobulin deficiency after renal transplantation. Acta-Hepato-Gastroenterol 22:304–309.

Chapter 8

Excessive Immunosuppression

Jeremiah J. Twomey

Introduction

Early interest in immunity concentrated on the effector apparatus. Clinical disorders of the immune system were generally ascribed to deficiencies or abberations of effector systems. Evidence that the effector apparatus is stringently regulated has greatly expanded current understanding in immunology. Immune responses are modulated by complex positive and negative systems that promote or suppress them. Perturbations of these regulatory systems can derange immune function. This chapter deals with excessive immune suppression as a cause for immunodeficiencies. The potential consequences of defective suppression are discussed in Chapter 10, which deals with autoimmunity.

It is evident that immune reactivity is controlled by a number of diverse mechanisms. The complexity of overall immune suppression is best appreciated from experimental models. These studies have been facilitated by the availability of inbred animal strains, especially of mice. However, improved cell identification and separation techniques have led to important new discoveries in the field of immune regulation in man. We are not yet at the stage of meaningful comparisons between human and mouse suppressor systems, although many parallels are emerging.

Immune responses are suppressed by products released from lymphocytes and macrophages. These products include antibodies, interferon, prostaglandins and various mediators. Suppression that primarily involves lymphocytes is generally conducted by specific subpopulations of T cells and, in the mouse, at least, involves a sequence of interactions between antigenically distinct T cell subpopulations. The technology with which to identify subpopulations of similar interest within the monocyte-macrophage series is not yet available, although considerable progress has recently been made toward that goal (see Chapter 3). The situation is further complicated by evidence that macrophages participate in some predominently T lymphocyte suppressor systems and vice versa.

This chapter first examines physiologic aspects of immune suppression. This is necessary so as to gain better insight into the changes that take place with disordered states of immunologic control. Attention is directed primarily to human systems involving lymphocytes, macrophages and their mediator products. Mechanisms responsible for excessive suppression of lymphocyte responses in culture are described. The potential relevance of these in vitro abnormalities to their associated immunodeficiencies in vivo is examined. Other substances, such as lipoproteins (Waddell et al., 1976) and products of cancer cells (Reinacle-Bonnet et al., 1976) that also suppress lymphocyte responses, are not discussed, in the interest of brevity.

When discussing regulatory T lymphocytes, it has become customary to refer to helper and suppressor subpopulations depending upon whether their effects upon effector cells promote or suppress reactivity. If cells of the monocyte-macrophage series are to be given equal status with T cells in immune regulation, then their positive and negative effects upon effector cells are equally deserving of verbal recognition. It seems reasonable that these regulatory effects of monocytes be referred to in terms similar to those that have received broad recognition with regulatory T cells. Thus, in this chapter, monocytes that promote lymphocyte responses are called helper monocytes and those that lower lymphocyte responses are called suppressor monocytes. It must be pointed out that help in the case of monocytes is complex and involves at least two stages; these are antigen presentation to lymphocytes and release of interleukin I (see Chapter 3). In the present context, suppression is reserved for systems in which the monocyte has a prominent role in bringing about inhibition of lymphocyte responses. This does not include a facilitating role in primarily T cell regulatory systems or lowering of immune responses through cytotoxic mechanisms.

Suppression Primarily Effected by T Lymphocytes

Experimental Models

A detailed discussion of the various experimental models of T lymphocyte suppressor systems exceeds the scope of this chapter. Intense ongoing efforts on this subject call for frequent additions and modifications (Cantor and Gershon, 1979; Tada and Okumura, 1980; Germain and Benacerraf, 1981). Nevertheless, these diligent studies provide an invaluable perspective on how to address immune regulation in man. First, various immune responses in the mouse are regulated by a number of suppressor T cell systems that, on the surface at least, appear quite distinct from one another. Perhaps additional studies will show that these differences can be partially reconciled. Second, T cell suppression results from a sequence of interactions between distinct T cell subpopulations; the identity of some of these subpopulations has not yet been established. Third, the suppressor T cell sequence involves the release of various inhibitory mediators. Finally, products determined by Ir gene loci participate in T cell suppression.

Research largely pioneered by Cantor and Boyse (1976) has shown that functionally distinct murine T lymphocytes express different membrane antigens. Ly 1^+, 2^+, 3^+ cells include cells that are relatively immature in functional development. It is uncertain whether Ly 1^+, 2^+, 3^+ cells become Ly 2^+, 3^+ cells themselves or activate other lymphocytes that already express, or acquire, the Ly 2^+, 3^+ phenotype to effect immunosuppression. Conversely, Ly 1^+ cells are generally considered helper lymphocytes. Unfortunately, the situation is more complex. It has recently been suggested that Lyt antigens are related more closely to the major histocompatibility complex than to discrete functional characteristics of the cells (Swain, 1980). Furthermore, help and suppression require broader definition to include the modulation of immune regulation itself. For example, Ly 1^+, I-J^+ helper cells activate suppressor cells. The effectors of suppression are usually Ly 2^+, I-J^- and are themselves subject to countersuppression by Ly 2^+, I-J^+ cells (Gershon et al., 1981). Thus, regulatory systems are also subject of both positive and negative controls and, as such, have qualities of effector activities themselves.

As might be expected, immune response (Ir) gene products enter into the picture. Here, too, variations are evident. T cells that release soluble immune response suppressor (SIRS), a mediator which suppresses the mixed leukocyte reaction, must be homologous at the I-C locus with the proliferating responser cells for suppression to occur (Rich and Rich, 1976). In another system involving primary antibody responses to alloantigens, similarity is needed at the I-A locus (Sorenson and Pierce, 1981). Antigenic determinants associated with the Ir locus are also present in various mediators involved in immunosuppression.

Mediators play an important part in T cell suppression, both in activating the final suppressor cell and in bringing about suppression of effector cells. Little is known about how these mediators work, although recent biochemical characterization should provide useful clues. The final mediators of suppression may also operate upon different target cells. Concanavalin A-activated T cells release suppressor mediators that suppress proliferation of antibody-producing cells in some systems (Rich and Pierce, 1973) and macrophages in others (Tadakuma and Pierce, 1976). Concanavalin A-activated T cells have also been reported to suppress only antibody responses that require helper T cell participation, implying that helper T cells are targets for this form of suppression (Ekstedt et al., 1977). Thus, it would seem that mitogen-activated T cell suppressor systems release a number of mediators that act upon different target cells involved in the effector apparatus. Factors that select different targets for suppressing mediators remain to be determined.

It must be remembered that mitogens are polyclonal activators. Specific immune responses are suppressed in some suppressor T cell systems that are activated by antigen (Eardley and Gershon, 1976). Obviously, antigenic stimulation is the biologic prototype of immunologic induction. In at least some systems, the potency of the antigenic challenge determines whether effector or suppressor cells are predominantly activated (Ramshaw et al., 1980). Cellular and humoral effector systems may react in opposing fashion to high and low antigenic stimulation. Regulatory mechanisms may also determine the type of immunoglobulin response evoked by antigen. For example, lymphoid cells, primarly in Peyer's patches, promote IgA but suppress IgG responses to ingested protein antigens (Richman et al., 1981).

It is apparent that incisive analyses of the various experimenal models of immune suppression must await clear identification of all cells that participate in the different cell-cell sequences, complete characterization and biological understanding of the various mediators and thorough testing to determine the range of immune responses that are modulated by individual suppressor systems. In addition, since some tissues, such as the spleen, may be richer in suppressor T cells than others (Rocklin et al., 1979), suppression should be tested in identical fashion using cells from different lymphoid organs.

Human T Cell Suppression

Suppression that is primarily effected by T cells is as complex in man as it is in rodents. Partially defined T cell subpopulations interact with one another to bring about suppression in a fashion that is reminiscent of mouse models. The specificity of suppression varies considerably in different test systems, presumably related to the number of suppressor clones that are activated. In some systems, suppression is restricted by a need for histocompatibility between suppressor and effector cells. Suppression is usually brought about by mediators.

The membrane characteristics of T lymphocyte subpopulations engaged in suppression are discussed in Chapter 1 and are addressed only briefly here. About 75% of circulating T cells have membrane receptors for the Fc fragment of IgM (T_μ cells) and 20% have receptors for the Fc fragment of IgC (T_γ cells). The concept that T_μ cells help and T_γ cells suppress immune responses (Moretta et al., 1977) needs modification. While T cell proliferation in mixed leukocyte cultures is suppressed by concanavalin A-activated T_γ cells, both T_γ and T_μ cells activated in this fashion suppress T cell proliferation stimulated with phytohemagglutinin and immunoglobulin synthesis stimulated with pokeweed mitogen (Herscowitz et al., 1980).

More recently, T lymphocyte subpopulations have been recognized through their membrane antigens. About 20% of circulating T cells react with an equine anti-human thymocyte globulin and are termed TH_2^+ (Reinherz et al., 1979). A similar percentage of T cells from peripheral blood are $T5^+/T8^+$ as identified by monoclonal antibodies (Morimoto et al., 1981). The TH_2^+ and $T5^+/T8^+$ cells represent the same or closely related T lymphocyte subpopulations and play an important role in T cell suppression. About 40% of T lymphocytes that are TH_2^- react with an antibody in serum from patients with active juvenile rheumatoid arthritis (JRA) (Reinherz et al., 1979). TH_2^-/JRA^- T cells are clearly helper cells. Lymphocytes from acutely ill patients who are JRA seropositive lack JRA^+ T cells and their cultured mononuclear leukocytes release increased amount of immunoglobulins, perhaps because of reduced regulation (Strelkauskas et al., 1978). This suggests that the TH_2^-/JRA^+ T cells as well as the TH_2^+/JRA^- T cells are capable of suppressing immunoglobulin synthesis.

The fact that two antigenically distinct types of T cells engage in immune suppression suggests that different T cell subpopulations interact with one another in order to accomplish inhibition. Alternatively, suppression may be accomplished by more than one T cell system. Evidence that promotion is needed from $T4^+$ helper cells to activate $T5^+/T8^+$ suppressor cells establishes the occurrence of T−T cell interactions in human as well as murine systems (Thomas et al., 1981; Morimoto et al., 1981). However, various classes of immune responses are suppressed by different subpopulations of T lymphocytes. For example, concanavalin A-activated T cells that suppress terminal B cell differentiation are steroid- and radiosensitive, while those that suppress T cell proliferation are not (Lobo and Spencer, 1979). It remains to be determined if there is a relationship between suppressor T lymphocytes that do and do not require prior activation (Saxon et al., 1977; Bluming et al., 1979) to cause suppression. Perhaps, the latter become activated early in the incubation period of systems which they suppress. Indeed, T cell suppression probably becomes increasingly selective until it reaches the clonal level where antigen-activated T cells only suppress responses to that particular antigen (Heijnen et al., 1981). This breakdown is analogous to effector cells which are first grouped into broad classes such as T and B cells and eventually into exquisitely specialized clones that effect specific functions.

The apparent heterogeneity of T cell suppression is evident from the various mediators through which they exercise regulation. Concanavalin A-activated T cells release two clearly distinct low molecular weight mediators, one of which suppresses B cells directly (Fleisher et al., 1981); the other suppresses T cells (Greene et al., 1981). After activation with concanavalin A, T cells release large amounts of interferon (Kadish et al., 1980). Interferon inhibits T cell proliferation (Johnson et al., 1975), which is an important component of many immune responses.

The suppressive activity of supernates from concanavalin A-activated cultures is greatly reduced by removing interferon with immobilized interferon antibody. This has lead Kadish et al. (1980) to suggest that interferon is an important mediator of suppression released by concanavalin A-activated T cells. It has recently been suggested that this suppressor system operates through a reverse mechanism whereby mediators needed to activate effector cells are removed by concanavalin A-activated T cells (Palacios and Moller, 1981). These investigators showed that the number of membrane receptors for interleukin 2 is greatly increased after T cells are activated with concanavalin A. These activated T cells critically depleted culture media of interleukin 2 through absorption. Thus, effector cells are deprived by mitogen-activated T cells of the activating signal given by interleukin 2. It was possible to prevent suppression by concanavalin A-activated T cells by presaturating their receptor sites with exogenous interleukin 2. Finally, T cell suppression may operate through direct cell-cell contact in some instances (Innes et al., 1979).

It is not known why different mechanisms, many involving well documented mediators, participate in suppression that is predominently effected by T cells. This may be necessary because of the large number and variety of immune responses that require regulation. The fact that macrophage participation is crucial for some systems (Raff et al., 1978) but not for others (Bernbaum and Swick, 1978) may have relevance to these variations. In addition, genetic restriction at the HLA-D locus has been observed in a few suppressor systems (Engleman et al., 1979). Concanavalin A-activated T cells suppress T lymphoproliferation (Shou et al., 1976), polyclonal immunoglobulin (Schwartz et al., 1977) and specific antibody responses (Heijnen et al., 1981), T lymphocytotoxicity (Bernbaum and Swick, 1978), natural killer cytotoxicity and antibody dependent cytotoxicity (Nair and Schwartz, 1981). There is need to identify the specificity and range of these seemingly unrelated T cell suppressor systems.

The apparent complexity of T cell suppression leaves it vulnerable to a number of disorders that could inhibit the immune system excessively. Excessive stimulation of systems that activate T cell suppression could lower normal immune reactivity. An imbalance between different T lymphocyte subpopulations could result in a relative excess of those engaged in suppression. An intrinsic abnormality of suppressor T cells could amplify their inhibitory effects to an excessive degree. Effector cells may become unusually sensitive to T cell suppression. The various T suppressor systems probably function normally in harmony with one another; this balance could be deranged with disease. We now have considerable information about the cells and mediators involved in human T cell suppression. This information can be applied to pinpoint the pathophysiology of various clinical situations where the immune systems is suppressed excessively.

Suppression Primarily Effected by the Monocyte-Macrophage Series

Immune responses are also suppressed by mechanisms that primarily involve the monocyte-macrophage series. These suppressor systems are not as well understood as their T cell counterparts. This partly reflects our poorer understanding of the subpopulations that comprise the monocyte-macrophage series. The plethora of systems used to study suppression by macrophages hampers comprehension, as in the case of T lymphocyte suppression. Yet, monocyte-macrophage suppression is remarkably potent and may have considerable clinical application. It has been implicated in the pathophysiology of some immunodeficiencies and offers an alternative regulatory mechanism when T cell suppression is deficient.

When high numbers of normal human monocytes are added to cultures, various immune responses are profoundly suppressed. These responses include T and B lymphoproliferation, terminal B cell differentiation, protein (including immunoglobulin) synthesis and switching from IgM to IgG production (Laughter and Twomey, 1977; Knapp and Baumgartner, 1978; Bobak and Whisler, 1980). The predominant suppressor cell adheres to foreign surfaces; is, or accompanies, a cell rich in cytoplasmic esterase; requires viability as is illustrated by its inactivation with carrageenin; is not injured by complement-fixing T cell antibody; and is a hardy cell that remains active after prolonged culture and is both steroid- and radioresistant (Laughter and Twomey, 1977: Rice et al., 1979).

We have recently cloned human monocytes from bone marrow precursors. Cloned cells that suppressed were phagocytic, esterase rich, expressed a number of monocyte-related membrane antigens, produced lysozyme and secreted C_3 and C_4 (Capra, personal communication), which identifies them with the monocyte-macrophage series. Cloned monocytes suppressed both before and after they lost membrane DR antigens during prolonged culture. Suppression by freshly collected monocytes also does not require the presence of DR membrane antigens (Knapp and Baumgartner, 1978). The apparent independence of suppression by monocytes from products of the immune response genetic locus contrasts with their requirement for helper monocytes to promote lymphocyte responses. This independence from DR determinants probably explains why monocytoid suppression is not donor specific.

The monocyte-macrophage series is probably comprised of a number of subpopulations analogous to lymphocytes (see Table 3.3). It is possible to separate helper from suppressor macrophages that regulate cytotoxic T cells using velocity sedimentation gradients (Lee et al., 1979). Human monocytes that secrete prostaglandins can also be separated from the other monocytes that do not secrete appreciable amounts of prostaglandins by their bouyant densities (Picker et al., 1980). Prostaglandins act as mediators that modulate lymphocyte responses (vide infra). We

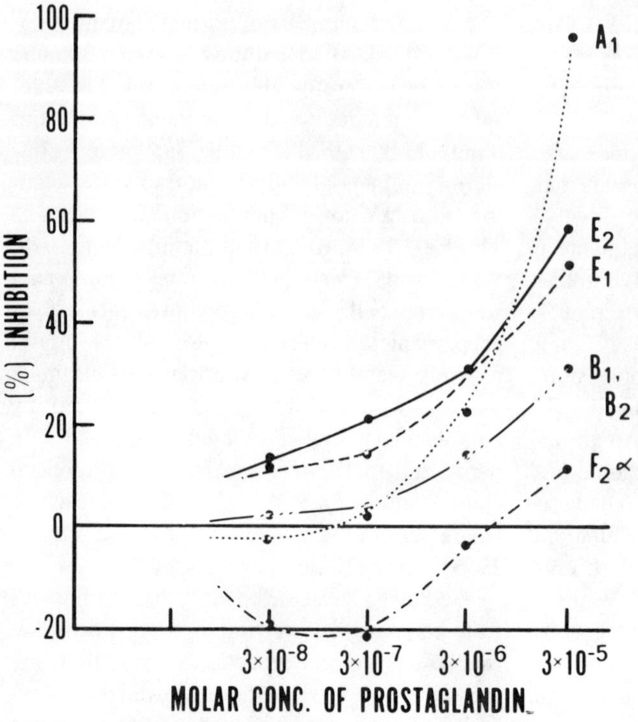

Fig. 8.1 Modulation of ³H-thymidine incorporation in the mixed leukocyte reaction by adding exogenous prostaglandins to the cultures. Cultures were of mononuclear leukocytes from allogeneic donor pairs and endogenous prostaglandin synthesis was inhibited with 1 μg/ml of indomethacin.

have recently produced monocyte lines derived from single bone marrow colonies initially grown in agar. These monocyte lines either promoted or suppressed the mixed leukocyte reaction, but never did both at different monocyte concentrations, as is the case with the combination of various monocyte subpopulations of whole blood. This apparent distinction of suppressor from helper monocytes seems logical; otherwise, individual monocytes would modulate immune responses in opposing directions.

The relative distribution of lymphocyte subpopulations varies in different tissues. Suppressor T lymphocytes are in particular abundance in spleens from experimental animals (Rocklin et al., 1979). The relative numbers of different monocyte-macrophage subpopulations may also vary from tissue to tissue, as is illustrated by the five-fold higher percentage of Ia positive macrophages in the spleen than in the peritoneal cavity of mice (Beller and Unanue, 1980). Both peripheral blood monocytes and pulmonary alveolar macrophages from man promote the mixed leukocyte reactions at lower concentrations and suppress it at higher concentrations. However, we have only observed help with spleen macrophages at up to a 50% total cell concentration. These preliminary clinical observations are supported by similar observations made on experimental animals (Youdin, 1979; Ting and Rodrigues, 1980). It is interesting that the spleen, which is rich in suppressor T lymphocytes, seems to be deficient in suppressor macrophages.

Suppression of immune responses in a number of experimental models is only achieved after macrophage activation. Mouse peritoneal macrophages, when activated with *C. parvum*, release hydrogen peroxide, which is a potent inhibitor of T cell proliferation (Metzger et al., 1980). However, suppression is not an inevitable consequence of macrophage activation. For example, mouse peritoneal macrophages activated with mineral oil do not suppress (Varesio and Holden, 1980). Suppression by human monocytes may not require activation. We did not demonstrate increased ³H-glucosamine uptake by monocytes that severely suppress T cell proliferation. This apparent independence of suppression by monocytes from activation may contribute to the apparent lack of specificity of the suppression caused by monocytes. However, it remains possible that human monocytes also suppress through mechanisms that call for activation. Conceivably, these systems could include the release of hydrogen peroxide, interferon or greater quantities of prostaglandins.

It is well known that prostaglandins modulate immune responses both in vivo and in vitro (Goldyne, 1977). We added various prostaglandins in pharmacological concentrations to mixed leuckocyte cultures in which endogenous prostaglandins synthesis was inhibited with 1μg/ml indomethacin. Prostaglandins E_1 and E_2 were moderately suppressive of ^{3}H-thymidine incorporation, while prostaglandin $F_{2\alpha}$ enhanced responses except at high concentrations (Fig. 8.1). Suppression by E series prostaglandins is mediated through a shortlived subpopulation of T lymphocytes (Goodwin et al., 1978a). It is not known if normal suppression by monocytes through other mechanisms involves an intermediary T cell, although T cells seem to participate in suppression of B cell colony formation by normal monocytes (Bobak and Whisler, 1980) and abnormal suppression of proliferation by monocytes with systemic fungal infections. Endogenous prostaglandins produced by mononuclear leukocytes also suppress immune responses, as is evidenced by the increase in these responses when endogenous prostaglandin synthesis is blocked with indomethacin (Goodwin et al., 1977a). This suggests that prostaglandins that inhibit lymphocyte responses predominate over others than enhance responses. Prostaglandins produced by mononuclear cells are predominently derived from adherent phagocytes. That is not surprising, since macrophage membranes are exceptionally rich in arachidonic acid (Scott et al., 1980), which is the substrate for prostaglandin synthesis. The synthesis of prostaglandins is stimulated by phagocytosis, lymphokines, certain bacterial products, ionophore A23187 and colchicine (Gemsa et al., 1980).

Proliferation is an integral component of many immune responses. Lymphoproliferation is modulated by cyclic nucleotides, being inhibited by an accumulation of cyclic AMP. Thus, the accumulation of cyclic AMP stimulated by prostaglandins may be central to their inhibition of those immune responses that are dependent upon proliferation. That is the opposite to circumstances that promote null lymphocyte differentiation which is positively influenced by a partial buildup of cyclic AMP. Recent evidence suggests that E series prostaglandins have a crucial intermediary role in T lymphocyte differentiation stimulated by thymic extracts through generating cyclic AMP (Garaci et al., Twomey, unpublished 1981). We have confirmed this observation and have shown that indomethacin blocks induction of T lymphocyte differentiation antigens with various inducing agents, presumably through inhibiting prostaglandin synthesis. Thus, lymphocyte differentiation and immunologic activation of lymphocytes that are already differentiated are not necessarily under parallel regulatory control.

Monocytes or macrophages are needed to process lymphocyte responses to antigens (Twomey et al., 1970). When lymphocytes severely depleted of monocytes from paired allogeneic donors were cocultured, a mixed lymphocyte reaction did not take place (Fig. 8.2). Monocytes harvested from mononuclear cells at an 86 to 94% purity by adherence to cold-insoluble globulins were then added to cultures. An optimal response was achieved with the addition of 11% fresh monocytes. At higher monocyte concentrations, the reaction was progressively suppressed. The added presence of indomethacin (or other inhibitors of the cyclo-oxygenase pathway) amplified ^{3}H-thymidine incorporation at lower monocyte concentrations but did not alter inhibition in the presence of high numbers of monocytes. Thus, a second suppressor mechanism that seems independent of prostaglandins exists in the presence of relatively high numbers of monocytes. This second mechanism is distinguished from that related to prostaglandins by resisting inactivation by cyclo-oxygenase inhibitors, suppressing preincubated as well as fresh lymphocytes, causing suppression later into the culture period and being much more potent (Rice et al., 1979).

Attempts in our laboratory to recover a mediator from cultures spontaneously suppressed by high numbers of human monocytes have been unsuccessful. Yet, when suppressive numbers of monocytes are separated from the reaction under test by a cell-impermeable membrane, they are as inhibitory as when comingled with the reacting cells (Laughter et al., 1981). The likeliest explanation is that this form of monocytoid suppression is mediated by an extremely labile mediator. The identity of this labile mediator of <1000 daltons is not known. Other more stable suppressive monokines have been described with certain diseases (Stobo, 1977), but not under physiological conditions.

Thus, the monocyte-macrophage series in man is capable of profound negative, as well as positive, influence upon immune responses. Preliminary evidence suggests that only some of these cells exercise suppression and that suppressor subpopulations are not equally distributed in different tissues. Suppression is effected by a number of mediators including prostaglandins of the E series, a labile low molecular weight poorly defined substance and, possibly, classical interferon as well. This type of suppression must be distinguished from predominently T cell suppression that requires macrophage participation.

Physiologic Elevations of Immunosuppression

Infancy

Infants are clearly at increased risk from infections. Various T lymphocyte responses are reduced, with the exception of proliferative responses to phytohemagglutinin or alloantigens (Stiehn et al., 1979). Helper T lymphocytes also function normally (Tosato et al., 1980). Immunoglobulin synthesis by B lymphocytes is defective and maturation of humoral immune responses is impaired after the stage of delta chain production and before the switch in synthesis from IgM to IgG or IgA (Durandy et al., 1979). These deficiencies are partially due to immaturity of the effector apparatus. There is also evidence that immune responses are suppressed excessively during the neonatal period.

Attention focused initially upon T cell suppression. Cord blood was found to have a relative excess of Tγ cells (Miyawaki et al., 1979). Immune responses by adult lymphocytes are suppressed excessively by cord blood T cells (Morito et al., 1979; Tosato et al., 1980). These suppressor T cells are steroid and radiosensitive and inhibit helper T cells rather than effector B cells. This spontaneous suppression by cord blood T cells resembles adult suppressor T cells after activation with concanavalin A (Durandy et al., 1979). Thus, there is credible evidence that cord blood T lymphocytes are excessively suppressive of responses by normal adult lymphocytes.

However, this situation becomes less clear after closer scrutiny. Elevated suppression persists for months after circulating Tγ cells decline to normal numbers (Miyawaki et al., 1979). Suppression during the neonatal period has been identified with non-Tγ cells (Durandy et al., 1979). The relative number of cord blood T cells bearing OKT8 membrane antigen, which is associated with suppression, is not elevated (Hayward and Kurmek, 1981). Thus, if T cell suppression is increased during infancy, it must be due to elevated suppression by normal numbers of suppressor lymphocytes or an accumulation of a subpopulation of suppressor cells that cannot be identified by techniques that are currently available. Furthermore, the biologic relevance of studies where cord blood cells are shown to suppress adult lymphocytes is open to question. These cells may suppress lymphocytes from adult donors, but not neonatal lymphocytes (Olding et al., 1977).

Alternatively, immune responses may be suppressed excessively during the neonatal period by the monocyte-macrophage series. Cord blood monocytes respond to chemotactic stimuli (Hawes et al., 1980) and produce classical interferon as effectively as monocytes from adult donors (Bryson et al., 1980). They also probably are able to suppress immune responses as effectively as do adult monocytes. While cord blood has an absolute monocytosis, this is relatively less than the concomitant lymphyocytosis. Thus, the number of monocytes relative to lymphocytes in mononuclear cell preparations is likely to be lower with cord blood than with adult blood. The possibility that cord blood monocytes are relatively more suppressive qualitatively than adult monocytes should be investigated.

Experimental data suggest that cells other than T lymphocytes or the monocyte-macrophage series may suppress excessively during the neonatal period. Spleens from neonatal mice have been reported to contain a suppressor cell that may be unique to that period of life. This cell lacks characteristics of T cells, B cells, NK cells or macrophages and suppresses both T cell dependent and independent responses (Calkins and Stutman, 1978; Rodrigues et al., 1979).

Pregnancy

There is no doubt that fetal tissues bear paternal transplantation antigens. Yet, most fetuses survive gestation and are not rejected by their mothers. This remarkable tolerance could result from a number of mechanisms. a) The mother's immune system may not become sensitized to paternal antigens. b) The mother's immune system may be selectively suppressed so that it does not reject the fetus. c) The placenta may be a strategically located site of intense immune suppression. d) The placenta may serve as an immunologic barrier between mother and fetus. e) Components of the mother's effector apparatus that pass through the placenta may be eliminated by the fetus before doing harm. This section discusses these possibilities.

There is evidence that maternal immune reactivity is lowered during pregnancy. The frequency of positive tuberculin skin tests is reduced and allograft rejection is prolonged (Finn et al., 1972; Andersen et al., 1962). While lymphoproliferative responses to phytohemag-

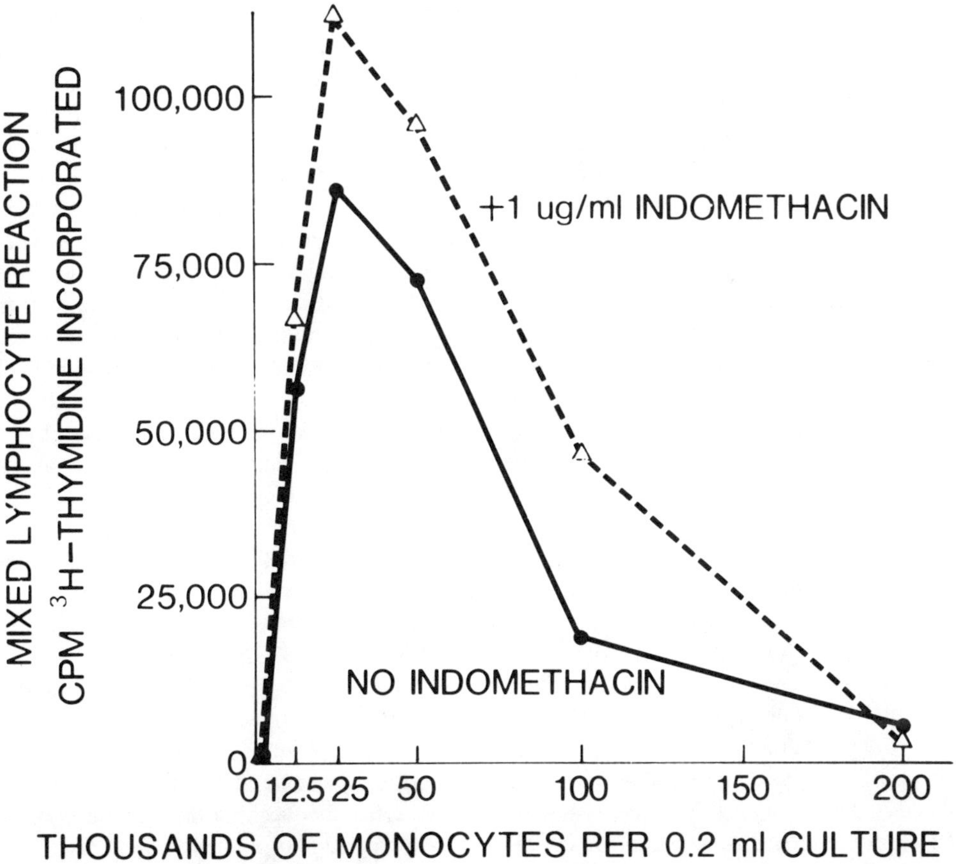

Fig. 8.2 The effects of different numbers of fresh monocytes upon the mixed lymphocyte reaction are shown. No response occurred with severe monocyte depletion. The reaction was promoted with lower numbers but suppressed by higher numbers of monocytes. Amplification of the response with indomethacin was only apparent at relatively low monocyte percentages.

glutinin are normal, the subsequent capacity of these transformed cells to generate lymphocyte colonies in soft agar is reduced (Stahn et al., 1978). Nevertheless, pregnant women do not experience a pattern of infections suggestive of clinically significant immunodeficiency.

Evidence that fetal cells bearing paternal antigens do cross the placental barrier (Herzenberg et al., 1978) indicates that the mother's immune system is given the opportunity to become sensitized to fetal antigens. After exposure to cord blood, maternal lymphocytes respond earlier than paternal lymphocytes to tissue antigens of their progeny (Moen et al., 1980). This suggests that mothers are at least partially sensitized to fetal alloantigens during pregnancy. That their immune systems recognize and respond to these antigens is evidenced by the increasing frequency of antibodies mothers develop to paternal antigens with successive pregnancies (Billingham, 1980). They also acquire cellular cytoxicity to fetal tissues (Chardonnens and Jeannet, 1979). Yet, these maternal responses to fetal tissues do not appear to compromise pregnancy. Indeed, experimental pregnancies were not harmed after females were sensitized with paternal antigens before conception (Larman et al., 1962). Thus, pregnant females can, and do, become sensitized to fetal tissues without apparent ill effect. This suggests that maternal immunity to the unborn is prevented from harming fetal tissues during pregnancy.

The production of cytotoxic lymphocytes in mixed leukocyte cultures is accompanied by lymphoproliferation. Thus, proliferative responses by maternal T lymphocytes to cord blood cells are of considerable interest to the immunobiology of pregnancy. There are reports of multiparous women who acquire T cells that selectively suppress mixed leukocyte responses to paternal cells (McMichael and Sasazuki, 1977). However, these are the exception rather than the rule. When pregnant serum is excluded from the culture medium, maternal lymphocytes usually proliferate briskly in coculture with cord blood cells (Moen et al., 1980). There is experimental evidence that the development of cytotoxic lymphocytes from committed precursors is selectively suppressed during pregnancy (Clark et al., 1980). This suppression may be greatest in regional lymph nodes draining the uterus (Clark and McDermott, 1978). In man, the increase in Tγ relative to Tμ lymphocytes during pregnancy (Hirahara et al., 1980) may have bearing upon this suppression.

A number of biological products mediate suppression during pregnancy. Pregnant women have elevated levels of circulating immune complexes (Masson et al., 1977). These complexes may saturate Fc receptors on the maternal side of the placenta, thereby interfering with the transfer of maternal antibodies across the placenta (Jenkenson et al., 1976; Billingham, (1980). Some immunosuppressive molecules are produced in large quantities by the placenta. These include progesterone (Clemens et al., 1979), gonadotrophins, somatotrophins (Hammerstrom et al., 1979) and prostaglandins (Billingham, 1980). Maternal responses to I region antigens are selectively suppressed by α_1-fetoprotein (Peck et al., 1978), which diffuses across the placenta into the maternal circulation. The origins of α-globulins (Okamura et al., 1980) and amine oxidase, which converts polyamines into immunosuppressive aminoaldehydes (Gaugas and Curzen, 1978) are not known. Therefore, it seems that a number of normal biologic products appear in increased amounts during pregnancy and contribute to the suppression of immune reactivity the mother.

There are obvious advantages to having the immunosuppressive effect predominently located at the feto-maternal interface, while retaining systemic immunocompetence by the mother. Some of these immunosuppressants are produced in, and are probably most active at, the placenta. These include progesterone, gonadotrophins and prostaglandins. Trophoblasts themselves express unique antigens that are also found on lymphoblasts that are specifically activated in the mixed leukocyte reaction (McIntyre and Faulk, 1979). These antigens are found in chromatographic fractions that selectively suppress the mixed leukocyte reaction.

Does the placenta offer an antigenically neutral interface between mother and unborn child or block passage of maternal immunity into the fetal circulation? It would appear that trophoblasts do not express HLA or Ia antigens (Faulk et al., 1977). However, they express other unique antigens that pose the risk of abortion if they become targets of immunologic attack (Beer et al., 1972). Obviously, the presence of these trophoblastic antigens could negate the advantage of trophoblasts lacking traditional transplantation antigens. This re-emphasizes the importance of local immune suppression at the placental level.

There is little doubt that the placental barrier is incomplete and that maternal blood enters the fetal circulation (Rigby et al., 1964; Billingham, 1980). However, volumes of blood transferred may be small. In general, maternal blood enters the circulation of immunologically immature fetuses. Yet, immune responses to alloantigens are well developed relatively early during fetal development (Stiehn et al., 1979) and may be able to dispose of small quantities of maternal cells. Alternatively, maternal immune responses may be suppressed in fetal tissues.

The usual tolerance throughout pregnancy by immunologically normal mothers to their fetuses is apparent. A number of maternal, placental and fetal adjustments probably contributes to this success. It seems likely that the net effect of these mechanisms is largely concentrated at the feto-maternal interface. These changes leave no permanent effect upon maternal immunologic competence and are readily reintroduced with subsequent pregnancies.

Old Age

The waning of immunologic vigor with old age is reviewed in Chapter 5. The importance of this immunologic senescence is illustrated by the shorter life expectancy among aged individuals who fail to respond when skin tested with recall antigens (Roberts-Thomson et al., 1974). The possibility that elevated suppression contributes to immunologic aging is examined in this section.

There is good evidence that immune suppression is elevated in aged mice. These mice develop Ly 2^+ cells in their spleens that interacts with Ly 1^+ cells, causing nonspecific suppression which is not found with younger mice (Callard et al., 1980). These T cells require priming and are Ia^+ (Segre and Segre, 1976), suggesting that they function in an activated state. In aged mice, suppression was greater with spleen cells than with cells from other tissues (Gerbase-DeLima et al., 1975), suggesting that suppression acquired with old age is not evenly distributed throughout the body.

Absolute blood lymphocyte counts do not decline in man with advanced age (Zacharski et al., 1971). A decline in E rosetting T lymphocytes with old age has been observed by some (Diaz-Jouanen et al., 1975), but not by others (Weksler and Hutteroth, 1974). There is a report that the relative number of circulating Tγ cells, which has been associated with suppression, is elevated in aged subjects (Gupta and Good, 1979). When activated with concanavalin A, T lymphocytes from elderly donors are more suppressive of proliferation by autologous lymphocytes than in similar experiments done with suppressing and responding cells from young adults (Antel et al., 1978).

Activated suppressor T cells from elderly individuals are not overly active when the responding cells are from young adult donors (Hallgren and Yunis, 1977; Rice et al., 1979). Obviously it is the suppressive effect of these cells upon immune responses by autologous aged cells, and not the allogeneic young donor cells, that has biological significance to the elderly.

The recovery of lymphocytes after isopyknic flotation of blood is not reduced with advanced age (Weksler and Hutteroth, 1974). Yet, we recover a higher percentage of monocytes in mononuclear cell fractions from donors over age 70 years (27 ± 10%) than from donors under age 40 years (18 ± 7%); there was no material difference in monocyte percentages in whole blood from the young and aged donors. Thus, the monocyte yield from aged blood in mononuclear cell preparations is elevated to suppressive levels when added to our culture system.

This may explain why mononuclear leukocytes from older donors are more suppressive than similar cells obtained from younger donors when tested in the mixed leukocyte reaction (Rice et al., 1979). T lymphocytes from aged humans are exceptionally sensitive to suppression by prostaglandins (Goodwin and Messner, 1979). In addition, macrophages from aged mice release increased quantities of prostaglandin E (Rosenstein and Strausser, 1979).

Thus, there is good evidence that suppression contributes to immunologic senescence, probably in combination with lowered reactivity of the effector apparatus. On the surface, this seems at variance with the increased frequency of autoimmune phenomena and the difficulty of inducing tolerance with advanced age (see Chapter 5). This becomes more worrisome, when one considers the evidence that incriminates defects of suppressor systems in the pathophysiology of autoimmune disease (see Chapter 10). However, autoimmunity can also be considered an expression of lowered self-tolerance. Furthermore, efforts have failed to implicate suppression in some models of tolerance. It is possible for immune suppression to be elevated on the one hand and tolerance to be defective on the other with advanced age. The manifestations of autoimmunity with old age may be products of lowered self-tolerance rather than abnormalities of immune regulation.

Abnormal Suppression by T Lymphocytes

The Chicken Model

The bursa of Fabricius is a lymphoepithelial organ intimately associated with the hind gut of fowl. Extensive studies have failed to identify its counterpart in mammals. The bursa in many ways parallels the thymus. It plays an important role in the development of humoral immunity in fowl, secretes one or more inducers of lymphocyte differentiation (Brand et al., 1976) and involutes with age. Humoral immunity does not develop after early bursetomy. Bursectomized chicks remain hypogammaglobulinemic, terminal B cell differentiation fails and B cell mass eventually declines (Glick et al., 1956; Waldemann et al., 1978). It, therefore, serves as a useful model for humoral immunodeficiency.
The situation with bursectomized birds is more complex than simple failure of B lymphocyte differentiation. Blaese et al. (1974) showed that marrow from bursectomized fowl caused lasting suppression of humoral immunity when grafted into normal adult syngeneic birds. Suppression was caused by T lymphocytes and lowered both thymic-dependent and independent antibody responses (Palladino et al., 1976). Furthermore, various dysglobulinemias could be produced by downward titration of the number of T cells from bursectomized fowl grafted into normal syngeneic birds. The potency of suppression of different immunoglobulin classes varied from bird to bird.

The exact role of the bursa of Fabricius remains unsolved. Does it bring about B cell maturation directly or does it indirectly permit B cell differentiation by preventing its suppression by T cells? Why do these suppressor T cells only develop when bursectomy is performed early in life, although they can suppress humoral immunity in mature as well as neonatal birds? Must prolonged B cell suppression, as well as intrinsic B cell defects, be considered as a potential cause of reduced B cell mass? Failure to identify a bursal equivalent in man makes it impossible to determine if this avian model of immunodeficiency has a clinical counterpart. If it does, it is most likely to have bearing upon immunoglobulin deficiencies of childhood origin. Abnormalities involving the thymus are more likely to underlie suppression when it is found with immunoglobulin deficiency at an older age.

Suppression of Humoral Immunity

A number of B cell abnormalities have been identified with common variable immunodeficiency (Geha et al., 1974). Waldemann et al. (1974) showed that immunoglobulin synthesis in culture is also suppressed by T lymphocytes from some patients with this syndrome. The combined data from three studies showed that mononuclear leukocytes from 50% of 49 patients suppressed immunoglobulin synthesis by normal B cells in coculture (Bloom et al., 1976; Waldemann et al., 1978; Morito et al., 1980). However, suppression specifically identified with T cells was established in only 5 out of 16 patients. In some other instances, monocytes may have been responsible for suppression (Sie-

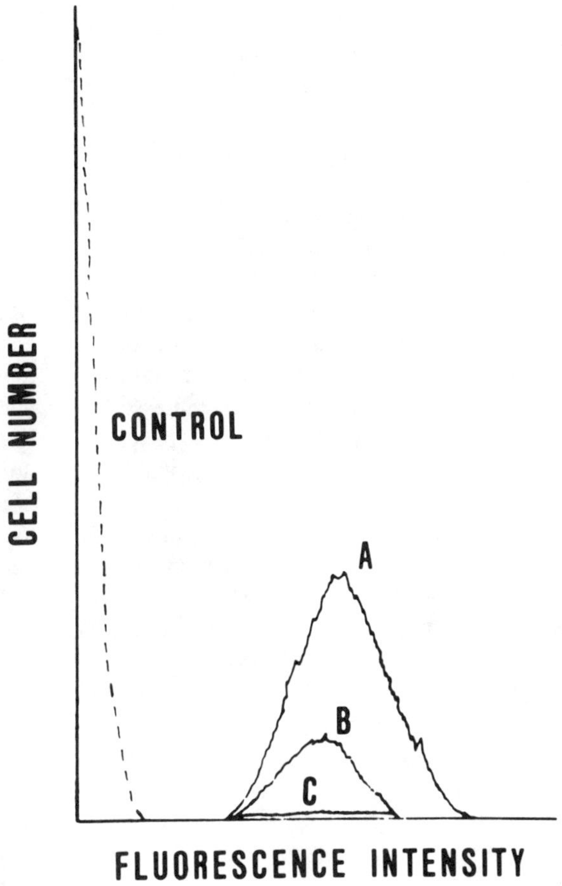

Fig. 8.3 Cytofluorograf curves of T cells that react with TH_2 antibody from a child with agammaglobulinemia (curve A), a normal donor (curve B) and a child with manifestations of autoimmunity (curve C). Adapted from Rheinherz, E.L. et al., 1979, New Engl J Med 301:1018, 1979. Reprinted by permission of the New England Journal of Medicine (301:1018, 1979).

gal et al., 1978). The suppressor T lymphocytes are Tγ cells; they are radiosensitive and in some, but not all, instances are steroid-sensitive. Suppression by T cells can also selectively inhibit IgA or IgG synthesis (Waldemann et al., 1978; Morito et al., 1980). These dysglobulinemias are reminiscent of selective suppression of various Ig classes by suboptimal numbers of T cells from bursectomized fowl.

The use of monoclonal antibodies that identify subpopulations of T lymphocytes has added considerable insight to the pathophysiology of immune deficiencies caused by dysregulation. Immunoglobulin deficiency has been associated with both an absolute deficiency (Reinherz and Schlossman, 1980) and functional impairment without numerical reduction (Reinherz et al., 1980b) of $T4^+$ helper T cells. Quantitative changes in T cell subpopulations that have been associated with suppression can also have clinical implications. Figure 8.3 illustrates the relationship between quantitative changes in TH_2^+lymphocytes (which probably correlate with $T5^+$, $T8^+$ cells and suppression) and disorders of immune regulation (Rheinherz et al., 1979). Profile B reflects the intensity of fluorescence and number of TH_2^+ T cells in normal blood. A child with agammaglobulinemia had greatly elevated numbers of circulating TH_2^+ cells (profile A). This patient had normal numbers of circulatng B cells, suggesting that the excess of TH_2^+ may have suppressed terminal B cell differentiation or that the TH_2^+ cell abnormality was not present long enough to affect B cell mass. These suppressor T cells, like those of patients with common variable immunodeficiency (Morito et al., 1980), were DR^+, suggesting that they were activated in vivo. In contrast, T cells from another child with an autoimmune disorder lacked TH_2^+ cells (profile

C). It remains to be shown that immunoglobulin deficiency can also result from increased suppressor activity by a normal number of suppressor T cells.

Infectious mononucleosis is an infectious disease in which the Epstein-Barr virus activates B lymphocytes and causes them to divide. The subsequent T lymphocytosis is believed to be a host response that helps terminate the infection. These T cells are abnormally suppressive of normal B cells in coculture (Tosato et al., 1979). This has recently been associated with an accumulation of Ia^{+} (activated) $T5^{+}$ (suppressor) T cells (Reinherz et al., 1980). The most beneficial effect of these $T5^{+}$ cells would probably be containment of infected B cells. They may also be responsible for the agammaglobulinemia that occasionally develops with infectious mononucleosis (Provisor et al., 1975). It is more difficult to explain why these suppressor cells accompany the plethora of autoantibodies that circulate during infectious mononucleosis. Perhaps this situation is analogous to old age, where suppression is high, but immune tolerance that is unrelated to suppression is low; reduced tolerance could lead to increased susceptibility to autoimmunity independent of regulatory control.

Suppression of Cellular Immunity

Engleman et al. (1979) showed that T cells from some patients with Hodgkin's disease suppress autologous lymphoproliferation in culture. We have confirmed this observation in 5 out of 11 untreated patients (Twomey et al., 1980). No coincidence was observed between abnormal spontaneous suppression by T cells and suppression by monocytes with Hodgkin's disease. Perhaps T cell suppression is caused by changes in the relative numbers of T cell subpopulations due to lymphocyte depletion; unbalanced depletion could lead to a net increase of suppressor cells in some cases. This possibility is supported by a report that the relative numbers of $T\gamma$ and $T\mu$ cells in peripheral blood may be altered with Hodgkin's disease (Romagnani et al., 1978). We do not know if these suppressor T cells circulate in an activated state, express T5 or T8 antigens or suppress B cell, as well as T cell, responses. They differ from the suppressor T cells that have been identified with humoral immunodeficiency by being restricted in function by the major histocompatibility locus.

Suppression of Hematopoiesis

Bacigalupo et al. (1980) have shown that $T\gamma$ cells from the blood of patients with aplastic anemia suppress colony formation from hematopoietic precursors in agar when cocultured with normal bone marrow. It seems important that aplastic anemia was ascribed to hepatitis and drug toxicity in some patients, making it unlikely that a coexistent thymoma contributed to the etiology. It is not known if bone marrow destruction led to the development of suppressor cells or the primary abnormality was the production of suppressor T cells, which then led to the bone marrow failure. These suppressor T cells probably contribute to bone marrow depression, in that prognosis is worse when the hypoplastic marrow is relatively rich in lymphocytes, and hematologic improvement has been observed after administering drugs that damage lymphocytes. There may be a relationship between T cells that suppress erythropoiesis and those that suppress immunoglobulin synthesis (Litwin and Zanzani, 1977).

Primary Tumors of Suppressor T Cells

The majority of lymphoproliferative disorders are B cell neoplasms. The fact that leukemic B cells usually produce membrane immunoglobulin, even if in reduced quantities, indicates that these neoplastic cells are capable of some functions ordinarily associated with normal B cells. Most Sezary cells express T4 antigen (Boumsell et al., 1981) and some function as helper cells when cocultured with normal B cells (Broder et al., 1979). However, one out of two patients with T cell chronic lymphocytic leukemia had $T8^{+}$ malignant cells, suggesting that they belonged with the suppressor subpopulation. In fact, Uchigama et al. (1978) showed that T cells from three out of six patients

Table 8.1 The frequency of elevated suppression of mixed lymphocyte culture response by mononuclear leukocytes from patients with Hodgkin's disease.

Subject Groups	Patients Tested (N)	MLR Suppressed (N)
Hodgkin's disease	30	16
Non-Hodgkin's lymphoma	30	0
Healthy subjects	100	0
Subgroups with Hodgkin's disease		
Clinical stages I and II	8	1
Clinical stages III and IV	22	15
Asymptomatic	12	4
Symptoms of disease activity	18	12
Favorable tumor histology	10	1
Unfavorable tumor histology	20	15

with subacute T cell leukemia did function as suppressor cells. Perhaps, Sezary syndrome is more likely to develop from cells of helper T cell lineage, while other T cell leukemias that more closely resemble lymphoytic leukemia are more closely identified with suppression. A childhood lymphoblastic leukemia of cells that activated suppressor T cells has been described (Broder et al., 1978). Correlations of detailed phenotypic and functional characteristics of T cell leukemias with the immunologic status of patients should provide useful information about the immunobiologic significance of these leukemic cells.

Commentary

The preceding studies, performed in vitro, seem to correlate well with their associated clinical syndromes. However, a word of caution is necessary. T cells from about 10% of apparently healthy individuals spontaneously suppress plaque-forming antibody responses in culture (Haynes and Fauci, 1979). In a genetically restricted system, Engleman et al. (1979) showed that a young man who had received thymic irradiation during childhood but appeared to be immunologically intact when studied had circulating T cells that profoundly suppressed proliferative responses by DR compatible T cells. Perhaps, greater numbers of or more potent inhibition by suppressor cells, coexistent functional impairments of effector cells, or selective genetic determinants that increase sensitivity of the effector apparatus to suppression are responsible for the suppression attaining clinically significant proportions.

Abnormal Suppression by Monocytes

Hodgkin's Disease

We reported that an adherent mononuclear leukocyte from 16 out of 30 patients with Hodgkin's disease suppressed T lymphoproliferation (Twomey et al., 1975). Others have substantiated this observation (Schechter and Soehnlen, 1978; Sibbett et al., 1978; Hillinger and Herzig, 1978). This is a disease-related and reversible phenomenon. Suppression is likeliest to be shown in patients who present with a poor prognosis. Thus, it is most frequent with a large tumor burden, symptoms of disease activity or tumors of mixed cellularity or lymphocyte depletion histology (Table 8.1). It has not been observed with non-Hodgkin's lymphoma.

There is little doubt that the cell responsible for this donor nonspecific spontaneous suppression is a monocyte. This is partially due to the release of prostaglandins which can be inhibited with indomethacin (Goodwin et al., 1977b). However, other mechanisms that do not seem to involve prostaglandin release also contribute to monocytoid suppression (Twomey et al, 1980). Perhaps the most important causative factor is that mononuclear cell preparations from these patients include elevated percentages of monocytes. That has particular relevance since, with normal cells, suppression by monocytes is proportional to the density of monocytes present in cultures (Laughter and Twomey, 1977). The basis for these high monocyte counts is not clear since monocytosis was not present in patient blood that provided mononuclear cell preparations and high monocyte counts in mononuclear cell preparations bore no relationship to the severity of lymphopenia in parent whole blood. Perhaps there is less loss of monocytes through adherence to containers during Ficoll-Hypaque separation of blood from patients with Hodgkin's disease than from normal subjects.

The fact that high monocyte counts, which are probably responsible for the suppression observed in culture, are only present in mononuclear cell fractions and not in whole blood calls in to question the clinical significance of these observations made in vitro. This challenge is extended by the observation that mononuclear cell preparations from untreated patients with Hodgkin's disease also suppress immunoglobulin synthesis in culture, although these patients do not have significant humoral immunodeficiency (Twomey et al., 1980). We do not believe that monocytes from patients with Hodgkin's disease are individually more suppressive than normal monocytes, although they may release increased amounts of prostaglandins (Bockman 1979). Undoubtedly, the overall immunodeficiency with Hodgkin's disease is complex and variable and includes lymphocyte depletion, lymphocyte dysfunction and probably suppression independently involving both T cells and monocytes.

Multiple Myeloma

Multiple myeloma is a primary tumor of terminal B cell differentiation. Humoral immunodeficiency is a major cause of morbidity and mortality with this neoplasm. The pathophysiology of this acquired immunodeficiency is probably complex. Normal plasma cell mass is reduced. B cell differentiation is in part clonally restricted by RNA, presumably of tumor origin. Normal immunoglobulins are catabolized at an increased rate. In addition, monocytes in mononuclear cell fractions of blood from some patients suppress normal immunoglobulin synthesis in cocultures (Broder et al, 1975; Paglioroni and MacKenzie, 1976). Suppression has also been ascribed to a non-T, non-B lymphoid cell that does not adhere to foreign surfaces (Paglioroni and MacKenzie, 1980). These studies failed to establish that suppression contributed to the primary immunodeficiency of these patients.

We have recently conducted similar studies on 13 untreated patients and 12 patients who had received conventional chemotherapy for a number of months. Mononuclear cells from none of the 13 untreated patients suppressed pokeweed mitogen-stimulated immunoglobulin synthesis when cocultured with normal cells. In contrast, mononuclear cells from 8 of the 12 treated patients suppressed immunoglobulin synthesis in coculture by >50%. The two patient groups were about comparable clinically, apart from therapy. Those mononuclear cell preparations that suppressed contained elevated percentages of monocytes. The latter finding correlated with the severity of lymphopenia in whole blood which itself did not manifest monocytosis. Since lymphopenia is frequent with the therapeutic regimens employed, but not with multiple myeloma per se, one must conclude that the combination of lymphopenia, elevated monocyte percentages in mononuclear cell fractions and suppression of immunoglobulin in culture is primarily related to therapy and not to multiple myeloma itself. Therefore, caution is urged in ascribing humoral immunodeficiency with multiple myeloma to abnormal suppression by cells of the monocyte-macrophage series.

Sarcoidosis

Sarcoidosis is a granulomatous disease of unknown etiology. It features various defects of cell mediated immunity and increased production of polyclonal immunoglobulins. Goodwin et al. (1979) produced in vitro data that implicate suppression by monocytes in the pathophysiology of the immunodeficiency with sarcoidosis. However, ongoing work in our laboratory questions the clinical relevance of these observations. On the surface, monocytoid cell suppression of PHA responses was more frequent and more marked among anergic than other patients. Closer scrutiny showed that this was due to lymphopenia being more severe among seriously ill and, therefore, anergic patients. This lymphopenia in whole blood led to higher monocyte percentages in mononuclear cell fractions, as with the treated myeloma, and did not seem directly related to the clinical condition of the patients. Furthermore,suppression in culture involved immunoglobulin synthesis, as well as T cell responses. This contrasts with the hypergammaglobulinemia often found with sarcoidosis.

Systemic Fungal Infections

Stobo et al. (1976, 1977) studied five patients with systemic fungal infections who had cutaneous anergy and reduced T cell proliferative responsiveness in culture. They showed that monocytes from these patients released a mediator which reacted with a subpopulation of low density short lived T cells. These cells in turn suppressed other effector T lymphocytes. Their studies have a number of important clinical implications. Monocytoid suppression operated through release of a mediator which did not require compatibility at the DR locus with target T cells. It illustrated a sequence of cell-cell interactions commencing with monocytes and ending with T cell suppression. Suppressor T cells activated in this way differed in the targets of their suppression from those responsible for excessive suppression of immunoglobulin synthesis reported with common variable immunodeficiency. It remains to be seen if a similar system exists under physiological conditions.

Commentary

There is ample evidence that a subpopulation of monocytes suppresses immune responses. Under optimal conditions, this suppression is remarkably potent and involves more than one mediator. Elevated suppression of T and B cell responses in culture has been ascribed to monocytes with a number of conditions that are frequently accompanied by immunodeficiency. The important issue is whether this suppression by monocytes demonstrated *in vitro* contributes to the pathophysiology of the associated clinical immunodeficiencies.

In each of the preceding examples of elevated suppression by monocytes in culture, inhibition of lymphocyte responses could be ascribed to a monocytosis in mononuclear cell preparations from the patients. Yet, whole blood from these patients had a normal monocyte content. This suggests that observations made with mononuclear cell fractions in vitro may not be representative of circumstances in vivo. Studies using monocyte concentrates suggest that monocytes from these patients are not abnormally suppressive qualitatively. Obviously, monocyte suppression directly related to iatrogenic lymphopenia cannot be considered an integral part of the immunopathology of multiple myeloma. Furthermore, suppression of immunoglobulin synthesis in culture by mononuclear cells from patients with Hodgkin's disease or sarcoidosis is at variance with the usual state of humoral immunity found in vivo with these conditions.

Yet, teleologically, it seems strange that such a potent system would not have biologic importance. Some anatomical locations that are exposed to considerable antigenic challenge, such as the alveolar air spaces, have high numbers of macrophages with suppressive potential and relatively few lymphocytes. The macrophage to lymphocyte ratio in the lung is such that, if extrapolation from in vitro data is valid, macrophages should exercise considerable suppression. In situations where lymphocyte reactivity is marginal, lower levels of suppression brought about by fewer cells of the monocyte-macrophage series could tip the scales in the direction of immune unresponsiveness.

Evidence of monocyte-related suppression in culture where the monocyte content of mononuclear cell preparations equated with that of whole blood would support a clinical association. Such an association has been made with ideopathic membranous glomerulonephropathy (Ooi et al., 1980). Mononuclear cells from these patients produced subnormal amounts of immunoglobulin when cultured with pokeweed mitogen and suppressed immunoglobulin synthesis when cocultured with normal cells. Although these cell preparations included normal percentages of monocytes, suppression was ascribed to monocytes. This suggests that monocytoid suppression is qualitatively increased with this glomerulopathy.

More definitive evidence that monocyte-related suppression in vitro has clinical relevance is provided by improving immunologic reactivity in vivo using approaches that inhibit suppression by these cells. This evidence has been provided by inhibiting prostaglandin synthesis by prescribing cyclo-oxyganase inhibitors. Goodwin et al. (1978b) demonstrated improved responses in culture to PHA and recovery of delayed cutaneous responsiveness when two patients with common variable immunodeficiency were treated with indomethacin. We have restored delayed hypersensitivity in three patients in like fashion. One patient had Hodgkin's disease, a second had sarcoidosis and a third had atypical mycobacterial pulmonary infection. These preliminary observations should provide impetus to seek improved immunologic reactivity through lowering excessive suppression.

References

Andresen, R.H., and Monroe, C.W. 1962. Experimental study of the behavior of adult human skin homografts during pregnancy. Am J Obstet Gyn 84:1096–1103.

Antel, J.P., Weinrich, M., and Arnason, B.G.W. 1978. Circulating suppressor cells in man as a function of age. Clin Immunol Immunopathol 9:134–141.

Bacigalupo, A., Podesta, M., Mingari, M.C., Moretta, L., van Lint, M.T., and Marmont, A. 1980. Immune suppression of hematopoiesis in aplastic anemia: Activity of Tγ lymphocytes. J Immunol 125:1449–1453.

Beer, A.E., Billingham, R.E., and Yang, S.L. 1972. Further evidence concerning the autoantigenic status of the trophoblast. J Exper Med 135: 117–1184.

Beller, D.I., and Unanue, E.R. 1980. Ia antigens and antigen-presenting function of thymic macrophages. J Immunol 124:1433f–1438.

Bernbaum, G., and Swick, L. 1978. Human suppressor lymphocytes. Cell Immunol 40:16–27.

Billingham, R.E. 1980. The immunobiology of the maternal-fetal relationship. Mount Sinai J Med 47:550–560.

Blaese, R.M., Weiden, P.L., Koski, I., and Dooley, N. 1974. Infectious agammaglobulinemia transmission of immunodeficiency with grafts of agammaglobulinemia cells. J Exp Med 14:1097–1100.

Bloom, B.C., De laConcha, E.G., Webster, A.D.B., Janossy, G.J., and Asherton, G.L., 1976. Intracellular immunoglobulin production *in vitro* by lymphocytes from patients with hypogammaglobulinaemia and their effect on normal lymphocytes. Clin Exp Immunol 23:73–77.

Bluming, A.Z., Cohen, H.G., and Saxon, A. 1979. Angioimmunoblastic lymphadenopathy with dysproteinemia. Am J Med 67:421–428.

Bobak, D., and Whisler, R. 1980. Human B lymphocyte colony responses. J Immunol 125: 2764–2769.

Bockman, R.S. 1979. Prostaglandins and T lymphocyte colonies in Hodgkin's disease. Clin Res 27:381A (abstract).

Boumsell, L., Bernard, A., Reinherz, E.L., Nadler, L.M., Ritz, J., Coppin, H., Richard, Y., Dubertret, L., Valensi, F., Degos, L., Lemerle, J., Flandrin, G., Dausset, J., and Schlossman, S.F. 1981. Surface antigens on malignant Sezary and T-CLL cells correspond to those of mature T cells. Blood 57:526–530.

Brand, A., Gilmour, D.G., and Goldstein, G. 1976. Lymphocyte-differentiating hormone of bursa of Favricius. Science 193:319–321.

Broder, S., Humphrey, R., Durm, M., Blackman, M., Meade, B., Goldman, C., Strober, W., and Waldmann, T. 1975. Impaired synthesis of polyclonal (non-paraprotein) immunoglobulins by circulating lymphocytes from patients with multiple myeloma. N Engl J Med 293:887–892.

Broder, S., Poplack, D., Whang-Peng, J., Durm, M., Goldman, C., Muul, L., and Waldmann, T.A. 1978. Characterization of a suppressor cell leukemia. Evidence for the requirement of an interaction of two T cells in the development of human effector suppressor cells. N Engl J Med 298:66–72.

Broder, S., Uchiyama, T., and Waldmann, T.A. 1979. Current concepts in immunoregulatory T cell neoplasms. Cancer Treatment Reports 63: 607–612.

Bryson, Y.J., Winter, H.S., Gard, S.E., Fisher, T.J., and Shetim, E.R. 1980. Deficiency of immune interferon production by leukocytes of normal newborns. Cell Immunol 55:191–200.

Calkins, C.E., and Stutman, O. 1978. Changes in suppressor mechanisms during prenatal development in mice. J Exp Med 147:87–97.

Callard, R.E., Fazekas, B., Basten, A., and McKenzie, I.F.C. 1980. Immune function in aged mice. J Immunol 124:52–58.

Cantor, H., and Boyse, E.A. 1976. Regulation of cellular and humoral immune responses by T-cell subclasses. Coll Spring Harbor Symp Quant Biol 41:23–32.

Cantor, H., and Gershon, R.K. 1979. Immunological circuits: Cellular composition, Fed Proc 38: 2058–2064.

Chardonnens, X., and Jeannet, M. 1979. Lymphocyte-mediated cytotoxicity and humoral antibodies in human pregnancy. Int Arch Allergy Appl Immunol 61:467-471.

Clark, D.A., and McDermott, M.R. 1978. Impairment of host vs. graft reaction in pregnant mice. J Immunol 121:1389–1393.

Clark, D.A., McDermott, M.R., and Szewczuk, M.R. 1980. Impairment of host-versus-graft reaction in pregnant mice. Cell Immunol 52:106–118.

Clemens, L.E., Siiteri, P.K., and Stites, D.P. 1979. Mechanism of immunosuppression of progesterone on maternal lymphocyte activation during pregnancy. J Immunol 122:1978–1985.

Diaz-Jouanen, E., Strickland, R.G., and Williams, R.C. 1975. Studies of human lymphocytes in newborns and the aged. Am J Med 58:620–628.

Durandy, A., Fischer, A., and Griscelli, C. 1979. Active suppression of B lymphocyte maturation by two different new born T lymphocyte subsets. J Immunol 123:2644–2650.

Eardley, D.D., and Gershon, R.K. 1976. Induction of specific suppressor T cells *in vitro*. J Immunol 117:313–318.

Ekstedt, R.D., Waterfield, J.D., Nespoli, L., and Moller, G. 1977. Mechanism of action of suppressor cell *in vivo*; Concanavalin A activated suppressor cells do not directly affect B cells. Scand J Immunol 6:247–253.

Engleman, E.G., Benike, C., Hoppe, R.T., and Kaplan, I.T.S. 1979. Suppressor cells of the mixed lymphocyte reaction in patients with Hodgkin's disease. Transplant Proc 11:1827–1829.

Engleman, E.G., and McDevitt, H.O. 1978. A suppressor T cell of the mixed lymphocyte reaction specific for the HLA-D region in man. J Clin Invest 61:828–838.

Faulk, W.P., Sanderson, A.R., and Temple, A. 1977. Distribution of MHC antigens in human placental chorioma vitti. Transplant Proc. 9:1379–1384.

Finn, R., Hill, C.A., Govan, A.J., Ralfs, I.G., and Gurney, F.J. 1972. Immunological responses in pregnancy and survival of fetal homograft. Brit Med J 3:150–152.

Fleisher, T.A., Greene, W.C., Uchiyama, T., Goldman, C.K., Nelson, D.L., Blaese, R.M., and Waldmann, T.A. 1981. Characterization of a soluble suppressor of human B cell immunoglobulin biosynthesis produced by a continuous human suppressor T cell line. J Exp Med 154:156–167.

Garaci, E., Rinaldi-Garaci, C., del Gobbo, V., Favalli, C., Santoro, G., and Jaffe, B. 1981. A synthetic analog of prostaglandin E_2 is able to induce *in vivo* theta antigen on spleen cells of adult thymectomized mice. Cell Immunol 62:8–14.

Gaugas, J.M., and Curzen, P. 1978. Polyamine interaction with pregnancy serum in suppression of lymphocyte transformation. Lancet 1:18–21.

Geha, R.S., Schneeberger, E., Merler, E., and Rosen, F.S. 1974. Heterogeneity of acquired or common variable agammaglobulinemia. N Engl J Med 291:1–6.

Gemsa, D., Kramer, W., Brenner, M., Till, G., and Resch, K. 1980. Induction of prostaglandin E release from macrophages by colchicine. J Immunol 124:376–380.

Gerbase-DeLima, M., Meredith, P., and Walford, R.C. 1975. Age related changes including synergy and suppression in the mixed lymphocyte reaction in long-lived mice. Fed Proc 34:159–161.

Germain, R.N., and Benacerraf, B. 1981. A single major pathway of T lymphocyte interactions in antigen-specific immune suppression. Scand J Immunol 13:1–10.

Gershon, R.K., Eardley, D.D., Duram, S., Green, D.R., Shen, F.W., Yamauchi, K., Cantor, H., and Murphy, D.B. 1981. Contrasuppression, a novel immunoregulatory activity. J Exp Med 153: 1533–1546.

Gershon, R.K., Lance, E.M., and Kondo, K. 1974. Immunoregulatory role of spleen localizing thymocytes. J Immunol 112:546–554.

Glick, B., Chang, T.S., and Jaap, R.G. 1956. The bursa of Fabricius and antibody production. Poultry Science 35:224–225.

Goldyne, M.E. 1977. Prostaglandins and the modulations of immunological responses. Int J Derm 16:701–712.

Goodwin, J.S., Bankhurst, A.D., and Messner, R.P. 1977a. Suppression of T cell mitogenesis by prostaglandin: Existence of a prostaglandin producing suppressor cell. J Exp. Med 146:1719–1734.

Goodwin, J.S., Bankhurst, A.D., Murphy, S.A., Selinger, D.S., Messner, R.P., and Williams, R.C., Jr. 1978a. Partial reversal of the cellular immune defect in common variable immunodeficiency with indomethacin. J Clin Lab Immunol 1:197–199.

Goodwin, J.S., DeHoratius, R., Israel, H., Peake, G.T., and Messner, R.P. 1979. Suppressor cell function in sarcoidosis. Ann Int Med 90:169–173.

Goodwin, J.S., and Messner, R.P. 1979. Sensitivity of lymphocytes to prostaglandin. J Clin Invest 64:434–439.

Goodwin, J.S., Messner, R.P., Bankhurst, A.D., Peake, G.T., Saiki, G., and Williams, R.C. 1977b. Prostaglandin producing suppressor cells in Hodgkin's disease. N Engl J Med 297:963–968.

Goodwin, J.S., Messner, R.P., and Peake, G.T. 1978b. Prostaglandin suppression of mitogen-stimulated lymphocytes *in vitro*. J Clin Invest 62:753–760.

Greene, W.C., Fleisher, T.A., and Waldmann, T.A. 1981. Soluble suppressor supernatants elaborated by concanavalin A activated human mononuclear cells. J Immunol 126:1185–1191.

Gupta, S., and Good, R.A. 1979. Subpopulations of human T lymphocytes. J Immunol 122:1214–1219.

Hallgren, H.M., and Yunis, E.J. 1977. Suppressor lymphocytes in young and aged humans. J Immunol 118:2004–2008.

Hammerstrom, L., Fuch, T., and Smith, C.I.E. 1979. The immunodepressive effect of human glucoproteins in the nonrejection process during pregnancy. Acta Obstet Gyn Scand 58:417–422.

Hawes, C.S., Kemp, A.S., and Jones, W.R. 1980. *In vitro* parameters of cell-mediated immunity in the human neonate. Clin Immunol Immunopathol 17: 530–536.

Haynes, B.F., and Fauci, A.S. 1979. Activation of human B lymphocytes. J Immunol 123:1189-1198.

Hayward, A.R., and Kurmek, J. 1981. Newborn T cell suppression: Early appearance, maintenance in culture and lack of growth factor suppression. J Immunol 126:50–53.

Heijnen, C.J., Uytdehaag, F.C. Pot, C.H., and Ballieux, R.E. 1981. Antigen specific human T cell factors. J Immunol 126:503–507.

Herscowitz, H.B., Sakane, T., Steinberg, A.D., and Green, I. 1980. Heterogeneity of human suppressor cells induced by concanavalin A as determined in simultaneous assays of immune function. J Immunol 124:1403–1410.

Herzenberg, L.A., Bianchi, D.W., Schroder, J., Cann, H.M., and Iverson, G.M. 1978. Fetal cells in the blood of pregnant women; Detection and enrichment by fluorescence-activated cell sorting. Proc Natl Acad Sci 76:1453–1455.

Hillinger, S.M., and Herzig, G.P. 1978. Impaired cell-mediated immunity in Hodgkin's disease and mediated by suppressor lymphocytes and monocytes. J Clin Invest 61:1620–1627.

Hirahara, G., Gorai, K., Tanaka, Y., and Shiojime, Y. 1980. Cellular immunity in pregnancy; Subpopulations of T lymphocytes bearing Fc receptors for IgG and IgM in pregnant women. Clin Exp Immunol 41:353–357.

Innes, J.B., Kuntz, M.M., Young, T.K., and Weksler, M.E. 1979. Induction of suppressor activity in the autologous mixed lymphocyte reaction and in cultures with concanavalin A. J Clin Invest 64:1608–1613.

Jenkenson, E.J., Billington, W.D., and Elson, J. 1976. Detection of receptors for immunoglobulin on human placenta by EA rosette test. Clin Exp Immunol 23:456–461.

Johnson, H.M., Snuth, B.G., and Baron, S. 1975. Inhibition of the primary *in vitro* antibody response by interferon preparations. J. Immunol 114: 403–409.

Kadish, A.S., Tansey, F.A., Yu, G.S., Doyle, A.T., and Bloom, B.R. 1980. Interferon as a mediator of human lymphocyte suppression. J Exp Med 151: 637–650.

Knapp, W., and Baumgartner, G. 1978. Monocyte-mediated suppression of human B lymphocyte differentiation *in vitro*. J Immunol 121:1177–1183.

Larman, J.T., Dinerstein, J., and Fikoig, S. 1962. Homograft immunity in pregnancy: Lack of harm to the fetus from sensitization of the mother. Ann NY Acad Sci 99:706–716.

Laughter, A.H., Rice, L., and Twomey, J.J. 1981. Suppression of lymphocyte responses to monocytoid cells does not require cell-cell contact. Cell Immunol 60:440–452.

Laughter, A.H., and Twomey, J.J. 1977. Suppression of lymphoproliferation by high concentrations of normal human mononuclear leukocytes. J Immunol 119:173–179.

Lee, K.C., Kay, J., and Wong, M. 1979 Separation of functionally distinct subpopulations of Corynebacterium parvum-activated macrophages with predominently stimulatory or suppressive effect on the cell mediated cytotoxic T cell response. Cell Immunol 42:28–41.

Litwin, S.D., and Zanzani, E.D. 1977. Lymphocytes suppressing both immunoglobulin production and erythroid differentiation in hypogammaglobulinemia. Nature 266:57–58.

Lobo, P.I., and Spencer, C.E. 1979. Inhibition of humoral and cell-mediated immune responses in man by distinct suppressor cell systems. J Clin Invest 63:1157–1163.

Masson, P.L., Delire, M., and Cambiaso, C.L. 1977. Circulating immune complexes in normal human pregnancy. Nature 266:542–543.

McIntyre, J.A., and Faulk, W.P. 1979. Trophoblast modulation of maternal allogeneic recognition. Proc Natl Acad Sci USA 76:4029–4032.

McMichael, A.J., and Sasazuki, T. 1977. A suppressor T cell in the human mixed lymphocyte reaction. J Exp Med 146:368–380.

Metzger, Z., Hoffeld, J.T., and Oppenheim, J.J. 1980. Macrophage mediated suppression. J Immunol 124:983–988.

Miyawaki, T., Seki, H., Kubo, M., and Taniguchi, N. 1979. Suppressor activity of T lymphocytes from lymphocytes from infants assessed by coculture with unfractionated adult lymphocytes in the pokeweed mitogen system. J Immunol 123:1092–1099.

Moen, T., Moen, M., Palbo, V., and Thorsby, E. 1980. *In vitro* feto-maternal responses at delivery; No gross changes in MLC and PLT responsiveness. J Reprod Immunol 2:213–224.

Moretta, L., Webb, S.R., Grossi, C.E., Lyndyard, P.M., and Cooper, M.D. 1977. Functional analysis of two human T-cell subpopulations; Help and suppression of B-cell responses by T-cells bearing receptors for IgM and IgG. J Exp Med 146:184–200.

Morimoto, C., Reinberg, E.L., and Schlossman, S.F. 1981. Regulation of *in vitro* primary anti-DNP antibody production by functional subsets of T lymphocytes in man. J Immunol 127:69–73.

Morito, T., Bankhurst, A.D., and Williams, R.C. 1979. Studies of human cord blood and adult lymphocyte interactions with *in vitro* immunoglobulin production. J Clin Invest 64:990–995.

Morito, T., Bankhurst, A.D., and Williams, R.C., Jr. 1980. Studies of T and B cell interactions in adult patients with combined immunodeficiency. J Clin Invest 65:422–431.

Nair, M.P.N., and Schwartz, S.A. 1981. Suppression of natural killer activity and antibody-dependent cellular cytotoxicity by cultured human lymphocytes. J Immunol 126:221–2229.

Okamura, K, Kuramoto, M., Hamazaki, Y., Takahashi, K., and Suzuki, M. 1980. Immunosuppressive factors in pregnancy serum: A preliminary report. Tohoku J Exp Med 130:11–23.

Olding, L.B. Murgita, R.A., and Wigzell, H. 1977. Mitogen stimulated lymphoid cells from human newborns suppress the proliferation of maternal lymphocytes across a cell impermeable membrane. J Immunol 119:1109–1114.

Ooi, B.S., Ooi, Y.M., Hsu, A., and Hurtubise, P.E. 1980. Diminished synthesis of immunoglobulin by peripheral lymphocytes of patients with idiopathic membranous glomerulonephropathy. J Clin Invest 65:789–797.

Paglioroni, T., and MacKenzie, M.R. 1976. Studies on the pathogenesis of an immune defect in multiple myeloma. J Clin Invest 59:1120–1133.

Paglioroni, T., and MacKenzie, M.R. 1980. Multiple myeloma: An immunologic profile. J Immunol 124:2563–2570.

Palacios, R., an Moller, G. 1981. T cell growth factor abrogates concanavalin A induced suppressor cell function. J Exp Med 153:1360–1365.

Palladino, M.A., Lerman, S.P., and Thorbecke, G.J. 1976. Transfer of hypogammaglobulinemia in two inbred chicken strains by spleen cells from bursedonized donors. J Immunol 116:1673–1676.

Peck, A.B., Murgita, R.A., and Wigzell, H. 1978. Cellular and genetic restrictions in the immunoregulatory activity of alphafetoprotein. J Exper Med 147:667–683.

Picker, L.J., Raff, H.V., Goldyne, M.E., and Stobo, J.D. 1980. Metabolic heterogeneity among human monocytes and its modulation by PGE_2. J Immunol 124:2557–2562.

Provisor, A.J., Iacuone, J.J., Chilcote, R.R., Neiburger, R.G., Crussi, F.C., and Bacher, R. 1975. Acquired agammaglobulinemia after life-threatening illness with clinical and laboratory features of infectious mononucleosis in three related male children. N Engl J Med 293:62–65.

Raff, H.V., Cochrum, K.C., and Stobo, J.D. 1978. Macrophage-T cell interactions in the con A induction of human suppressive T cells. J Immunol 121:2311–2315.

Ramshaw, I.A., Woodsworth, M., Wright, K., and McKenzie, I.F.C. 1980. Induction of suppressor T cells of antibody formation under conditions that preferentially stimulate DTH. J Immunol 125:197–201.

Reinacle-Bonnet, M.M., Pommier, G.J., Kaplanski, S., Rance, R.J., and Depieds, R.C. 1976. Inhibition of normal allogeneic lymphocyte mitogenesis by a soluble inhibitor extracted from human colonic carcinoma. J Immunol 117:1145–1151.

Reinherz, E.L., Geha, R., Wohl, M.E., Morimoto, C., Rosen, F.S., and Schlossman, S.F. 1980a. Immunodeficiency associated with loss of T4+ 'nducer T cell function. N Engl J Med 303:811–816.

Reinherz, E.L., O'Brien, C., Rosenthal, P., and Schlossman, S.F. 1980b. The cellular basis for viral-induced immunodeficiency; Analysis by monoclonal antibodies. J Immunol 125: 1269–1274.

Reinherz, E.L., and Schlossman, S.F. 1980. The differentiation and function of human T lymphocytes. Cell 19:821–827.

Reinherz, E.L., Strelkauskas, A.J., O'Brien, C., and Schlossman, S.F., 1979. Phenotypic and functional distinctions between the TH_2^+ and JRA^+ T cell subsets in man. J Immunol 123:83–86.

Rice, L. Laughter, A.H., and Twomey, J.J. 1979. Three suppressor systems in human blood that modulate lymphoproliferation. J Immunol 122: 991–996.

Rich, R.A., and Pierce, C.W. 1973. Biological expressions of lymphocyte activation. II. Generation of a population of thymus derived suppressor lymphocytes. J Exp Med 137:649–657.

Rich, S.S., and Rich, R.R. 1976. Regulatory mechanisms in cell-mediated immune responses. J Exp Med 143:672–677.

Richman, L.K., Graeff, A.S., Yarchoan, R., and Strober, W. 1981. Simultaneous induction of antigen specific IgA helper T cells and IgG suppressor T cells in the murine Peyer's patches after protein feeding. J Immunol 126:2079–2083.

Rigby, P.G. Hanson, T.A., and Smith, R.S. 1964. Passage of leukemia cells across the placenta. N Engl J Med 271:124–127.

Roberts-Thomson, I.C., Whittingham, S., Youngchaiyud, U., and Mackay, I.R. 1974. Aging, immune response and mortality. Lancet 2:368–371.

Rocklin, R.E., Greeneder, D.K., and Melmon, K.L. 1979. Histamine-induced suppressor factor (HSF): Further studies on the nature of the stimulus and the cell which produces it. Cell Immunol 44:404–415.

Rodriguez, G., Anderson, G., Wigzell, H., and Peck, A.B., 1979. Non-T cell nature of the naturally occurring spleen associated suppressor cells present in the newborn mouse. Eur J Immunol 19:737.

Romagnani, S., Maggi, E., Biagiotti, R. 1978.

Altered proportion of Tμ and Tγ cell subpopulations in patients with Hodgkin's disease. Scand J Immunol 7:511–514.

Rosenstein, M.M., and Strausser, H.R. 1979. Macrophage-induced T cell mitogen suppression with age. J Retic Soc 27:159–166.

Saxon, A., Stevens, R.H., and Ashman, R.F. 1977. Regulation of immunoglobulin production in human peripheral blood leukocytes; Cellular interactions. J Immunol 118:1872–1879.

Schecter, G.P., and Soehnlen, F. 1978. Monocyte-mediated inhibition of lymphocyte blastogenesis in Hodgkin's disease. Blood 52:261–271.

Schwartz, S.A., Shou, L., Good, R.A., and Chou, Y.S. 1977. Suppression of immunoglobulin synthesis and secretion by peripheral blood lymphocytes from normal donors. Proc Natl Acad Sci 74:2099–2103.

Scott, W.A., Zrike, J.M., Hamill, A.L, Kempe, J., and Cohn, Z.A. 1980. Regulation of arachidonic acid metabolites in macrophages. J Exp Med 152:324–335.

Segre, D., and Segre, M. 1976. Humoral immunity in aged mice. J Immunol 116:735–738.

Shou, L., Schwartz, S.A., and Good, R.A. 1976. Concanavalin A activated suppressor cells in normal human peripheral blood lymphocytes. J Exp Med 143:1100–1108.

Sibbett, W.L, Bankhurst, A.D., and Williams, R.C. 1978. Studies of cell populations mediating mitogen hyporesponsiveness in patients with Hodgkin's disease. J Clin Invest 61:55–63.

Siegal, F.P., Siegal, M., and Good, R.A. 1976. Suppression of B-cell differentiation by leukocytes from hypogammaglobulinemic patients. J Clin Invest 58:109–2.

Siegel, F.P., Siegal, M., and Good, R.A. 1978. Role of helper, suppressor and B-cell defects in the pathogenesis of hypogammaglobulinemias. N Engl J Med 299:172–178.

Sorenson, C.M., and Pierce, C.W. 1981. Haplotype-specific suppression of antibody responses *in vitro*. I. Generation of geneticaly restricted suppressor T cells by neonatal treatment with semiallogeneic spleen cells. J Exp Med 154:35–47.

Stahn, R., Fabricius, A.A., and Hartleitner, W. 1978. Suppression of human T-cell colony formation during pregnancy. Nature 276:831–832.

Stiehn, E.R., Winter, H.S., and Bryson, Y.J. 1979. Cellular (T cell) immunity in the human newborn. Pediatrics 64:814–821 (Suppl).

Stobo, J.D. 1977. Immunosuppression in man: Suppression by macrophages can be mediated by interactions with regulatory T cells. J Immunol 119:918–924.

Stobo, J.D., Paul, S., Van Scoy, R.E., and Hermans, P.E. 1976. Suppressor thymus-derived lymphocytes in fungal infections. J Clin Invest 57:319–328.

Strelkauskas, A.J., Callery, R., McDowell, J., Yves, B., and Schlossman, S.F. 1978. Direct evidence for loss of human suppressor cells during active autoimmune disease. Proc Natl Acad Sci 75: 5150–5154.

Swain, S.L. 1980. Association of Ly phenotypes, T cell function and MHC recognition. Fed Proc 39:3110–3113.

Tada, T., an Okumura, K. 1980. The role of antigen specific T cell factors in the immune response. Adv Immunol 28:1–87.

Tadakuma, T., and Pierce, C.W. 1976. Site of action of soluble immune response suppressor (SIRS) produced by concanavalin A activated spleen cells. J Immunol 117:967–972.

Thomas, Y., Sosman, J., Jrigoyen, D., Friedman, S.M., Kung, P.C., Goldstein, G., and Chess, L. 1981. Functional analysis of human T cell subsets defined by monoclonal antibodies. J Immunol 125:2402–2408.

Ting, C.C., and Rodrigues, D. 1980. Immunoregulatory circuit among macrophage subsets for T cell-mediated cytotoxic response to tumor cells. J Immunol 124:1039–1044.

Tosato, G., Magrath, I., Koski, I., Dooley, N., and Blaese, M. 1979. Activation of suppressor T cells during Epstein-Barr virus induced infectious mononucleosis. New Engl J Med 301:1018–1021.

Tosato, G., Magrath, I.T., Koski, I.R., Dooley, N.J., and Blaese, R.M. 1980. B cell differentiation and immunoregulatory T cell function in human cord blood lymphocytes. J Clin Invest 66:383–388.

Twomey, J.J., Laughter, A.H., Farrow, S., and Douglass, C.C. 1975. Hodgkin's disease, an immunodepleting and immunosuppressive disorder. J Clin Invest 56:467–475.

Twomey, J.J., Laughter, A.H., Rice, L., and Ford, R. 1980. Spectrum of immunodeficiencies with Hodgkin's disease. J Clin Invest 66:629–637.

Twomey, J.J., Sharkey, O., Brown, J.A., Laughter, A.H., and Jordan, P.H. 1970. Cellular requirements for the mitotic response in allogeneic mixed leukocyte cultures. J Immunol 104: 845–853.

Uchigama, T., Sagawa, K., and Takatsuki, K. 1978. Effect of adult T-cell leukemia cells on pokeweed mitogen-induced normal B-cell differentiation. Clin Immunol Immunopathol 10:24–34.

Waddell, C.C., Taunton, O.D., and Twomey, J.J. 1976. Inhibition of lymphoproliferation by hyperlipoproteinemic plasma. J Clin Invest 58:950–954.

Waldmann, T.A., Durm, M., Broder, S., Blockman, M., Blaese, R.M., and Strober, W. 1974. Role of suppressor T cells in pathogenesis of common variable hypogammaglobulinemia. Lancet 2: 609–613.

Waldmann, T.A., Blaese, R.M., Broder, S., and Krakaur, R.S. 1978. Disorders of suppressor immunoregulatory cells in the pathogenesis of immunodeficiency and autoimmunity. Annals Int Med 88:226–238.

Waldmann, T.A., Durm, M., Broder, S., Blockman, M., Blaese, R.M., and Strober, W. 1974. Role of suppressor T cells in pathogenesis of common variable hypogammaglobulinemia. Lancet 2: 609–613.

Weksler, M.E., and Hutteroth, T.H. 1974. Impaired lymphocyte function in aged humans. J Clin Invest 53:99–104.

Youdin, S. 1979. Enhancing and suppressive effects of macrophages on T lymphocyte stimulation *in vitro*. Cell Immunol 45:377–388.

Zacharski, L.R., Elveback, L.R., and Linman, J.W. 1971. Leukocyte counts in healthy adults. Am J Clin Path 56:148–150.

Chapter 9

Immune Complexes, Anti-Immunoglobulins, and Disease

R.D. Rossen

Introduction

When functioning in an optimally regulated manner, antibodies produced by the immune system effectively immobilize foreign sustances, or antigens, and initiate a train of events which degrade and dispose of those antigens with minimal injury to the host. Frequently, however, because of a massive or persistent antigen load or because the response to the antigen is inadequately controlled, tissue injury occurs.

The events which occur when complement-fixing antibodies encounter antigens deposited in specific tissue sites (the Arthus reaction) or antigens introduced into the circulation (serum sickness) have been carefully documented and reviewed (Cochrane and Koffler, 1973; Germuth and Rodriguez, 1973; Haakenstad and Mannik, 1977; Mannik, 1980; Theofilopoulos and Dixon, 1979; Theofilopoulos, 1980; Williams, 1980a and 1980b). The physical union of antigen and antibody by themselves does not cause inflammation. Acute inflammation results from the activation of complement with the liberation of anaphylotoxins from the third and fifth components, and in some cases, from the aggregation of platelets, which is a consequence of interactions between platelet Fc receptors and aggregated immunoglobulin and antigen.

Release of the anaphylotoxins, C_{3a} and C_{5a}, from complement causes histamine release from mast cells and basophils and results in increased vascular permeability. Chemotaxis of polymorphonuclear (PMN) leukocytes to the site of complement activation also occurs (Cochrane and Koffler, 1973). Further degradation of the third component of complement (C_3), with release of C_{3e}, mobilizes PMN from the bone marrow (Ghebrehiwet and Muller-Eberhard, 1979), accounting perhaps for the leukocytosis which is often seen in immune complex (IC) diseases. Phagocytosis of immune complexes is triggered by interactions between immunoglobulin Fc and PMN Fc receptors. It is facilitated by interactions between the C_{3b} and C_{3d} fragments of the third complement component in immune complexes and the C_3 receptors on granulocytes. During phagocytosis these cells may release intracellular proteolytic enzymes (Atkinson and Frank, 1980; Atkinson and Rosse, 1980). These enzymes break down connective tissue and nucleic acids and may activate the kinin system. Activation of this system also increases vascular permeability. In addition, vascular permeability may increase following release of 5-hydroxytryptamine from platelets.

Changes in regional blood flow may also result from microthrombi, a consequence of platelet or leukocyte aggregation (Fauci et al.,

1978; Lawley and Frank, 1980; Wiggins and Cochrane, 1981).

Release of platelet-activating factor from circulating basophils, which is a consequence of the interaction of antigen with IgE antibodies bound to basophil cell-surface Fc receptors, may also cause platelet aggregation and release of platelet amines (Cochrane and Koffler, 1973).

Additional tissue injury may result from the phenomenon of bystander lysis, in which the activated $C_{5,6,7}$ complex binds to tissue sites which are not targets of the antigen antibody reaction that originally stimulated complement fixation. Activated $C_{5,6,7}$ can bind C_8 and C_9, completing the effector limb of the complement cascade (Thompson and Lachman, 1970; Atkinson and Frank, 1980).

Retraction of endothelial cells from the vascular basement membranes, which is a consequence of histamine release, may expose anionic (negatively charged) sites in these membranes to circulating C_{1q}, a cationic protein, and other polycations in the blood and facilitate preferential deposition of circulating cationic proteins and antigens (Cochrane and Koffler, 1973; Gallo et al., 1981; Lawley and Frank, 1980; Kelley and Cavallo, 1980). Antigens localized in the membranes can subsequently serve as a site for attachment of circulating antibodies and initiate immunologic assault on the membranes at that time (Izui et al., 1977a). Immunoglobulin deposits in such sites can also serve as foci for localization of anti-immunoglobulins, thereby increasing the quantity of antibody deposited in the vessel wall (Rossen et al., 1975, 1977). DNA, a polyanion, also has a selective affinity for collagen and can preferentially deposit in vascular basement membranes exposed to the bloodstream (Izui et al., 1976). Later development of circulating antibodies specific for DNA can result in deposition of antibody in sites where DNA previously localized (Izui et al., 1977a; Fournie et al., 1980).

Development of new methods for identifying IC in body fluids and further research into the interactions of IC with the cellular elements of the immune system during the past 7 years has expanded the catalogue of diseases in which circulating IC occur and provided new information about the mechanisms which regulate these interactions. Recent reviews have summarized much of the current knowledge about these methods and their applications (Barnett et al. 1979; Lambert et al, 1978; Lawley and Frank, 1980; Nydegger, 1979; Theofilopoulos and Dixon, 1979; Theofilopoulos, 1980). A brief summary of the rationale for these methods is presented here.

Methods for Detecting Soluble Immune Complexes in Biological Fluids

A number of the methods for identifying soluble IC can detect as little as 6 μg of aggregated immunoglobulin per ml of serum or other body fluid. All methods have in common the ability to distinguish soluble aggregates containing Ig or Ig bound to components of complement from monomeric Ig. For diagnosis and monitoring of specific diseases, techniques that recognize IC which incorporate specific antigens relevant to the disease process are preferred. Thus the host response to gastrointestinal carcinoma can be efficiently evaluated by measuring both free carcinoembryonic antigen (CEA) and CEA bound to antibody (Kapsopoulou-Dominos and Anderer, 1979a and b; Staab et al., 1980a and b; Staab and Anderer, 1980). However, in the majority of the conditions in which circulating IC have been identified, the antigen(s) in the complex remain unknown. Therefore, techniques which identify IC by distinctive physical and biologic characteristics have the greatest application. Widespread use of these methods has demonstrated that serum IC can even be found in sera of apparently healthy donors (Theofilopoulos et al., 1977).

Considering their biologic diversity, it is not surprising that there is no one best method by which to detect soluble IC (Lambert et al., 1978). A variety of methods, each of which recognizes a different characteristic of soluble IC, is therefore used in most clinical studies. Even so, one must bear in mind that circulating

Table 9.1 · Special Characteristics of Immune Complexes which Permit Their Identification in Biological Fluids.

	Comments
A. Physical characteristics	
Size, poor solubility at unphysiologic temperatures (cryoprecipitation) or in polymer solutions (polyethylene glycol precipitation).	Aggregation of Ig by heating or other denaturing influences may cause false positives.[a]
B. Interactions with specific proteins	
C1q, conglutinin, anti-immunoglobulins, staphylococcal protein A.	Assays can be adapted to nephelometry or standard radioimmunoassay formats using radiolabeled ligands or ligands insolubilized on surfaces of tubes or in the wells of microtiter trays.
C. Interactions with specific cell receptors	A principle disadvantage of all these methods is the possible presence of antibodies in test sera which react with cell surface proteins on the detector cell.[a]
1. Fc receptors on macrophages, granulocytes, platelets, L1210 murine leukemia cells.	
2. Complement (C1q, C_{3b}, C_{4b}, C_{3d}, etc.) receptors on B cells, group O, Rh positive, human erythrocytes.	
D. Simultaneous	IC may be selectively adsorbed by permitting these to react with immobilized antibodies to complement (C). Ig associated with the bound C may then be detected with labeled antibodies specific for the Ig.
Presence of immunoglobulin and complement components in the same macromolecular aggregate.	

[a]Many of the cellular receptors react with both IC and monomeric Ig. The complex formed with immunoglobulin aggregates is often more avid, however, reflecting the effects of multipoint binding created by the close array of Fc determinants C1q or C_3 fragments, etc., which are present in an immune complex. To verify that the reactant is indeed an immune complex, it is important to use size separation techniques to demonstrate that the putative immune complex, has the physical characteristics of a macromolecular aggregate containing Ig.

IC is a feature of very dynamic disease processes and, as a result, measurements of IC at only one point in time may not reflect crucial events which determine the outcome of these diseases. Table 9.1 shows special characteristics of immune complexes which permit their identification in biological fluids.

Commentary on Methods for Detecting Soluble IC

Many of the cell receptors and proteins used as selective binding agents for IC react with both immunoglobulin aggregates and monomeric Ig. However, interactions formed by these with immunoglobulin aggregates are often more avid, reflecting the effects of multipoint binding created by the close array of Fc determinants, C_{1q} and C_3 fragments, etc., which are present in immune complexes. To verify that these truly have properties of IC, it is important to use size separation techniques to demonstrate that they have the macromolecular characteristics of Ig-containing aggregates.

Perhaps some of the most versatile tests for immune complexes are those which employ C_{1q}, conglutinin or anti-C_3 immobilized on the walls of tubes or the wells of microtiter plates (Casali et al., 1977; Devey et al., 1980; Eisenberg et al., 1977; Hay et al., 1976; Zubler and Lambert, 1978). Immunoglobulin aggregates which contain bound complement will adhere to these ligands. After monomeric immunoglobulins are washed away, radiolabeled or peroxidase-labeled antibodies, specific for human immunoglobulins, are added to quantitate bound immunoglobulin (Ig) by radiometric or ELISA techniques. Staphylococcal protein A may also be used to detect soluble IC in sera (Farrell et al., 1975; McDougal et al., 1979).

Complement-fixing aggregates can also be identified by measuring their ability to consume complement (Gupta et al., 1979). Measurement of anticomplementary activity has been used in a number of clinical investigations to detect soluble IC in sera. However, meticulous care must be taken with the collection and storage of samples to be assayed for anticomplementary activity. This technique is exquisitely sensitive to immunoglobulin aggregates created by freez-

Table 9.2 Receptor-Ligand Interactions which May Influence Clearance of Immune Complexes from the Circulation.

A. Interactions with bound complement components	
C Component	Cells
C1q	B lymphocytes
C_{3b}/C_{4b}	Erythrocytes, B lymphocytes, macrophages, neutrophils,[a] eosinophils
C_{3d}	B lymphocytes, eosinophils
B. Interactions with Fc fragments of Ig	
IgG	Platelets, B and T lymphocytes, neutrophils, macrophages, eosinophils; mast cells and basophils
IgM	B and T lymphocytes
IgA	B and T lymphocytes and neutrophils
IgE	B and T lymphocytes, basophils and mast cells

[a]Neutrophils may also have a receptor for C_{5b}.

ing, thawing or other manipulations which denature Ig. Tests for serum anticomplementary activity also require prior heat inactivation (56°C for 30 minutes) of the sample, a treatment which can cause some immunoglobulin aggregation (Soltis et al., 1979).

Because freezing of sera at ≥ -20°C may also aggregate Ig, storage at -70°C or lower until the day of testing is important for preserving activity of samples to be tested for IC by any assay.

In addition to methods which directly demonstrate circulating immunoglobulin aggregates, it is often possible to detect breakdown products of C_3 or C_{1q} in sera and other body fluids as indicators of ongoing intravascular complement activation and consumption (Zubler and Lambert, 1978).

Effect of Complement on Soluble IC

Surprisingly, complement can dissociate or partly dissociate certain IC. Solubilization requires factor B, properdin, factor D, C_3 and magnesium ion. Thus it appears to be a property of the alternate complement pathway (Miller and Nussenzweig, 1974, 1975; Rajnavolgyi et al., 1978; Takahaski et al., 1978).

Evidence for and against the Idea that the Soluble IC Detected in Sera is Responsible for Disease

Soluble IC can be found in sera of people with a variety of conditions, including some who are apparently healthy (Theofilopoulos et al., 1977; Morgan et al., 1979; Williams, 1980a and b). To demonstrate involvement of circulating IC in a disease, it is necessary to show localization of immunoglobulin in affected organs by immunofluorescence or comparable immunohistologic techniques in sites showing evidence of acute inflammation. Establishing evidence of IC-mediated tissue injury is sometimes difficult (Cohen et al., 1979; Lawley et al., 1980). IC may circulate intermittently (Rossen et al., 1976). Sites in which IC has localized may also serve as foci for subsequent deposition of anti-immunoglobulins or antigens which are not related or only partly related to the immune mechanisms which initiated the disease in the first place (Fleuren et al., 1980a and b; Rossen et al., 1975; 1977; Izui and Eisenberg, 1980).

A model of IC-mediated disease, recently described by Izui et al. (1976, 1977a) illustrates the problems involved in relating circulating IC to tissue injury (Fournie et al., 1980). Injection of bacterial lipopolysaccharides intravenously in mice results in release of DNA from leukocytes and secondarily in the induction of anti-DNA antibodies. The circulating DNA localize in renal glomerular basement membranes for which DNA has a selective affinity. Thereafter anti-DNA antibodies, entering the circulation, bind to the DNA in the glomerular capillaries. This in situ immune complex formation initiates typical immune complex-mediated complement-dependent inflammatory reactions. Although circulating immune complexes are also present in this model, their composition is thought to be different from that of IC deposited in the glomeruli.

There has been ample verification from other studies that immune complexes can deposit in situ and that such focal accretions of immune complexes may be an important cause of tissue injury (Fleuren et al., 1980; Magil et al., 1981; Makker and Moorthy, 1981; Michels et al., 1980). Even in systemic lupus erythematosus (SLE), circulating DNA-anti-DNA complexes may be infrequent, suggesting that in situ deposition of IC may be an important mechanism of tissue injury in this disease as well (Izui et al., 1977b).

Interactions of Immune Complexes with Cellular Elements of the Immune System

Many tests for soluble IC take advantage of the fact that cellular elements of the immune system have specific receptors which preferentially bind soluble IC. These cell-surface receptors normally serve important biological functions. They facilitate intracellular communications required for regulation of both humoral and cellular immune responses, as well as facilitate removal of soluble complexes from blood and other body fluids. Table 9.2 shows receptor-ligand interactions which may influence clearance of immune complexes from the circulation.

Factors governing interactions of cells with soluble and particulate IC have recently been reviewed in detail by Theofilopoulos and Dixon (1979). Certain generalizations about these may explain how IC is removed from the plasma and why certain IC circulates longer than others. First, in order for IC to bind to cellular Fc receptors, the CH_3 domain of IgG must be intact (Haakenstad and Mannik, 1974, 1976). Damage by proteolytic enzymes (plasmin, trypsin, pepsin, etc.) which can hydrolyze peptides in the CH_3 domain reduces the affinity of IC for phagocytic cells and prolongs the time that the IC persist in the circulation. Second, the forces which bind IC to cell-surface Fc and C3 receptors are weak (Griffin, 1980), but large Ig-containing aggregates and particles heavily coated with antibody and complement have many points at which they can interact with the receptors on phagocytes. The sum of these many weak interactions, sometimes called multipoint binding, results in a firm attachment of the IC to these cells. Third, cooperative interactions between receptors for Fc and complement, principally the receptors for C_{3b}, C_{3d} and C_{4b}, are important for optimal removal of IC from body fluids (Atkinson and Rosse, 1980). The complement receptors on cells promote apposition of IC to the surface of phagocytic cells. Fc receptor-ligand interactions promote their internalization (phagocytosis) (Miller and Nussenzweig, 1974). Fourth, in the case of IgM antibody-coated cells, clearance from the circulation may be a temporary event. Recirculation of the antibody-coated cells can occur after degradation of the cell-bound C_{3b} to C_{3d} by complement regulatory proteins, C_{3b} inactivator (C_3INA) and beta-1-H (Schreiber and Frank, 1972a and b; Frank et al., 1977). Fifth, interactions of IC with cell surface complement and Fc receptors are not only important for uptake and removal of IC from body fluids (Kurlander, 1980), they may also activate functions in the cell which promote degradation of the IC and release enzymes which injure surrounding tissues. These include intracellular lysozomal enzymes (Keisari and Witz, 1973). These enzymes may cleave fresh C_3, prolonging and possibly intensifying the inflammatory response. Prostaglandins may modulate these inflammation-producing events. PGE_1 administration, for example, ameliorates experimental IC nephritis (Kelley et al., 1979; Kelley and

Winkelstein, 1980; Kunkel et al., 1979; Winkelstein and Kelley, 1980). Sixth, IC may exit from the circulation through leaky vascular membranes caused by the release of histamine and the SRS-A leukotrienes from mast cells and basophils. Seventh, cells in the placenta, the renal glomerulus and the choroid plexus have specific receptors for Fc and or C. (Theofilopoulos and Dixon, 1979; Gleicher and Theofilopoulos, 1980; Harbeck et al., 1979). These receptors may cause selective adherence of IC to such tissues.

Granulomatous Disease and Immune Complexes

One of the most intriguing observations which has come from the survey of diseases for circulating immune complexes is that these may be detected in conditions characterized by granulomatous inflammation. For example, IC has been demonstrated in sera of patients with sarcoidosis by both the Raji cell and the monoclonal rheumatoid factor radioimmunoassays (Gupta et al., 1977; Hedfors and Norberg, 1974). Complexes were found predominantly in sera of patients with stage three sarcoidosis, that is, those who have pulmonary infiltration without hilar adenopathy. Complexes were also found in 30% of sera from patients with stage 1 and stage 2 disease, especially in those with extrapulmonary sarcoidosis.

It is not clear whether these complexes are involved in the pathophysiology of the granulomatous inflammation or whether they are an epiphenomenon; perhaps they are another example of the abnormal immune responses which have been identified in this disease. The studies of Gupta indicate that the complexes are predominately 15S, although some are more rapidly sedimenting.

Other abnormalities in immune responses have been observed in sarcoidois. Hypergammaglobulinemia and low titers of rheumatoid factors are seen in less than one-half the patients. Particularly in studies from the United States, serum complement levels may be elevated.

Some of the defects in cellular immune function in sarcoidosis may be attributed to serum factors which could be IC. Kantor et al. (1976) demonstrated that sera of patients with sarcoidosis depress normal lymphocyte function. When cells from sarcoid patients are cultured in the absence of autologous plasma, normal function returns.

A monocyte chemotactic defect has been identified in sarcoidosis (Campbell, 1977). Preincubation of normal donor monocytes in plasma from sarcoidosis patients also depressed their chemotactic response, an effect not observed when plasma from normal donors was used with these cells.

Monocytes and macrophages from sarcoidosis patients, when separated from donor plasma, have either normal or supernormal functional abilities. They kill bacteria and yeast normally in vitro. They can also collaborate with T cells to promote specific responses to antigens.

Skin window techniques have been used in sarcoidosis patients to study neutrophil chemotaxis. Migration of leukocytes into the skin window was diminished as compared to normal controls (Gange et al., 1977). Neutrophil chemotaxis in vitro was also decreased. Serum from patients with sarcoidosis inhibited the chemotaxis of cells from normal donors as well. Since immune complexes inhibit leukotactic responses, it is likely that the IC in the sera is responsible for these defects.

Circulating IC has also been identified in Wegener's granulomatosis, a necrotizing granulomatous vasculitis involving both medium size veins and arteries. Immunoglobulin and complement deposits in renal glomeruli are a feature of the segmental nephritis seen in this disease. As in sarcoidosis, the role of immune complexes in the pathophysiology of the disease is not known. The IC could represent a response to the agent(s) responsible for triggering the granulomatous vasculitis. However, it is just as likely that the granulomatous lesions and the circulating IC in these diseases are byproducts of some more fundamental disorder in immunological regulation.

Even when a condition is clearly caused by an infectious agent, nonspecific activation of the humoral immune response can occur, resulting in the production of large quantities of immunoglobulins which have no apparent role in the host defense against that agent (Lambert et al., 1981).

It is often difficult to sort out those components of the host response which are appropriate from those directed against autologous tissue damaged by the disease process. Some beautiful effects may represent a generalized nonspecific activation of the elements of the immune system. Moreover, the functions of the thymic-dependent and the humoral limbs of the immune response are inextricably intertwined. Considering this inter-dependence and the fact that activated B cells can generate lymphokines similar to those elaborated by T cells when responding to specific antigens, it may be particularly difficult in granulomatous disease with circulating IC to determine whether mononuclear cells infiltrating tissues were triggered initially by B cell or T cell responses to the agents which provoked the disease in the first place (Yoshida et al., 1973).

Effects of IC on the Functions of the Cells of the Immune System

IC formation and accumulation in the cortical sinuses of lymph nodes and at the surface of primary follicles is an important mechanism for trapping antigen and stimulating secondary immune responses. However, encounters of IC with lymphoid elements may also suppress activation of these cells (Kontiainen and Mitchison, 1975; Oberbarnscheidt and Kolsch, 1978). Ig aggregates can bind to Fc receptors on B cells, sterically blocking their antigen receptors (Gorczynski et al., 1975; Oberbarnscheidt and Kolsch, 1978). Such interactions can induce migration or ''capping'' of the Fc cell surface receptors. They may also inhibit the DNA synthesis normally induced by incubation with bacterial lipopolysaccharides (LPS). Encounters with IC inhibit release of antibodies from B cells and can stimulate release of soluble suppressor factors which inhibit the maturation of B cell precursors. IC may also interact with specific Fc receptors for IgM or IgG on non-B lymphoid cells (Rabinovitch et al., 1975; Ryan et al., 1975). In short, adherence of IC to mononuclear cells (Griffin, 1980), to B cells or to T cells appears to influence crucial cell-cell interactions necessary to generate specific immune responses (Soderberg and Coons, 1978; Morgan et al., 1978). IC may also interfere with phagocytosis (Ito et al., 1979). Finally, idiotype and anti-idiotype IC influences regulatory interactions between opposing pairs of cells which produce these complementary antibodies (Eichmann, 1978; Rowley et al., 1980).

The biologic effects of IC on immune function have been studied intensively in the course of research which has sought to identify and evaluate the mechanisms which can prevent host immune responses from destroying spontaneous and transplantable tumors (Gorczynski et al., 1975; Jose and Seshardi, 1974; Prather and Lausch, 1976; Sjogren et al., 1971; 1972). Circulating IC suppresses recruitment of new tumor-specific lymphocytes by the mechanisms mentioned above. IC can also interfere with antibody-dependent cellular cytotoxicity (ADCC) (Shaw et al., 1978). IC immobilized on surfaces can inhibit macrophage phagocytosis of antibody-coated target cells (Rabinovitch et al., 1975; Saksela et al., 1976; Walker et al., 1979). This effect is not observed with fluid phase IC nor in the presence of complement. Thus it is not self evident that this effect is important in vivo. Nevertheless, these and the previously mentioned studies suggest that soluble IC in the circulation, or in the extravascular tissue spaces, may influence interactions which are crucial for the normal functioning of the immune system. Table 9.3 shows factors which influence formation, circulation and tissue deposition of immune complexes.

Table 9.3 Factors which Influence Formation, Circulation and Tissue Deposition of Immune Complexes.

A. Properties of the antibodies
  1. Immunoglobulin class or subclass
  2. Relative quantity of antibody
  3. Heterogeneity and affinity of the antigen-binding sites
  4. Net surface charge

B. Properties of antigens
  1. Net surface charge
  2. Valence
  3. Quantity
  4. Resistance to hydrolysis

C. Properties of the complex of Ab and Ag
  1. Ab:Ag ratio
  2. Ability to fix complement
  3. Size

D. Properties of the host including genetic considerations
  1. Activity of the phagocytic system
  2. Activity of the complement system
  3. Presence or absence of a concurrent immediate (IgE-mediated) hypersensitivity response to antigens which induced immune complex production.

Factors which Influence Formation, Tissue Localization and Persistence of Immune Complexes

There are a number of factors (Table 9.3) which influence the rate of formation of IC, IC survival in the circulation, tendency to localize in specific tissues sites and persistence in tissues, once they have deposited. With antigens which have many sites to bind antibody, the average affinity (or avidity) of the antibodies and their relative abundance significantly influences the size of the complexes. Large complexes formed in antibody excess readily fix complement and present a close array of Fc fragments to phagocytic cells that facilitates interactions with their Fc receptors and promotes phagocytosis. Soluble complexes are preferentially removed by the mononuclear phagocytic system of the liver and, secondarily, the spleen (Haakenstad and Mannik, 1974; 1976; 1977; Haakenstad et al., 1976). Complexes formed on the surfaces of circulating cells are taken up preferentially by phagocytes in the spleen, when coated with IgG antibodies, and in the liver, when coated with IgM antibodies.

Complexes formed with antibodies of low average affinity may result in immune complex disease more frequently than those formed with high affinity antibody. Soothill and Steward (1971) noted that mice of the SwR/5 and B10D2 new strain were prone to develop nephritis following lymphocytic choriomeningitis virus infection. These strains produced antibodies of lower average affinity to human serum albumin and transferrin than did the AJAX and C3H strains, in which spontaneous nephritis develops infrequently. They later showed that the rate of elimination of soluble protein antigens differs in various immunized strains (Alpers et al., 1972). Animals which produce mainly high affinity antibodies eliminate antigen rapidly. Moreover, the rate of elimination of complexed antigen is a feature of the antibody, not the host. Complexes formed with passively transferred low affinity antibodies are cleared slowly even when injected in strains which normally produce high affinity antibodies to that antigen. Similarly, high affinity antibody results in rapid elimination of soluble protein antigens when passively infused in strains which normally produce low affinity antibody (Germuth et al., 1979a and b).

In mice selectively bred for production of either high or low affinity antibodies, repeated injection of human serum albumin under conditions optimal for the development of chronic serum sickness nephritis (Devey and Steward, 1980) results in relatively more immune complex deposits in the glomeruli of mice which produce the low affinity antibodies (Steward, 1979). In these mice, the immune complexes were deposited mainly in the glomerular basement membrane whereas, in mice which produce high affinity antibodies, the complexes deposit mainly in the mesangium. The numbers of animals used in the studies of Steward (1979) were relatively small and, possibly as a result, no significant differences were observed in the numbers dying from renal disease. Nevertheless, by extrapolation to human disease and to the more widely used rabbit model of chronic serum sickness nephritis, one would expect that those developing glomerular basement membrane deposits would be more likely to develop irreversible structural lesions.

Surprisingly, high affinity antibodies were eluted from the IC deposited in the kidneys of mice producing low average affinity antibody (Steward, 1979). Either the minority of high affinity antibody produced by these mice formed sufficiently stable IC to deposit in the glomeruli or the high affinity antibodies were better equipped to survive the reagents used to elute these kidneys. These results are consistent with those reported by Winfield et al. (1977) who studied the affinity of anti-DNA antibodies in kidney eluates of patients with SLE.

Other Factors Which Affect the Severity of IC Disease

The ability of complement to promote inflammation and to opsonize IC for phagocytosis has been discussed previously. Its ability to dissociate IC has also been mentioned. The importance of this second role for complement in IC-mediated diseases is unclear at present. It may be a homeostatic mechanism which limits the size of IC that can persist in the circulation.

The magnitude, intensity and duration of the host response to antigens entering the circulation may be related to the nutritional status of the host. For example, starved animals with IC mediated-disease survive longer than those fed ad libitum (Safai-Kutti et al., 1980).

Aging, with its attendant disintegration of normal immunoregulatory mechanisms, may also be a factor which adversely influences immune complex diseases. C1q binding immune complexes are most frequently detected in sera of the older patients with chronic idiopathic glomerulonephritis and cancer (Rossen et al., 1979).

If the antigenic stimulus does not persist or if the antibody response lapses, the tissue injury which results from circulating IC is limited (Germuth and Rodriguez, 1973). Recurrent antigen infusions, however, in the face of a stable or increasing antibody response or an impaired mononuclear phagocytic system may precipitate or worsen immune complex diseases. Indeed, the level of function of this phagocytic system may be crucial to the outcome of IC diseases.

The Mononuclear Phagocyte System and IC Disease

So long as the phagocytic capacity comfortably exceeds the quantity of complexes in the circulation, glomerular deposits of IC do not develop and IC localization in vessel walls is presumably limited to deposits formed in situ (Cochrane and Koffler, 1973; Germuth and Rodriguez, 1973). The complexes that are preferentially removed from the circulation by the mononuclear phagocytic system contain more than two antigen and more than two antibody molecules (Haakenstad and Mannik, 1974, 1977). As the dose of IC is increased, clearance velocity and rate of hepatic localization reaches a maximum. Beyond that maximum, significant glomerular deposition occurs and immune complex disease in other highly vascularized tissues such as the lung may develop (Brentjens et al., 1974; Ward, 1979).

Conservation of normal antibody structure is crucial for rapid clearance of IC. Prior reduction and alkylation of the antibodies prolongs survival of IC in the circulation and reduces uptake in the liver. IC prepared with reduced and alkylated antibodies fix guinea pig complement poorly and do not adhere well to macrophages in vitro (Haakenstad and Mannik, 1976; Haakenstad et al, 1976). It is likely that this treatment impairs interactions of the IgG Fc fragment with cellular Fc receptors and also with the attachment of C1q to Ig in the IC. IC can bind and activate plasminogen, which can then hydrolyze components in the IC (Ungar et al, 1953). Evidence for this type of degradation of circulating IC has been seen in studies of naturally occurring idiotype-anti-idiotype complexes present in normal donor sera (Morgan et al., 1979).

Clearance of IC prepared with reduced and alkylated antibodies may also be delayed because the increase in vascular permeability which normally follows injection of IC does not occur (Haakenstad and Mannik, 1976). Presumably the injection of IC in the circulation is normally followed by an anaphylactoid reaction, triggered by intravascular activation of the complement cascade or the generation of platelet activating factor from circulating basophils sensitized with IgE antibodies specific for the same antigens.

Kidney localization of IC prepared with reduced and alkylated antibodies is greater than with IC prepared with intact antibodies (Haakenstad et al., 1976; Mannik, 1980). Moreover, IC prepared with reduced and alkylated antibodies bound more C3 and the C3 deposits persisted longer than in mice injected with IC containing unmodified antibodies. By electron microscopy, both unmodified and reduced and alkylated IC deposited initially in the fenestrae of glomerular endothelial cells. Subsequently, IC collected in the mesangial matrix. IC prepared with intact antibodies are quickly removed, whereas those prepared with reduced and alkylated antibodies persist much longer in the mesangial matrix.

The agency which removed IC from the mesangium was not identified, but it did not appear to be the mesangial cell itself (Haakenstad et al., 1976). Nevertheless, mesangial cell accumulation of IC adversely influences glomerular filtration (Michels, 1980; Schneeberger et al, 1979; Suzuki et al., 1979). Augmentation or at least preservation of mononuclear cell function is necessary to prevent overload of the mesangial compartment (Hoffsten et al., 1979; Holdsworth et al., 1980).

The role of the mononuclear phagocyte system in modifying the ability of circulating IC to cause glomerulonephritis has been further illuminated by studies of Barcelli et al. (1981). They showed that clearance of soluble IC can be increased and glomerular deposition reduced by activation of the mononuclear phagocyte system with *Corynebacterium parvum*. This activation not only resulted in increased uptake of radiolabeled IC by the liver and spleen; it also enhanced degradation of the circulating IC as shown by release of the radiolabel from the antibody. However, reticuloendothelial activating agents, like *C. parvum*, are antigenic and can sometimes provide an immune response which by itself causes IC-mediated tissue injury (Mitcheson et al., 1980). Reversal of impaired splenic phagocytic function in patients with immune complex nephritis and vasculitis can also be achieved with plasma exchange therapy (Lockwood et al., 1979).

Genetic Influences

The importance of genetic influences on the development of IC diseases has already been discussed in presenting the work of Steward and Soothill.

The work of Biozzi (1980), Feingold (1976) and Stiffel (1977) has emphasized the complexity of the genetic influences which regulate the quantity of antibody produced to specific antigenic stimuli. Only some of these genes are linked to the major histocompatibility gene complex; others involved in these regulatory events assort independently. However, studies of autologous immune complex glomerulonephritis in inbred rats suggest that susceptibility to nephritis may be strongly influenced by genes linked to the major histocompatibility complex

(Stenglein et al., 1978). Six inbred strains (Lewis, AS, BDV, L.BDV, AS2 and L.AS2) frequently develop proteinuria and immunohistological changes indicative of glomerulonephritis following a single injection of a primary tubular epithelial fraction emulsified in Freund's complete adjuvant. The BN, AVN and DA strains of rats do not develop nephritis when immunized with this antigen. Possible linkage of this host response to genes within the rat major histocompatibility gene complex (H-1) was suggested by preliminary experiments in F1 and backcross hybrids between nephritis-prone and nephritis-resistant strains. Animals which were homozygous for the H-1$^{n/n}$ haplotype (BN strain) did not develop nephritis. Susceptibility to disease appeared to be associated with homozygous inheritance of the H-1$^{l/l}$ haplotype and with heterozygous inheritance of the H-1$^{n/l}$ haplotype. The segregation of disease with H-1 type was not exact, however. Inheritance patterns suggested multifactorial genetic control of this response.

Genetic influences controlling the onset and development of immune complex glomerulonephritis are presumed to be highly complex, similar perhaps in complexity to those which influence the serologic and immunohistologic features of murine SLE (Raveche et al., 1981; Theofilopoulos, 1980).

In man, inherited complement deficiencies are often detected in patients with auto-antibody and immune complex disease (Thompson et al., 1980). A number of diseases involving immunologic dysfunction, including IC diseases in man, are also associated with the inheritance of specific HLA antigens. Many of these, including Grave's disease, chronic active hepatitis, celiac disease, myasthenia gravis, dermatitis herpetiformis and other conditions, are associated with the inheritance of HLA B8. This HLA antigen is inherited along with HLA-DRw3 more frequently than one would expect from the population frequencies of the two genes. Lawley et al. (1981) recently observed that patients with dermatitis herpetiformis have an impaired ability to clear autologous erythrocytes coated with IgG antibody. Ninety percent or more of these patients have HLA B8 and the genetically linked allele HLA-DRw3.

This defect in Fc receptor function was further demonstrated by enumerating E rosetting cells which express Fc receptors. Healthy controls who inherited HLA-B8/DRw3 have a similar deficiency in Fc receptor-bearing E rosetting cells.

Healthy HLA-B8/-DRw3 donors also cleared IgG-coated erythrocytes slowly as compared to random normal controls. In addition, both normals with HLA-B8/DRw3 and patients with dermatitis herpetiformis had increased numbers of circulating B cells that spontaneously released immunoglobulin in vitro. Thus a genetically determined deficiency of Fc receptors or a defect in Fc receptor function in lymphoid cells appears to interfere not only with removal of immune complexes from the circulation but also with the regulation of antibody formation and/or release by B cells.

Patients with dermatitis herpetiformis and others with HLA-B8/-DRw3 associated diseases frequently have circulating immune complexes. Many of these patients also have hypergammaglobulinemia, which may be additional evidence of poor regulation of the humoral immune response system in these individuals.

Bartolotti (1981) has suggested that the Fc receptor defect and other abnormalities observed by Lawley et al. (1981) related to the inheritance of HLA-B8/-DRw3 may be due to an underlying defect in glycosylation. Possibly genes linked to B8 and DRw3 may cause the production of a defective glycosyl transferase. This enzyme might influence cell surface expression of carbohydrate residues crucial to the adequate functioning of the Fc receptor site or even to the overall structure of that site. The effects could be extensive, influencing lymphocyte homing as well as other important cell-to-cell interactions involved in the development and function of T cells, B cells and monocyte/macrophages.

Carbohydrates play an important role in the clearance of IgG-containing complexes from the circulation and may also be important in C3b-C3b receptor interactions (Thornburg et al., 1980). Processing and secretion of C4 in the mouse is also dependent on glycosylation (Roos et al., 1980).

In future attempts to understand the mechanisms which explain why people who inherit specific HLA antigens are more susceptible to certain diseases, it may be useful to examine in the broadest possible terms the biochemical processes involved in the functioning of the immune system.

Anti-immunoglobulins and Immune Complexes

Anti-immunoglobulins and Inflammation

Perhaps one of the important influences that determine the size of IC in the circulation are the anti-immunoglobulins. Anti-immunoglobulins (anti-Ig which react with antigens within the Fc, the $F(ab')_2$ fragment or other sites within IgG) have been identified as belonging to all Ig classes. The classical rheumatoid factor is an IgM antibody specific for antigens within Fc. Some anti-Ig are found in the circulation only as part of soluble IC. These are the intermediate sedimenting immune complexes, first recognized by Kunkel et al. (1961) in sera of patients with rheumatoid arthritis (RA). These have also been demonstrated in synovial fluids of rheumatoid patients (Nardella et al., 1981). Intermediate sedimenting complexes are composed of IgG and exhibit anti-Fc activity; they appear to be head-to-tail polymers of IgG specific for antigenic determinants in the CH_2 domain of that molecule (Pope et al., 1974; Nardella et al., 1981). The proposed structure of these complexes is shown in Figure 9.1. Interactions with native IgG which do not have anti-immunoglobulin activity terminate the polymer (Nardella et al., 1981). The relative abundance of native IgG in plasma may account for the smaller size of these complexes in plasma as compared to synovial fluids.

There is evidence both for and against the idea that IC containing anti-Ig causes tissue injury (Eisenberg et al., 1979; Fauci et al., 1978). On the other hand, it has been suggested that classical IgM anti-Fc rheumatoid factors might protect tissues against damage caused by circulating immune complexes (Lightfoot et al., 1969). Patients with rheumatoid arthritis frequently have circulating immune complexes (Zubler and Lambert, 1978), but they rarely have immune complex-mediated glomerulonephritis. Conceivably, circulating anti-immunoglobulins can protect the glomerulus by increasing the size of the soluble immune aggregates in the circulation to the point where they are preferentially cleared by fixed tissue phagocytes before they deposit in the glomeruli.

Although this is theoretically possible, there are a number of influences which determine the quantity of immunoglobulin which can deposit in the kidney. There is also evidence which suggests that anti-immunoglobulins can augment immunological injury caused by immunoglobulins previously deposited in glomerular

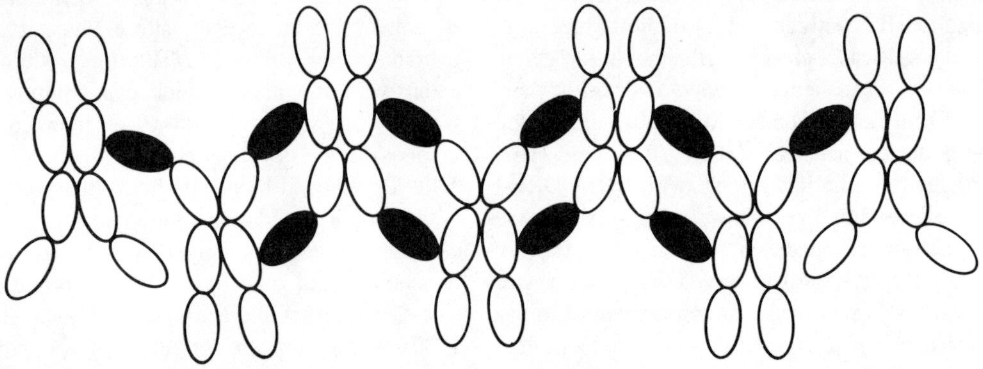

Fig. 9.1 Postulated structure of immune complexes made up of self-reacting IgG anti-IgG antibodies. The antigen-combining region of these molecules, shown in black, reacts with antigens present in the second constant domain of the IgG molecule. Once these anti-immunoglobulins encounter IgG which lack antigen receptors for other IgG, the polymerization stops.

capillaries and other vascular beds. Enhancement of antibody and complement-mediated tissue injury by anti-immunoglobulins has been demonstrated by injecting rheumatoid factors into animals previously treated with xenogeneic antikidney antibody (McCormick et al., 1969). Deposits of antibodies which can fix fluorescein-labeled aggregates of human IgG and isolated Ig Fc fragments have been detected in glomeruli of patients with idiopathic immune complex-mediated glomerulonephritis and SLE (Rossen et al., 1975, 1977). The quantity of immunoglobulin and complement in glomeruli which contain these anti-immunoglobulins is significantly greater than is found in patients with idiopathic glomerulonephritis whose tissues lack anti-immunoglobulin deposits. Renal insufficiency is also more frequent and microscopic evidence of glomerular inflammation and scarring more evident in patients whose glomeruli contain anti-immunoglobulins.

Anti-immunoglobulins, localized within glomeruli, can also interfere with attempts to identify other antigens in this tissue. Maggiore et al. (1981) studied three patients with mixed cryoglobulinemia and two with lupus nephritis who had glomerular immunoglobulin deposits which reacted with fluorescein-conjugated antibodies to hepatitis B virus (anti-HBsAg). These deposits failed to react with fluorescein-labeled anti-HBsAg when the antibody was digested to Fab′ fragments, but they did react with fluorescein-conjugated heat-aggregated IgG. This suggested that this tissue contained anti-immunoglobulins which could bind any fluorescein-labeled Fc-containing molecule, regardless of its specificity. Blocking studies with unlabeled anti-human IgM, -IgG and -IgA demonstrated that anti-IgM best blocked the binding of the fluorescein-labeled aggregated IgG. Thus, the anti-immunoglobulins deposited in these kidneys may have been classical IgM rheumatoid factors.

This work is cited in detail because it calls into question previous reports which contend that antigens have been identified in immune complexes based solely on a positive reaction with labeled antibodies specific for that antigen.

Anti-idiotypes

One particular species of anti-immunoglobulin mimics the "antigenic" properties of antigen. These are anti-idiotypes, which are antibodies that bind to antigenic sites within or adjacent to the antigen-combining site of other immunoglobulin molecules (Kunkel et al., 1963).

Naturally occurring soluble immune complexes which incorporate antibodies (idiotypes) and their respective anti-idiotypes have been demonstrated (Bankert and Pressman, 1976; Morgan et al., 1979). A general theory predicting many of the subsequently described interactions between these molecules has been elaborated by Niels Jerne (1974). The nature of the idiotypic determinants on immunoglobulin molecules, the characteristics of the anti-idiotypes which they elicit and the important role they play in immunoregulation have recently been reviewed (Eichmann, 1978; Rowley et al., 1980).

The term idiotype was first suggested by Oudin (1963), who observed that, "idiotypic specificities . . . (or) designated antigenic specificities of immunoglobulins (are) peculiar, first to antibodies against one given antigen, and secondly to one individual, or perhaps one group of individuals."

In the classically circular way in which immunological concepts develop, idiotypes were defined as antigens on specific antibody molecules which faithfully reflect the peculiarities of structure which allow these molecules to function as specific antibodies. Idiotypic antigens, not surprisingly, tend to be localized in the variable regions of the Fab′ fragment (Claflin and Davie, 1976).

Idiotypes are defined by antibodies (anti-idiotypes) (Gell and Kelus, 1964; Kelus and Gell, 1968) which fall into two categories, those which react with structures within the antigen combining site of the idiotype (Brient and Nisonoff, 1970) and those which react with antigens in the "framework" which supports or enfolds that antigen combining site (Grey et al., 1965; Claflin and Davie, 1976). Anti-idiotypes of the first type are easily demonstrated against antibodies to very small molecular weight haptenic determinants. In such cases the specificity of the anti-idiotype can be assessed by means of competitive inhibition studies with free hapten.

Anti-idiotypic antibodies have been raised by immunization across species barriers (Kunkel et al., 1963; Oudin and Michel, 1963), as well as in individuals who are genetically identical with the donor of the idiotypic antibody (Sakato and Eisen, 1975). They also occur spontaneously during the course of specific immune responses.

Since idiotypic antigens are almost invariably found within or adjacent to the antigen combining site of other immunoglobulins, antibodies which differ in immunoglobulin class (that is, antibodies which differ in the antigens determined by polypeptide sequences located in the Fc portion of the molecule) can possess identical idiotypes (Hopper, 1975; Capra and Kehoe, 1974).

Idiotypes are expressed in antigen receptors on the surface of B cells (Wernet et al., 1972). Progeny of a clone derived from a single B cell express the same idiotype even when the secreted product carries different isotypic (immunoglobulin class-specific) antigens (Gearheart et al., 1975).

Idiotypes, like other immunoglobulin polypeptides, are genetically determined (Yarmush, 1977). The inheritance of genes which influence certain idiotypes are linked to genes which determine structural polypeptides in adjacent constant regions of the Ig molecule. Crossreactions have been demonstrated among certain idiotypes (Kuettner et al., 1972; Leslie, 1979).

Understanding the structure of the antigen receptor on T cells recently has been advanced by the recognition that these cells share the same or very similar idiotypic markers as do B cells specific for the same antigen (Prange et al., 1977). This does not mean that the antigen receptor on T cells has necessarily the same overall structure as the cell surface immunoglobulins on B cells. The structure of that part of the antigen receptor of T cells equivalent to the constant domains of Ig molecules is only now beginning to be elucidated. It may contain polypeptides coded for by genes in the major histocompatibility gene complex (Sy et al., 1980B; Dietz et al., 1981).

Anti-idiotypes as Regulator Molecules

There is increasing evidence that anti-idiotype-idiotypic interactions play an important role in regulating antibody and cell-mediated immune responses (Trenkner and Riblett, 1975; Eichmann and Rajewsky, 1975; Eichmann, 1974, 1975, 1978; Aguet et al., 1978; Binz and Wigzell, 1978). Injection of guinea pig IgG_1 non-complement fixing anti-idiotypes enhances production of antibodies expressing the complementary idiotype in mice (Eichmann, 1974; Eichmann and Rajewsky, 1975). In contrast, IgG_2 complement fixing anti-idiotypes suppress idiotype production (Eichmann, 1975). Suppression of idiotype production by anti-idiotypes generally requires intact Ig molecules. Fab or $F(ab')_2$ fragments of the anti-idiotype molecules do not suppress (Kohler et al., 1977; Pawlak et al., 1973).

There are qualitative differences among neonates and adults in their response to anti-idiotypic suppression (Strayer et al., 1974). Anti-idiotypes injected into neonatal mice suppressed production of the complementary idiotype for over 4 months. The equivalent quantity of anti-idiotype, injected into adults of the same strain, suppressed idiotype production only for 4 weeks. B cells from the adult recipients of the anti-idiotype produced antibodies expressing the idiotype eventually, whereas suppression of specific idiotype-bearing B cells by administration of anti-idiotypes appeared to be virtually indefinite in neonates.

Anti-idiotype suppression of specific antibody biosynthesis (Hart et al., 1972; Cosenza and Kohler, 1972) is mediated by at least two mechanisms (Eichmann, 1975; Rowley et al., 1981). These are blockade of antigen (idiotype) receptors by the anti-idiotype and induction of T suppressor cells. The first mechanism usually requires high doses of anti-idiotype, whereas the quantity required to stimulate suppressor cells is usually less (Hetzelberger and Eichmann, 1978).

Experimentally induced anti-idiotype-mediated regulation probably reflects, to some extent, certain of the normal mechanisms which control antibody biosynthesis. Anti-idiotypes

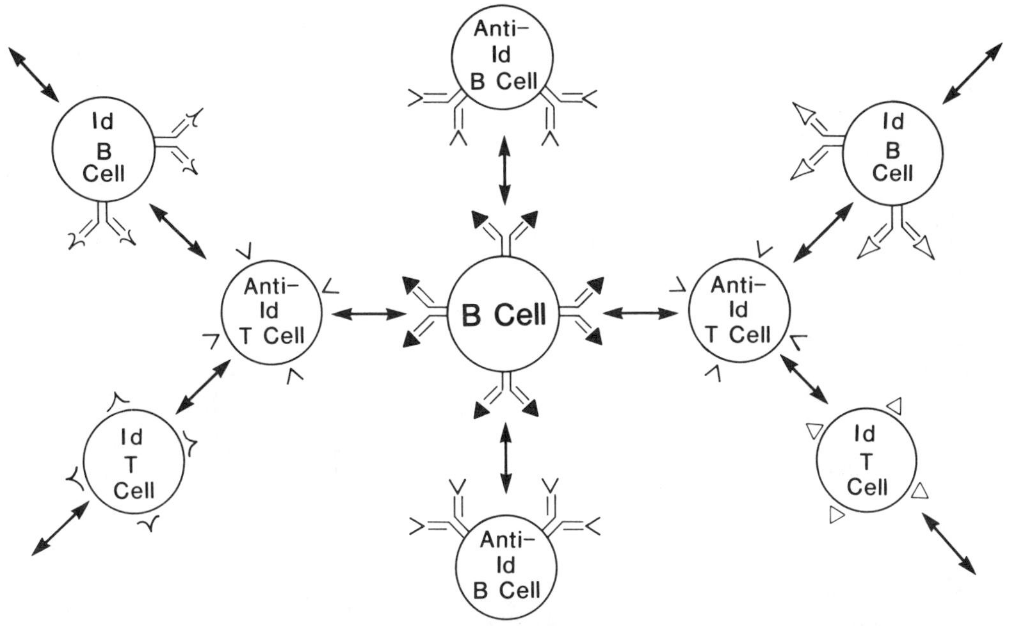

Fig. 9.2 B cell (in center) represents an expanding clone of antibody-producing cells. These stimulate both T and B cells which express complementary idiotypes. These in turn stimulate other B and T cells to produce clones which express idiotypes complementary to those produced by the first wave of anti-idiotypic cells. Note that the second wave of cells expresses antigen receptors which are structurally similar but slightly different from the antigen receptors present on the cell in the center. These peripheral second order cells are shown with slightly different antigen receptors to illustrate that idiotype-anti-idiotype interactions may be one mechanism for achieving diversification of the immune response.

can be detected during the course of induced or naturally occurring immune respones (Kluskens and Kohler, 1974; Bankert and Pressman, 1976; Morgan et al., 1979). Series of interacting antibodies have been traced at least through to the production of anti-anti-idiotypes, representing the expanding concentric network of cells which are stimulated by the introduction of antigen. The sequential changes in idiotype, anti-idiotype and anti-anti-idiotype bearing cells induced by antigen administration may be likened to the concentric rings of ripples produced by tossing a pebble into still water (Fig. 9.2).

Recent studies by Rowley et al. (1981) have demonstrated that anti-idiotypic antibodies, produced against an antigen-combining site structure (idiotype) specific for phosphoryl choline, profoundly suppress the host response to that antigen. This suppression does not seem to require the mediation of suppressor cells. Rather, the suppression appears to be initiated by the anti-idiotype alone and is prevented when small quantities of the antibody (idiotype) are already present at the time the anti-idiotype and antigen are administered. It is postulated that the anti-idiotype blocks antigen receptors for phosphoryl choline on B cells. Any free idiotype available at the time the anti-idiotype is administered forms antigen-antibody complexes with the anti-idiotype and thus protects new emerging B cells from the suppressive influences of the anti-idiotype.

Anti-idiotypic interactions among T cells are also intimately involved in regulating T cell-mediated hypersensitivity responses, including transplant rejection (McKearn et al., 1974; Aguet et al., 1978; Binz and Wigzell, 1978). Cell-mediated responses to haptens are also regulated by anti-idiotype-idiotype interactions. For example, intravenous administration of antibodies to azobenzene arsenate (ABA) coupled to syngeneic spleen cells in A/J mice generates T suppressor cells which specifically suppress the development of delayed hypersensitivity responses to ABA but do not suppress delayed type hypersensitivity to the unrelated hapten 2,4 dinitrofluorobenzene (Sy et al., 1979).

ABA-coupled syngeneic spleen cells also induce the generation of T suppressor cells. These cells are antigen-specific and share idiotypic determinants with the major crossreactive idiotype of antibodies specific for ABA in the A/J mouse (Sy et al., 1980). These T cells produce a molecule which expresses this idiotype, as well as antigens coded for by the I-J subregion of the major histocompatability complex. This molecule or factor (TsF) is capable of inducing a second set of specific suppressor cells endowed with anti-idiotypic receptors. These second order suppressor cells inhibit delayed hypersensitivity responses to ABA late in the immune response. Similar interactions between cells elaborating TsF molecules with idiotypic and anti-idiotypic components has been presented by Hirai and Nisonoff (1980).

A recent report concerning these interacting sets of suppressor T cells and their soluble suppressor factors indicates that there is still a third T suppressor cell involved in this chain. The third suppressor cell expresses an idiotype similar to that on the first of the series of suppressor cells. Once activated, this third cell will suppress T effector cells other than those which express the major idiotype which initiated this response (Sy et al., 1981).

The mode of encounter with antigen is crucial for the generation of suppressor cells which control delayed hypersensitivity responses. For example, in the above-mentioned system, intravenous injection of haptenated spleen cells activates first order suppressor cells. The third order T suppressor cells are activated by subcutaneous administration of the haptenated spleen cells. It is not clear whether antigen alone or antigen plus a second signal, possibly provided by histocompatablity gene-encoded cell surface determinants, is required for the activation of either suppressor cell.

These results indicate nevertheless that a highly complex series of regulatory events involving idiotypes and anti-idiotypes regulates specific immune responses. Development and retention of clones producing certain anti-idiotypes may explain some of the derangements in immune function seen with advancing age (Szewczuk and Cambell, 1980). The capacity of newborns to produce certain specific immune responses may likewise be influenced by the idiotypic array present in the maternal circulation during development in utero (Wikler et al., 1980).

Anti-idiotypes in Clinical Immunology

Idiotype-anti-idiotype interactions may also influence human immune responses. Morgan et al. (1979) demonstrated that normal donor sera frequently contain hidden antibodies cytotoxic for certain tumor cells. These antibodies normally circulated as one component of a 24 to 26S complex. The other component was an IgG antiglobulin specific for antigens residing in the Fab′ fragment of the cytotoxin. Presumably these anti-immunoglobulins were naturally occurring anti-idiotypes.

Nasu et al. (1980) demonstrated that sera from normal donors as well as patients with a variety of infectious and collagen vascular diseases contained antibodies reactive with $F(ab')_2$ fragments of IgG. These antibodies, detected by a solid phase radioimmunoassay, were particularly abundant in sera of patients wih rheumatoid arthritis. Sucrose density gradient ultracentrifugation studies demonstrated that these anti-Fab antibodies sedimented as >19S and between 19S and 7S in sera, suggesting that these were incorporated in a soluble immune complex in their normal environment. They postulated that these may be idiotype-anti-idiotype complexes.

Blocked or hidden anti-Fab′ antibodies have also been detected in supernatants of cultured human lymphocytes by a Farr-type radioimmunoassay (Birdsall and Rossen, 1982). In these studies, ^{125}I-Fab′ was added to the culture supernatants prior to acidification. After dropping the pH to ≤ 3, the culture supernatants were returned to pH 7.4 and assayed for anti-Fab′ activity by precipitating the antibody-bound ^{125}I-Fab′ with polyethylene glycol. Acidification-neutralization of the culture supernatants permitted detection of ten times more anti-Fab′ than was detectable without this treatment. The specificity of these anti-Fab′ antibodies was not determined, however. It remains to be seen whether these were combining site specific.

Abdou et al. (1981) have recently shown that sera obtained from patients with inactive SLE block the DNA binding activity of anti-DNA antibodies in sera from the same patient obtained at a previous time when the disease was active and the anti-DNA activity of the serum was high. The blocking activity resided in the $F(ab')_2$ fragment of IgG. These same blocking antibodies had no influence on the anti-tetanus toxoid activity of serum from a recently immunized allogeneic normal donor. Surprisingly, sera from laboratory workers who had contact with blood specimens from patients with SLE also had some anti-DNA antibody. Blocking antibodies from patients with SLE partially blocked the DNA-binding activity of these sera.

Sera collected from SLE patients when the disease was active did *not* contain C1q binding soluble immune complexes. In contrast sera from SLE patients with inactive disease, which contained the high levels of blocking antibodies, often contained C1q binding immune complexes (Abdou et al., 1981). Although further studies were not done to specifically determine if these complexes contained hidden anti-DNA antibodies, it seems probable that they may have included both anti-DNA (idiotype) and anti-anti-DNA (anti-idiotype).

It will be important to determine if similar blocking antibodies control the level of anti-T cell antibodies in SLE. Recent studies by Kumagai et al. (1981) have shown that antibodies to T cells in plasma of patients with SLE facilitate antibody-dependent cellular cytotoxic killing of autologous and normal donor T cells. These ADCC reactions were mediated principally by IgG, whereas the complement-dependent lymphocyte cytotoxins in SLE are usually cold-reactive (15°C) IgM. Anti-T cell antibodies influence immune responses in SLE (Twomey et al., 1978); similar immunoregulatory functions have been attributed to the circulating anti-T cell antibodies in New Zealand mice (Klassen et al., 1977). Studies which evaluate the relationship between these anti-T cell antibodies and anti-idiotypes specific for their antigen receptors to determine if they influence the cycling of anti-DNA and anti-anti-DNA in SLE may provide important new insights into the mechanisms which cause autoimmune responses in this disease.

There may come a day when anti-idiotypes to specific auto-antibodies or to antigens expressed on certain T cell subclasses may be used therapeutically in auto-allergic diseases to interrupt a cycle of idiotype-anti-idiotype interactions which produce unwanted autoimmune responses. Conceptually, this is no different than attempting to treat a lymphoma with infusions of a monoclonal antibody specific for antigenic determinants on the malignant cells. It may also be frustrated for the same reason. Products of the unwanted clone may form intravascular complexes with the injected anti-idiotype (Nadler et al., 1980). The ability to manipulate selectively aberrant T cell subsets or clones of B or T cells which are responsible for tissue injury is nevertheless a highly desirable goal. It would provide discrete control over disease processes which can now be treated only with corticosteroids and nonspecific cytoreductive agents.

Acknowledgments

This work was supported by the Veterans Administration Medical Center, Houston, Texas, and National Institutes of Health grants CA20543 and HL17269.

References

Abdou, N.I., Wall, H., Lindsley, H.B., Halsey, J.F., and Suzuki, T. 1981. Network theory in autoimmunity: In vitro suppression of serum anti-DNA antibody binding to DNA by anti-idiotypic antibody in systemic lupus erythematosus. J Clin Invest 67:1297–1304.

Aguet, M., Andersson, L.C., Andersson, R., Wight, E., Binz, H., and Wigzell, H. 1978. Induction of specific immune unresponsiveness with purified mixed leukocyte culture-activated T lymphoblasts as autoimmunogen. II. An analysis of the effects measured at the cellular and serological levels. J Exp Med 147:50–61.

Alpers, J.H., Steward, M.W., and Soothill, J.F. 1972. Differences in immune elimination in inbred mice. The role of low affinity antibody. Clin Exp Immunol 12:121–132.

Atkinson, J.P., and Frank, M.M. 1980. Complement, Ch. 8. In: Clinical Immunology, ed. C.W. Parker, pp. 219–271. W.B. Saunders; Phila., Pa.

Atkinson, J.P., and Rosse, W.F. 1980. Immunohematology, Ch. 30. In: Clinical Immunology, ed. C.W. Parker, pp. 930–981. W.B. Saunders; Phila., Pa.

Bankert, R.B., and Pressman, D. 1976. Receptor-blocking factor present in immune serum resembling auto-anti-idiotype antibody. J Immunol 117:457–462.

Barcelli, U., Rademacher, R., Ooi, Y.M., and Ooi, B.S. 1981. Modification of glomerular immune complex deposition in mice by activation of the reticuloendothelial system. J Clin Invest 67:20–27.

Barnett, E.V., Knutson, D.W., Abrass, C.K., Chia, D.S., Young, L.S., and Liebling, M.R. 1979. Circulating immune complexes: Their immunochemistry, detection, and importance. Ann Int Med 91:430–440.

Bartolotti, S.R. 1981. Defective Fc-receptor functions with the HLA B8/DRw3 haplotype. N Engl J Med 305:346.

Binz, H., and Wigzell, H. 1978. Induction of specific immune unresponsiveness with purified mixed leukocyte culture-activated T lymphoblasts as autoimmunogen. III. Proof for the existence of autoidiotypic killer T cells and transfer of suppression to normal syngeneic recipients by T or B lymphocytes. J Exp Med 147:63–76.

Biozzi, G., Siqueira, M., Stiffel, C., Ibanez, O.M., Mouton, D., and Ferreira, V.C.A. 1980. Genetic selections for relevant immunological function. In: Progress in Immunology IV, ed. M. Fougereau and J. Dausset, pp. 432–457. Academic Press; New York.

Birdsall, H.H., and Rossen, R.D. 1982. Production of antibodies specific for Fc, Fab′, and SKSD in vitro by peripheral blood cells from patients with rheumatoid arthritis and normal donors: Identification of immune complexes in culture supernatants containing hidden antibodies reactive with Fab′ fragments of IgG. J Clin Invest. 69:75–84.

Brentjens, J.R.,O'Connell, D.W., Pawlowski, I.B., Hsu, K.C., and Andres, G.A. 1974. Experimental immune complex disease of the lung: The pathogenesis of a laboratory model resembling certain human interstitial lung diseases. J Exp Med 140:105–125.

Brient, B.W., and Nisonoff, A. 1970. Quantitative investigations of idiotypic antibodies. IV. Inhibition by specific haptens of the reaction of anti-hapten antibody with its anti-idiotypic antibody. J Exp Med 132:951–962.

Campbell, P.B. 1977. Defective monocyte leukotaxis in sarcoidosis. Possible relationship to a plasma factor. Amer Rev Resp Dis 116:251–259.

Capra, J.D., and Kehoe, J.M. 1974. Structure of antibodies with shared idiotype: The complete sequence of the heavy chain variable regions of two immunoglobulin M anti-gamma globulins. Proc Nat Acad Sci USA 71:4032–4036.

Casali, P., Bossus, A., Carpentier, N.A., and Lambert, P.-H. 1977. Solid-phase enzyme immunoassay or radioimmunoassay for the detection of immune complexes based on their recognition by conglutinin: Conglutinin-binding test. A comparative study with ^{125}I-labelled C1q binding and Raji-cell RIA tests. Clin Exp Immunol 29:342–354.

Claflin, J.L., and Davie, J.M. 1976. Specific isolation and characterization of antibody directed to binding site antigenic determinants. J Immunol 114:70–75.

Cochrane, C.G., and Koffler, D. 1973. Immune complex disease in experimental animals and man. Adv Immunol 16:185–264.

Cohen, S.L., Fisher, C., Mowbray, J.F., Hopp, A., and Burton-Kee, J. 1979. Circulating and deposited immune complexes in renal disease and their clinical correlation. J Clin Pathol 32:1135–1139.

Cosenza, H., and Kohler, H. 1972. Specific suppression of the antibody response by antibodies to receptors. Proc Nat Acad Sci USA 69:2701–2705.

Devey, M.E., and Steward, M.W. 1980. The induction of chronic antigen-antibody complex disease in selectively bred mice producing either high or low affinity antibody to protein antigens. Immunol 41:303–311.

Devey, M.E., Taylor, J., and Steward, M.W. 1980. Measurement of antigen-antibody complexes in mouse sera by conglutinin, C1q and rheumatoid factor solid phase binding assays. J Immunol Methods 34:191–203.

Dietz, M.H., Sy, M.-S., Benacerraf, B., Nisonoff, A., Greene, M.I., and Germain, R.N. 1981. Antigen and receptor driven regulatory mechanisms. VII. H-2 restricted anti-idiotypic suppressor factor from efferent suppressor T cells. J Exp Med 153:450–463.

Eichmann, K. 1974. Idiotype suppression. I. Influence of the dose and of the effector functions of anti-idiotypic antibody on the production of an idiotype. Eur J Immunol 4:296–302.

Eichmann, K. 1975. Idiotype suppression. II. Amplification of a suppressor T cell with anti-idiotypic activity. Eur J Immunol 5:511–517.

Eichmann, K. 1978. Expression and function of idiotypes on lymphocytes. Adv Immunol 26:195–254.

Eichmann, K., and Rajewsky, K. 1975. Induction of T and B cell immunity by anti-idiotypic antibody. Eur J Immunol 5:661–666.

Eisenberg, R.A., Theofilopoulos, A.N., and Dixon, F.J. 1977. Conglutinin and immune complexes. Use of bovine conglutinin for the assay of immune complexes. J Immunol 118:1428–1434.

Eisenberg, R.A., Thor, L.T., and Dixon, F.J. 1979. Serum-serum interactions in autoimmune mice. Arthritis Rheum 22:1074–1081.

Farrell, C., Sogaard, H., and Svehag, S.-E. 1975. Detection of IgG aggregates or immune complexes using solid-phase C1q and protein A-rich *Staphylococcus aureus* as an indicator system. Scand J Immunol 4:673–680.

Fauci, A.S., Haynes, B.F., and Katz, P. 1978. The spectrum of vasculitis. Clinical, pathologic, immunologic, and therapeutic considerations. Ann Int Med 89:660–676.

Feingold, N., Feingold, J., Mouton, D., Bouthillier, Y., and Stiffel, C. 1976. Polygenic regulation of antibody synthesis to sheep erythrocytes in the mouse: A genetic analysis. Eur J Immunol 6:43–51.

Fleuren, G.J., Grond, J., and Hoedemaeker, P.J. 1980a. The pathogenetic role of free-circulating antibody in autologous immune complex glomerulonephritis. Clin Exp Immunol 41:205–217.

Fleuren, G., Grond, J., and Hoedemaeker, P.J. 1980b. In situ formation of subepithelial glomerular immune complexes in passive serum sickness. Kidney Int 17:631–637.

Fournie, G.J., Mignon-Conte, M.A., Lule, J., Gayval-Taminh, M., Hass, S., Bauriand, R., and Conte, J.J. 1980. Immune complex glomerulonephritis in mice infected with *E. coli*. Clin Exp Immunol 42:77–85.

Frank, M.M., Schreiber, A.D., Atkinson, J.P., and Jaffe, C.J. 1977. Pathophysiology of immune hemolytic anemia. Ann Int Med 87:210–222.

Gallo, G.R., Caulin-Glaser, T., and Lamm, M.E. 1981. Charge of circulating immune complexes as a factor in glomerular basement membrane localization in mice. J Clin Invest 67:1305–1313.

Gange, R.W., Carrington, P., Black, M.M., and McKerron, R. 1977. Defective neutrophil migration in sarcoidosis. Lancet ii:379–381.

Gearhart, P.J., Sigal, N.H., and Klinman, N.R. 1975. Production of antibodies of identical idiotype but diverse immunoglobulin classes by cells derived from a single stimulated B cell. Proc Nat Acad Sci USA 72: 1707–1711.

Gell, P.G.H., and Kelus, A.S. 1964. Anti-antibody or clone-product? Nature 201:687–689.

Germuth, F.G., Jr., and Rodriguez, E. 1973. Immunopathology of the Renal Glomerulus. Little Brown; Boston.

Germuth, F.G., Jr., and Rodriguez, E., Lorelle, C.A., Trump, E.I., Milano, L., and Wise, O. 1979a. Passive immune complex glomerulonephritis in mice: Models for various lesions found in human disease. I. High avidity complexes and mesangiopathic glomerulonephritis. Lab Invest 41:360–365.

Germuth, F.G., Jr., Rodriguez, E., Lorelle, C.A., Trump, E.I., Milano, L.L., and Wise, O. 1979a. Passive immune complex glomerulonephritis in mice: Models for various lesions found in human disease. II. Low avidity complexes and diffuse proliferative glomerulonephritis with subepithelial deposits. Lab Invest 41:366–371.

Ghebrehiwet, B., and Muller-Eberhard, H.J. 1979. C3e: An acidic fragment of human C3 with leukocytosis-inducing activity. J Immunol 123:616–621.

Gleicher, N., and Theofilopoulos, A.N. 1980. Immune complexes (ICs) and pregnancy. Pregnancy as an IC-state or IC-disease and the influence of IC-diseases on pregnancy. Diag Gyn Obstet 2:7–31.

Gorczynski, R.M., Kilburn, D.G., Knight, R.A., Norbury, C., Parker, D.C., and Smith, J.B. 1975. Nonspecific and specific immunosuppression in tumor-bearing mice by soluble immune complexes. Nature 254:141–143.

Grey, H.M., Mannik, M., and Kunkel, H.G. 1965. Individual antigenic specificity of myeloma proteins: Characteristics and localization to subunits. J Exp Med 121:561–575.

Griffin, F.M., Jr. 1980. Effects of soluble immune complexes on Fc receptor and C3b receptor-mediated phagocytosis by macrophages. J Exp Med 152:905–919.

Gupta, R.C., Kueppers, F., DeRemee, R.A., Huston, K.A., and McDuffie, F.C. 1977. Pulmonary and extrapulmonary sarcoidosis in relation to circulating immune complexes. A quantification of immune complexes by two radioimmunoassays. Amer Rev Resp Dis 116:261–266.

Gupta, R.K., Golub, S.H., and Morton, D.L. 1979. Correlation between tumor burden and anticomplementary activity in sera from cancer patients. Cancer Immunol Immunother 6:63–71.

Haakenstad, A.O., and Mannik, M. 1974. Saturation of the reticuloendothelial system with soluble immune complexes. J Immunol 112:1939–1948.

Haakenstad, A.O., and Mannik, M. 1976. The disappearance kinetics of soluble immune complexes prepared with reduced and alkylated antibodies and with intact antibodies in mice. Lab Invest 35:283–292.

Haakenstad, A.O., and Mannik, M. 1977. The biology of immune complexes, Ch. 11. In: Autoimmunity, ed. N. Talal, pp. 278–362. Academic Press; New York.

Haakenstad, A.O., Striker, G.E., and Mannik, M. 1976. The glomerular deposition of soluble immune complexes prepared wih reduced and alkylated antibodies and with intact antibodies in mice. Lab Invest 35:293–301.

Harbeck, R.J., Hoffman, A.A., Hoffman, S.A., and Shucard, D.W. 1979. Cerebrospinal fluid and the choroid plexus during acute immune complex disease. Clin Immunol Immunopathol 13:413–425.

Hart, D.A., Wang, A., Pawlak, L.L., and Nisonoff, A., 1972. Suppression of idiotypic specificities in adult mice by administration of antiidiotypic antibody. J Exp Med 135:1293–1300.

Hay, F.C., Nineham, L.J., and Roitt, I.M. 1976. Routine assay for the detection of immune complexes of known immunoglobulin class using solid phase C1q. Clin Exp Immunol 24:396–400.

Hedfors, E., and Norberg, R. 1974. Evidence for circulating immune complexes in sarcoidosis. Clin Exp Immunol 16:493–496.

Hetzelberger, D., and Eichmann, K. 1978. Idiotype suppression. III. Induction of unresponsiveness to sensitization with anti-idiotypic antibody: Identification of the cell types tolerized in high zone and in low zone, suppressor cell-mediated, idiotype suppression. Eur J Immunol 8:839–846.

Hirai, Y., and Nisonoff, A. 1980. Selective suppression of the major idiotypic component of an anti-hapten response by soluble T cell derived factors with idiotypic or anti-idiotypic receptors. J Exp Med 151:1213–1231.

Hoffsten, P.E., Swerdlin, A., Bartell, M., Hill, C.L., Venverloh, J., Brotherson, K., and Klahr, S. 1979. Reticuloendothelial and mesangial function in murine immune complex glomerulonephritis. Kidney Int 15:144–159.

Holdsworth, S.R., Neale, T.J., and Wilson, C.B. 1980. The participation of macrophages and monocytes in experimental immune complex glomerulonephritis. Clin Immunol Immunopathol 15:510–524.

Hopper, J.E. 1975. Comparative studies on monotypic IgM lambda and IgG kappa from an individual patient. I. Evidence for shared V_H idiotypic determinants. J Immunol 115:1101–1107.

Ito, S., Mikawa, H., Shinomiya, K., and Yoshida, T. 1979. Suppressive effect of IgA soluble immune complexes on neutrophil chemotaxis. Clin Exp Immunol 37:436–440.

Izui, S., and Eisenberg, R.A. 1980. Circulating anti-DNA-rheumatoid factor complexes in MRL/1 mice. Clin Immunol Immunopathol 15:536–551.

Izui, S., Lambert, P.-H., Fournie, G.J., Turler, H., and Miescher, P.A. 1977a. Features of systemic lupus erythematosus in mice injected with bacterial lipopolysaccharides. Identification of circulating DNA and renal localization of DNA-anti-DNA complexes. J Exp Med 145:1115–1130.

Izui, S., Lambert, P.-H., and Miescher, P.A. 1976. In vitro demonstration of a particular affinity of glomerular basement membrane and collagen for DNA. A possible basis for a local formation of DNA-Anti-DNA complexes in systemic lupus erythematosus. J Exp Med 144:428–443.

Izui, S., Lambert, P.-H., and Miescher, P.A. 1977b. Failure to detect circulating DNA-anti DNA complexes by radioimmunological methods in patients with systemic lupus erythematosus. Clin Exp Immunol 30:384–392.

Jaffe , C.J., Vierling, J.M., Jones, E.A., Lawley, T.J., and Frank, M.M. 1978. Receptor specific clearance by the reticuloendothelial system in chronic liver diseases. Demonstration of defective C3b-specific clearance in primary biliary cirrhosis. J Clin Invest 62:1069–1077.

Jerne, N.K. 1974. Towards a network theory of the immune system. Ann Immunol (Inst. Pasteur) 125C: 373–389.

Jose, D.G., and Seshadri, R. 1974. Circulating immune complexes in human neuroblastoma: Direct assay and role in blocking specific cellular immunity. Int J Cancer 13:824–833.

Kantor, F.S., Dwyer, J.M., and Mangi, R.J. 1976. Sarcoid. J Invest Dermatol 67:470–476.

Kapsopoulou-Dominos, K., and Anderer, F.A. 1979a. Circulating carcinoembryonic antigen immune complexes in sera of patients with carcinomata of the gastrointestinal tract. Clin exp Immunol 35:190–195.

Kapsopoulou-Dominos, K., and Anderer, F.A. 1979b. An approach to the routine estimation of circulating carcinoembryonic antigen immune complexes in patients with carcinomata of the gastrointestinal tract. Clin Exp Immunol 37:25–32.

Keisari, Y., and Witz, I.P. 1973. Degradation of immunoglobulins by lysosomal enzymes of tumors. I. Demonstration of the phenomenon using mouse tumors. Immunochemistry 10:565–570.

Kelley, V.E., and Cavallo, T. 1980. Glomerular permeability: Focal loss of anionic sites in glomeruli of proteinuric mice with lupus nephritis. Lab Invest 42:59–64.

Kelley, V.E., and Winkelstein, A. 1980. Effect of prostaglandin E1 treatment on murine acute glomerulonephritis. Clin Immunol Immunopathol 16:316–323.

Kelley, V.E., Winkelstein, A., and Izui, S. 1979. Effect of prostaglandin E on immune complex nephritis in NZB/W mice. Lab Invest 41:531–537.

Kelus, A.S., and Gell, P.G.H. 1968. Immunological analysis of rabbit antibody systems. J Exp Med 127:215–234.

Klassen, L.W., Krakauer, R.S. and Sternberg, A.D. 1977. Selective loss of suppressor cell function in New Zealand mice induced by NTA. J Immunol 119:830–837.

Kluskens, L., and Kohler, H. 1974. Regulation of immune response by autogenous antibody against receptor. Proc Nat Acad Sci USA 71:5083–5087.

Kohler, H., Richardson, B.C., Rowley, D.A., and Smyk, S. 1977. Immune response to phosphorylcholine. III. Requirement of the Fc portion and equal effectiveness of IgG subclass in anti-receptor antibody-induced suppression. J Immunol 119:1979–1986.

Kontiainen, K.S., and Mitchison, N.A. 1975. Blocking antigen-antibody complexes on the T-lymphocyte surface identified with defined protein antigens. I. Lymphocyte activation during in vitro incubation before adoptive transfer. Immunol 28:523–533.

Kuettner, M.G., Wang, A., and Nisonoff, A. 1972. Quantitative investigations of idiotypic antibodies. VI. Idiotypic specificity as a potential genetic marker for the variable regions of mouse immunoglobulin polypeptide chains. J Exp Med 135:579–595.

Kumagai, S., Steinberg, A.D., and Green, I. 1981. Antibodies to T cells in patients with systemic lupus erythematosus can induce antibody-dependent cell mediated cytotoxcity against human T cells. J Clin Invest 67:605–614.

Kunkel, H.G., Muller-Eberhard, H.J., Fudenberg, H.H., and Tomasi, T.B. 1961. Gamma globulin complexes in rheumatoid arthritis and certain other conditions. J Clin Invest 40:117–129.

Kunkel, H.G., Mannik, M., and Williams, R.C. 1963. Individual antigenic specificity of isolated antibodies. Science 140:1218–1219.

Kunkel, S.L., Thrall, R.S., Kunkel, R.G., McCormick, J.R., Ward, P.A., and Zurier, R.B. 1979. Suppression of immune complex vasculitis in rats by prostaglandin. J Clin Invest 64:1525–1529.

Kurlander, R.J. 1980. Reversible and irreversible loss of Fc receptor function of human monocytes as a consequence of interaction with immunoglobulin G. J Clin Invest 66:773–781.

Lambert, P.-H., Berney, M., and Kazyumba, G. 1981. Immune complexes in serum and in cerebrospinal fluid in African trypanosomiasis. J Clin Invest 67:77–85.

Lambert, P.-H., Dixon, F.J., Zubler, R.H., Agnello, V., Cambiaso, C., Casali, P., Clarke, J., Cowdery, J.S., McDuffie, F.C., Hay, F.C., MacLennan, I.C.M., Masson, P., Muller-Eberhard, H.J., Penttinen, K., Smith, M., Tappeiner, G., Theofilopoulos, A.N., and Verroust, P. 1978. A WHO collaborative study for the evaulation of eighteen methods for detecting immune complexes in serum. J Clin Lab Immunol 1:1–15.

Lawley, T.J., and Frank, M.M. 1980. Immune complexes and immune complex diseases, Ch. 6. In: Clinical Immunology, ed. C.W. Parker, pp. 143–172. W.B. Saunders, Phila.

Lawley, T.J., Hall, R.P., Fauci, A.S., Katz, S.I., Hamburger, M.I., and Frank, M.M. 1981. Defective Fc-receptor functions associated with the HLA-B8/DRw3 haplotype. N Engl J Med 304:185–192.

Lawley, T.J., James, S.P., and Jones, E.A. 1980. Circulating immune complexes: Their detection and potential significance in some hepatobiliary and intestinal diseases. Gastroenterology 78:626–641.

Leslie, G.A. 1979. Expression of a cross reactive idiotype on the IgG_{2c} subclass of rat anti-streptococcal carbohydrate antibody. Mol Immunol 16:281–285.

Lightfoot, R.W., Jr., Drusin, R.E., and Christian, C.L. 1969. The interaction of soluble immune complexes with rheumatoid factors. NY Acad Sci 168:105–110.

Lockwood, C.M., Worlledge, S., Nicholas, A., Cotton, C., and Peters, D.K. 1979. Reversal of impaired splenic function in patients with nephritis or vasculitis (or both) by plasma exchange. N Engl J Med 300:524–530.

McCormick, J.N., Day, J., Morris, C.J., and Hill, A.G.S. 1969. The potentiating effect of rheumatoid arthritis serum in the immediate phase of nephrotoxic nephritis. Clin Exp Immunol 4:17–28.

McDougal, J.S., Redecha, P.B., Inman, R.D., and Christian, C.L. 1979. Binding of immunoglobulin G aggregates and immune complexes in human sera to *Staphylococci* containing protein A. J Clin Invest 63:627–636.

McKearn, T.J., Stuart, F.P., and Fitch, F.W. 1974. Anti-idiotypic antibody in rat transplantation immunity. I. Production of anti-idiotypic antibody in animals repeatedly immunized with alloantigens. J Immunol 113:1876–1882.

McKenzie, I.F.C., Clarke, A., and Parish, C.R. 1977. Ia antigenic specificities are oligosaccharide in nature: Hapten-inhibition studies. J Exp Med 145:1039–1053.

Maggiore, Q., Bartolomeo, F., Abbate, A.L., and Misefari, V. 1981. HBsAg glomerular deposits in glomerulonephritis: Fact or artifact? Kidney International 19:579–586.

Magil, A.B., Wadsworth, L.D., and Loewen, M. 1981. Monocytes and human renal glomerular disease: A quantitative evaluation. Lab Invest 44:27–33.

Makker, S.P., and Moorthy, B. 1981. In situ immune complex formation in isolated perfused kidney using homologous antibody. Lab Invest 44:1–5.

Mannik, M. 1980. Physicochemical and functional relationships of immune complexes. J Invest Dermatol 74:333–338.

Michels, L.D., Davidman, M., and Keane, W.F. 1980. The effects of chronic mesangial immune injury on glomerular function. J Lab Clin Med 96:396–407.

Miller, G.W., and Nussenzweig, V. 1974. Complement as a regulator of interactions between immune complexes and cell membranes. J Immunol 113:464–469.

Miller, G.W., and Nussenzweig, V. 1975. A new complement function: Solubilization of antigen-antibody aggregates. Proc Natl Acad Sci USA 72:418–422.

Mitcheson, H.D., Uff, J., Pussell, B.A., Brill, M., and Castro, J.E. 1980. Immune-complex disease in mice and humans given *C. parvum*. Br J Cancer 42:34–40.

Morgan, A.C., Jr., Rossen, R.D., and Twomey, J.J. 1979. Naturally occurring circulating immune complexes: Normal human serum contains idiotype-anti-idiotype complexes dissociable by certain IgG antiglobulins. J Immunol 122:1672–1680.

Morgan, E.L., Thoman, M.L., and Weigle, W.D. 1981. Enhancement of T lymphocyte functions by Fc fragments of immunoglobulins. I. Augmentation of allogeneic mixed lymphocyte culture reactions requires I-A or I-B subregion differences between effector and stimulator cell populations. J Exp Med 153:1161–1172.

Nadler, L.M., Stashenko, P., Hardy, R., Kaplan, W.D., Button, L.N., Kufe, D.W., Antman, K.H., and Schlossman, S.F. 1980. Serotherapy of a patient with a monoclonal antibody directed against a human lymphoma-associated antigen. Cancer Res 40:3147–3154.

Nardella, T.A., Teller, D.C., and Mannik, M. 1981. Studies on the antigenic determinants in the self-association of IgG rheumatoid factor. J Exp Med 154:112–125.

Nasu, H., Chia, D.S., Knutson, D.W., and Barnett, E.V. 1980. Naturally occurring human antibodies to the $F(ab')_2$ portion of IgG. Clin Exp Immunol 42:378–386.

Nydegger, U.E. 1979. Biologic properties and detection of immune complexes in animal and human pathology. Rev Physiol Biochem Pharmacol 85:63–123.

Nydegger, U.E. 1980. Soluble immune complexes in human disease. CRC Crit Rev Clin Lab Sci 12:123–170.

Oberbarnscheidt, J., and Kolsch, E. 1978. Direct blockade of antigen-reactive B lymphocytes by immune complexes. An "off" signal for precursors of IgM-producing cells provided by the linkage of antigen- and Fc-receptors. Immunol 35:151–157.

Oudin, J., and Michel, M. 1963. Une nouvelle forme d'allotypie des globulines γ du serum de lapin apparemment liee a la fonction et a la specificite anticorps. Compt Rend 257:805– 808.

Pawlak, L.L., Hart, D.A., and Nisonoff, A., 1973. Requirements for prolonged suppression of an idiotypic specificity in adult mice. J Exp Med 137:1442–1458.

Pope, R.M., Teller, D.C., and Mannik, M. 1974. The molecular basis of self association of antibodies to IgG (rheumatoid factors) in rheumatoid arthritis. Proc Natl Acad Sci USA 71:517–521.

Prange, C.A., Fiedler, J., Nitecki, D.E., and Bellone, C.J. 1977. Inhibition of T-antigen-binding cells by idiotypic antisera. J Exp Med 146:766–778.

Prather, S.O., and Lausch, R.N. 1976. Kinetics of serum factors mediating blocking, unblocking and antibody-dependent cellular cytotoxicity in hamsters given isografts of PARA-7 tumor cells. Int J Cancer 17:380–388.

Rabinovitch, M., Manejias, R.E., and Nussenzweig, V. 1975. Selective phagocytic paralysis induced by immobilized immune complexes. J Exp Med 142:827–838.

Rajnavolgyi, E., Fust, G., Kulics, J., Ember, J., Medgyesi, G.A., and Gergely, J. 1978. The effect of immune complex composition on complement activation and complement dependent complex release. Immunochemistry 15:887–894.

Raveche, E.S., Novotny, E.A., Hansen, C.T., Tjio, J.H., and Steinberg, A.D. 1981. Genetic studies in NZB mice. V. Recombinant inbred lines demonstrate that separate genes control autoimmune phenotype. J Exp Med 153:1187–1197.

Roos, M.H., Shreffler, D.C., and Kornfield, S. 1980. Role of glycosylation in the proteolytic processing and secretion of the fourth component of complement (SS protein) of the mouse. J Immunol 125:1869–1871.

Rossen, R.D., Reisberg, M.A., Sharp, J.T., Suki, W.N., Schloeder, F.X., Hill, L.L., and Eknoyan, G. 1975. Antiglobulins and glomerulonephritis: Classification of patients by the reactivity of their sera and renal tissue with aggregated and native human IgG. J Clin Invest 56:427– 437.

Rossen, R.D., Reisberg, M.A., Singer, D.B., Schloeder, F.X., Suki, W.N., Hill, L.L., and Eknoyan, G. 1976. Soluble immune complexes in sera of patients with nephritis. Kidney International 10:256–263.

Rossen, R.D., Reisberg, M.A., Singer, D.B., Suki, W.N., Duffy, J., Hersh, E.M., Schloeder, F.X., Hill, L.L., and Eknoyan, G. 1979. The effect of age on the character of immune complex disease: A comparison of the incidence and relative size of materials reactive with C1q in sera of patients with glomerulonephritis and cancer. Medicine 58:65–79.

Rossen, R.D., Rickway, R.H., Reisberg, M.A., Singer, D.B., Schloeder, F.X., Suki, W.N., Hill, L.L., and Eknoyan, G. 1977. Renal localization of antiglobulins in glomerulonephritis and after renal transplantation. Arthritis Rheum 20:947–961.

Rowley, D.A., Griffith, P., and Lorbach, I. 1981. Regulation by complementary idiotypes. Ig protects the clone producing it. J Exp Med 153:1377–1390.

Rowley, D.A., Kohler, H., and Cowan, J.D. 1980. An immunologic network. Contemp Top Immunobiol 9:205–230.

Ryan, J.L., Arbeit, R.D., Dickler, H.B., and Henkart, P.A. 1975. Inhibition of lymphocyte mitogenesis by immobilized antigen-antibody complexes. J Exp Med 142:814–826.

Safai-Kutti, S., Fernandes, G., Wang, Y., Safai, B., Good, R.A., and Day, N.K. 1980. Reduction of circulating immune complexes by calorie restriction in NZB X NZW/F1 mice. Clin Immunol Immunopathol 15:293–300.

Sakato, N., and Eisen, H.N. 1975. Antibodies to idiotypes of isologous immunoglobulins. J Exp Med 141:1411–1426.

Saksela, E., Pyrhonen, S., Timonen, T., Teppo, A.-M., Wager, O., and Penttinen, K. 1976. Blocking effect of rheumatoid factor on the in vitro cytotoxicity of lymphoid cells from carcinoma patients. Scand J Immunol 5:1075–1080.

Sarkar, M., Liao, J., Kabat, E.A., Tanabe, T., and Ashwell, G. 1979. The binding site of rabbit hepatic lectin. J Biol Chem 254:3170–3174.

Schneeberger, E.E., O'Brein, A., and Grupe, W.E. 1979. Altered glomerular permeability in Munich-Wistar rats with autologous immune complex nephritis. Lab Invest 40:227–235.

Schreiber, A.D., and Frank, M.M. 1972a. Role of antibody and complement in the immune clearance and destruction of erythrocytes. I. In vivo effects of IgG and IgM complement-fixing sites. J Clin Invest 51:575–582.

Schreiber, A.D., and Frank, M.M. 1972b. Role of antibody and complement in the immune clearance and destruction of erythrocytes. II. Molecular nature of IgG and IgM complement-fixing sites and effects of their interaction with serum. J Clin Invest 51:583–589.

Shaw, G.M., Levy, P.C., and LoBuglio, A.L. 1978. Human monocyte antibody-dependent cell-mediated cytotoxicity to tumor cells. J Clin Invest 62:1172–1180.

Sjogren, H.O., Hellstrom, I., Bansal, S.C., and Hellstrom, K.E. 1971. Suggestive evidence that the "blocking antibodies" of tumor-bearing individuals may be antigen-antibody complexes. Proc Natl Acad Sci USA 68:1372–1375.

Sjogren, H.O., Hellstrom, I., Bansal, S.C., Warner, G.A., and Hellstrom, K.E. 1972. Elution of "blocking factors" from human tumors, capable of abrogating tumor-cell destruction by specifically immune lymphocytes. Int J Cancer 9:274–283.

Soderberg, L.S.F., and Coons, A.H. 1978. Complement-dependent stimulation of normal lymphocytes by immune complexes. J Immunol 120:806–811.

Soltis, R.D., Hasz, D., Morris, M.J., and Wilson, I.D. 1979. Studies on the nature of heat-labile anti-complementory activity in human serum. Clin Exp Immunol 37:310-322.

Soothill, J.F., and Steward, M.W. 1971. The immunopathological significance of the heterogeneity of antibody affinity. Clin Exp Immunol 9:193–199.

Stabb, H.J., and Anderer, F.A. 1980c. Are circulating CEA immune complexes a prognostic marker in patients with carcinomata of the gastrointestinal tract? Brit J Cancer 42:26–33.

Staab, H.J., Anderer, F.A., Stumpf, E., and Fischer, R. 1980a. Rezidivprognosen bei Patienten mit Adenocarcinomen des Gastrointestinaltraktes auf der Basis von Carcinoembryonalem Antigen (CEA) und seinen zirkulierenden Immunokocomplexen. Klin Wochenscher 58:125–133.

Staab, H.J., Anderer, F.A., Stumpf, E., and Fischer, R. 1980b. Die Prognostische Bedeutung von Zirkulierenden Immunkopmlexen des Carcinoembryonalen Antigens (CEA) bei Patienten mit Adenokarzinomen des Gastrointestinaltraktes. J Clin Chem Clin Biochem 18:175–181.

Stenglein, B., Thoenes, G.H., and Gunther, E. 1978. Genetic control of susceptibility to autologous immune complex glomerulonephritis in inbred rat strains. Clin Exp Immunol 33:88–94.

Steward, M.W. 1979. Chronic immune complex disease in mice: The role of antibody affinity. Clin Exp Immunol 38:414–423.

Stiffel, C., Liacopoulos-Briot, M., Decreusefond, C., and Lambert, F. 1977. Genetic selection of mice for quantitative responsiveness of lymphocytes to phytohemagglutinins. Eur J Immunol 7:291–297.

Strayer, D.S., Cosenza, H., Lee, W.M.F., Rowley, D.A., and Kohler, H. 1974. Neonatal tolerance induced by antibody against antigen-specific receptor. Science 186:640–643.

Stuart, F.P., Scollard, D.M., McKearn, T.J., and Fitch, F.W. 1976. Cellular and humoral immunity after allogeneic renal transplantaton in the rat. V. Appearance of anti-idiotypic antibody and its relationship to cellular immunity after treatment with donor spleen cells and alloantibody. Transplantation 22:455–466.

Suzuki, Y., Kihara, I., Morita, T., Oite, T., and Yamamoto, T. 1979. Accelerated immune complex nephritis due to mesangial overloading in spontaneous hypertensive (SHR) rats. Japan J Exp Med 49:373–382.

Sy, M.-S., Bach, B.A., Brown, A., Nisonoff, A., Benacerraf, B., and Greene, M.I. 1979. Antigen and receptor-driven regulatory mechanisms. II. Induction of suppressor T cells with idiotype-coupled syngeneic spleen cells. J Exp Med 150:1229–1240.

Sy, M.-S., Dietz, M.H., Germain, R.N., Benacerraf, B., and Greene, M.I. 1980. Antigen and receptor-driven regulatory mechanisms. IV. Idiotype-bearing I− J+ suppressor T cell factors induced second order suppressor T cells which express anti-idiotypic receptors. J Exp Med 151:1183–1195.

Sy, M.-S., Nisonoff, A., Germain, R.N., Benacerraf, B., and Greene, M.I. 1981. Antigen and receptor-driven regulatory mechanisms. VIII. Suppression of idiotype-negative *p*-azobenzene arsonate specific T cells results from the interaction of an anti-idiotypic second order T suppressor cell with a crossreactive-idiotype-positive, *p*-azobenzene arsonate-primed T cell target. J Exp Med 153:1415–1445.

Szewczuk, M.R., and Campbell, R.J. 1980. Loss of immune competence with age may be due to auto-anti-idiotypic antibody regulation. Nature 286:164–166.

Takahashi, M., Takahashi, S., Brade, V., and Nussenzweig, V. 1978. Requirements for the solubilization of immune aggregates by complement. The role of the classical pathway. J Clin Invest 62:349–358.

Theofilopoulos, A.N., Andrews, B.S., Urist, M.M., Morton, D.L., and Dixon, F.J. 1977. The nature of immune complexes in human cancer sera. J Immunol 119:657–663.

Theofilopoulos, A.N. 1980. Evaluation and clinical significance of circulating immune complexes. Prog Clin Immunol 4:63–106.

Theofilopoulos, A.N., and Dixon, F.J. 1979. The biology and detection of immune complexes. Adv Immunol 28:89–220.

Theofilopoulos, A.N., McConahey, P.J., Izui, S., Eisenberg, R.A., Pereira, A.B., and Creighton, W.D. 1980. A comparative immunologic analysis of several murine strains with autoimmune manifestations. Clin Immunol Immunopathol 15:258–278.

Thompson, R.A., Haeney, M., Reid, K.B., Davies, J.G., White, R.H., and Cameron, A.H. 1980. A genetic defect of the C1q subcomponent of complement associated with childhood (immune complex) nephritis. N Engl J Med 303:22–24.

Thompson, R.A., and Lachmann, P.J. 1970. Reactive lysis: The complement-mediated lysis of unsensitized cells. I. The characterization of the indicator factor and its identification as C7. J Exp Med 131:629–641.

Thornburg, R.W., Day, J.F., Baynes, J.W., and Thorpe, S.R. 1980. Carbohydrate-mediated clearance of immune complexes from the circulation: A role for galactose residues in the hepatic uptake of IgG-antigen complexes. J Biol Chem 255:6820–6825.

Trenkner, E., and Riblet, R. 1975. Induction of antiphosphorylcholine antibody formation by anti-idiotypic antibodies. J Exp Med 142:1121–1131.

Twomey, J.J., Laughter A.H., and Steinberg, A.D. 1978. A serum inhibitor of immune regulation in patients with systemic lupus erythematosus. J Clin Invest 63:954–965.

Ungar, G., Damgaard, E., and Hummel, F.P. 1953. Activation of profibrinolysin by antigen-antibody reaction and by anaphylactoid agents, its relation to complement. J Exp Med 98:291–303.

Walker, L., Hay, F.C., and Roitt, I.M. 1979. Characteristics of complexes for arming and inhibiting effector cells for antibody-dependent cell-mediated cytotoxicity. Clin Exp Immunol 36:397–407.

Ward, P.A. 1979. Immune complex injury of the lung. Am J Pathol 97:85–92.

Wernet, P., Feizi, T., and Kunkel, H.G. 1972. Idiotypic determinants of immunoglobulin M detected on the surface of human lymphocytes by cytotoxicity assays. J Exp Med 136:650–655.

Wiggins, R.C., and Cochrane, C.G. 1981. Immune-complex-mediated biologic effects. N Engl J Med 304:518–520.

Wikler, M., Demeur, C., Dewasme, G., and Urbain, J., 1980. Immunoregulatory role of maternal idiotypes. Ontogeny of immune networks. J Exp Med 152:1024–1035.

Williams, R.C., Jr. 1980a. Immune complex-mediated rheumatic diseases: The evidence and the enigmas. Postgrad Med 68:124–131.

Williams, R.C., Jr. 1980b. Immune Complexes in Clinical and Experimental Medicine. Harvard University Press; Cambridge.

Winchester, R.J., Agnello, V., and Kunkel, H.G. 1970. Gamma globulin complexes in synovial fluids of patients with rheumatoid arthritis. Partial characterization and relationship to lowered complement levels. Clin Exp Immunol 6:689–706.

Winfield, J.B., Faiferman, I., and Koffler, D. 1977. Avidity of anti-DNA antibodies in serum and IgG glomerular eluates from patients with systemic lupus erythematosus. Association of high avidity and anti-native DNA antibody with glomerulonephritis. J Clin Invest 59:90–96.

Winkelstein, A., and Kelley, V.E. 1980. The effect of PGE_1 on lymphocytes in NZB/W mice. Clin Immunol Immunopathol 17:212–218.

Yarmush, M.L., Sogn, J.A., Mudgett, M., and Kindt, T.J. 1977. The inheritance of antibody regions in the rabbit: Linkage of an H-chain-specific idiotype to immunoglobulin allotype. J Exp Med 145:916–930.

Yoshida, T.H., Sonozaki, H., and Cohen, S. 1973. The production of migration inhibition factor by B and T cells of the guinea pig. J Exp Med 138:784–797.

Zubler, R.-H., and Lambert, P.H. 1978. Detection of immune complexes in human disease. Prog Allergy 24:1–48.

Chapter 10

Disorders of Immune Regulation

Josef S. Smolen and Alfred D. Steinberg

Introduction

In the past 15 years, cellular immunology has been born and has weathered growing pains; it is on the verge of becoming a mature discipline. Much of the success of investigations in cellular immunology is due to the availability of highly inbred mouse strains. As a result, a concept of immune regulation has emerged that has already proven to be more complex than other biological systems. The basis of immune regulation is the differentiation of stem cells into three major lineages of cells; these are T cells, B cells and macrophages. T cells are effector cells for cell-mediated immunity, whereas B cells are the effector cells for humoral immunity. (Details of these ontogenetic aspects have been discussed in Chapters 1 to 3.) The first demonstration of the complexity of the immune system stems from studies on antibody production. Not only could it be shown that a bone marrow-derived (B) cell was the antibody producing cell precursor, but also that a thymus-derived (T) cell had to "help" the B cell for optimal antibody production; accessory cells, macrophages and macrophage-like cells, were also necessary (Claman et al., 1966; Miller and Mitchell, 1968; Mosier and Coppleson, 1968). The later cells have been shown to present antigen to lymphocytes in association with self-determinants, thereby providing both processed antigen and a self-regulation structure necessary for lymphocyte triggering (Rosenthal and Shevach, 1973).

Immunology seemed complicated by the requirement for several different cells for optimal immune responses; however, an additional complexity was revealed by the observation that certain cells served, not to help in the generation of immune responses, but rather to suppress or regulate them downward (Gershon, 1974; Steinberg and Klassen, 1977; Germain and Benacerraf, 1980). These suppressive phenomena were actually demonstrated indirectly prior to the demonstration of helper phenomena. However, since many of the suppressor cell experiments ran counter to the intuition of most immunologists and were demonstrated in systems that had special requirements, the notion of suppressor cells did not gain wide acceptance until the accumulated evidence was overwhelming. Suppressor cells have been demonstrated for immune responses to many kinds of antigens: thymic-independent and thymic-dependent, soluble and particulate, inducers of antibody and of cell-mediated immunity, for the major immunoglobulin classes, for responses controlled by the major histocompatibility complex and for others. Thus, there appeared to be helper T cells, cytotoxic T cells, suppressor T cells, B cells and macrophages. However, evidence was available indicating that there were subpopulations of B cells (Moller, 1975; Huber et al., 1977; Ahmed et al., 1977). In addition, antibody could suppress immune responses (Uhr and Moller, 1968). Finally, it appeared possible that subpopulations of macrophages might also exist (Cowing et al., 1978; Raff et al., 1980). The increase in the number of cellular [and also humoral (Cohen et al., 1978)] participants in immune responses led to an appreciation of complexity without necessarily providing major advances in understanding. It was like a football game involving similar players who kept changing positions, or even teams, and in which none of the players wore uniforms. This unhappy state of affairs has been partially overcome by the development of antibodies reacting with functionally distinct lymphocyte subsets. With the aid of such antisera, at first against mouse T cell subsets, it was found that T cells which subserved helper or inducer functions could be distinguished from those which subserved suppressor and cytotoxic functions. The helper cell bears the Lyt 1 antigen and the suppressor/cytotoxic subset bears the Lyt 2 and 3 antigens (Cantor and Boyse, 1976). Recently it has been found that the latter cells also contain Lyt 1, but in distributions that were not detected by the original method of complement-dependent cytotoxicity (Ledbetter et al., 1980). Similar antisera have identified at least two B cell subsets (Huber et al., 1977; Ahmed et al., 1977).

The Complexity of the Immune System

As a result of the advances in mouse immunology, experiments defining the details of regulatory pathways indicated the degree of the complexity previously suggested. Thus, multiple cell-cell interactions appeared to be necessary to go from an antigenic signal to an effector suppressor cell. Such cellular interactions do not necessarily involve cells of only one functional family, but an inducer cell may activate a suppressor precursor cell to act as an effector suppressor cell. Moreover, a subset of such effector suppressor cells may, in turn, regulate inducer cells downward for both antibody-forming cells and suppressor precursor cells (Eardley et al., 1978). A schematic diagram of such a feedback inhibitory loop is presented in Figure 10.1. Finally, more than one kind of T cell appears to operate to provide for maximal helper function for B cells (Janeway, 1980). The production of a specific antibody is regulated by distinct *antigen* specific helper and suppressor cells and also by nonspecific suppressor effector cells. The antibody molecules produced, with their unique structures called idiotopes, are antigens themselves and can be recognized specifically. Thus B cells and T cells which have receptors for a particular idiotope may interact in a specific and selective manner with a specific family of antibody molecules (Eichmann, 1978), imposing additional regulatory effects upon the specific ongoing immune response.

In order to reconcile some of the partly divergent experimental results and to provide a framework for conceptualizing the immune response to an antigen, we have developed a tentative model of the immune response and its regulation in the mouse (Fig. 10.2). The suggestion that this is a simplified view of the immune system is not made with tongue in cheek. For example, we have omitted all of the macrophages which are necessary for the interactions among the various regulatory T cells; also, we have not discussed the nature of the various signals operating in cellular communication. In addition, we have not dealt with the whole range of B cell development, including some aspects of B cell tolerance. Finally, we have not indicated that the immune system, prior to encountering the new antigen, has been in a dynamic state of activity, the exact details of which may determine the overall responsiveness of the different circuits shown.

In the construction of Figure 10.2, we have drawn upon the experimental data and ideas of many groups of investigators. Although this figure is neither complete nor definitive, we would like to discuss it in some detail as a basis for understanding immune regulation. In a subsequent figure we will present an analogous human system and try to describe where defects in immune regulation might be associated with disease.

In Figure 10.2, an antigen either interacts directly with a B cell or, more commonly, is processed by antigen-presenting cells (here designated as a macrophage) prior to presentation to B cells. Whereas the antigen-presenting cells do not appear to require specific receptors for antigens, the B cells do. Similarly, T cells also interact with antigen via receptors which may be related to, but are not identical to, the specific receptors of B cells (Eichmann, 1978). The combination and interaction of macrophages, antigen, antigen-specific B cells and antigen-specific T cells lead to antibody production by the B cells and their progeny. T cells and B cells with specific receptors for the idiotype of the newly secreted antibody may interact with the antibody itself or with the identical idiotypic site on the antigen-specific cells. These anti-idiotype receptor-bearing cells are indicated in the diagram as anti-Id. One such T cell can act as helper cell for antibody production; other T cells may serve to regulate the ultimate magnitude of the antibody response. B cells with such receptors can produce anti-antibody, which is antibody specific for the anti-antigen (Ab1), called anti-idiotypic antibody (Ab_2). The production of such Ab_2 is T cell-dependent. Anti-idiotype antibody can then exert further immunoregulatory actions. However, it should be noted that antibody (Ab_1), itself or as an immune complex in association with antigen, can be a potent regulator of the immune response (Uhr and Moller, 1968; Rao et al., 1980; Hoffmann, 1980). Although all of the initiators of the various suppressor circuits are specific (that is, they involve either an antigen receptor or an idiotype receptor), the ultimate effector of the suppressor circuits (TS) may be antigen nonspecific (Germain and Benacerraf, 1980). A number of factors not shown in the diagram may determine the degree to which the various pathways are activated. A few will serve as illustrations. Presentation of the antigen in association with a strong adjuvant or polyclonal B-cell activator may initially divert the system toward increased antibody production. Exposure to a strong antigen immediately prior to stimulation may have already activated a large number of TS cells which would lead to a reduced response to the new antigen (antigenic competition). In addition, a variety of genetic effects must be superimposed; these may either favor or interdict a strong antibody response. Finally, prior exposure to the antigen in an immunogenic or priming state may have led to expansion of cells reactive with that antigen. In some circumstances, that prior exposure may lead to an emphasis of the helper pathways and a de-emphasis of the suppressive pathways; alternatively, prior exposure to the antigen in a tolerogenic form (such as exposure in a manner that prevents efficient antigen processing or by presentation on certain cell membranes) may lead to emphasis of the suppressive pathways. Our understanding of the cellular bases for such modifying factors varies from system to system. In many instances, such factors can be incorporated into the cells and pathways shown in Figure 10.2. Not shown are the various soluble

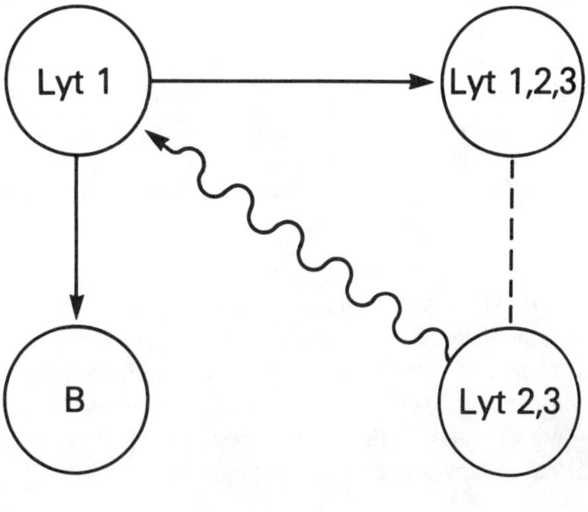

Fig. 10.1 Feedback inhibition of murine immune responses. An Lyt 1 (helper) cell, educated by antigen, acts in concert with an intermediary cell (Lyt 1,2,3) to give rise to a suppressor effector cell (Lyt 2,3) in the presence of antigen. The suppressor effector cell acts, either directly (as shown) or through an additional mechanism, to decrease the ability of Lyt 1 cells to help B cells. In addition (not shown), suppressor cells may act directly on B cells to inhibit their function. Various reactions also require macrophages (not shown).

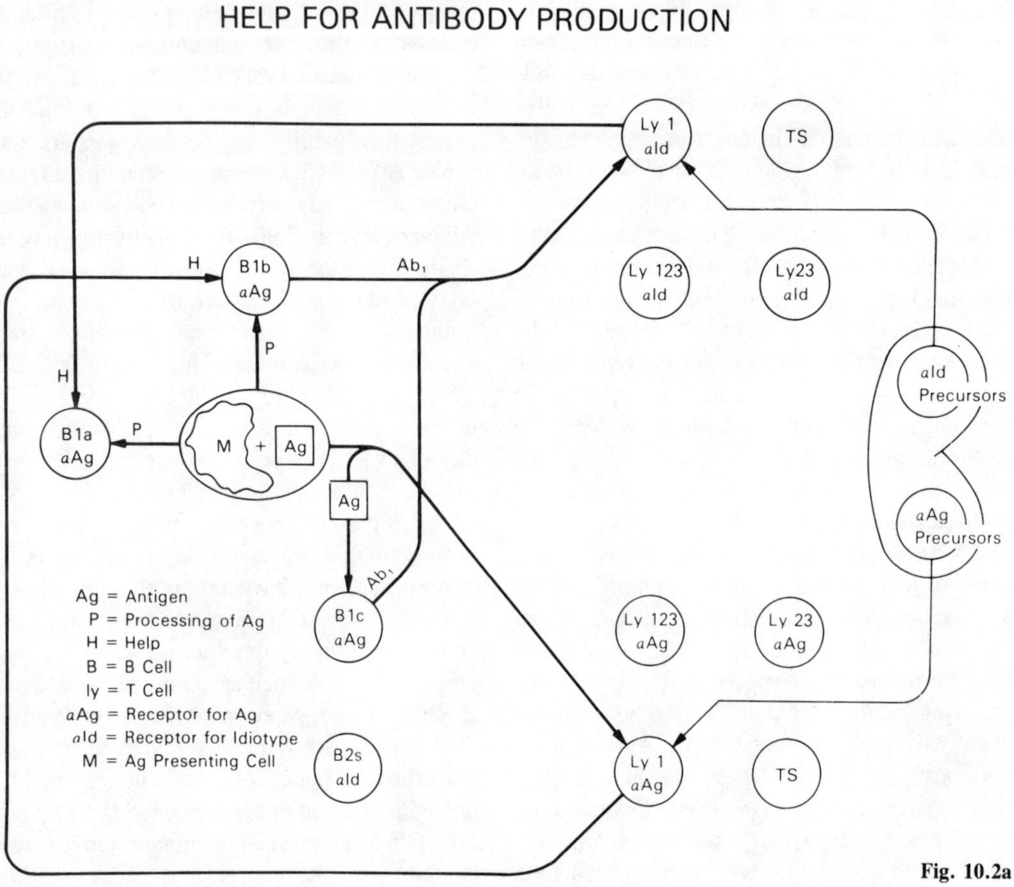

Fig. 10.2a

Fig. 10.2 Schematic diagram of immune regulation in the mouse. Pathways involved in helper function are shown in Figure 10.2a. Those involved in suppressor functions are shown in Figure 10.2b. Figure 10.2c represents a composite of the other two.

In these figures, the T cells are to the right. Precursor T cells give rise to T cells with receptors for antigen (Ag) or receptors for idiotype (αId). Lyt 1 αId T cells represent T cells which help T-dependent B cells. They can help in either the production of antibody to antigen or in the production of anti-idiotype antibody (Ab_2). In addition, they can act on Lyt 123 αAg T cells in feedback suppression. Similarly, Lyt 1 αAg T cells, in association with macrophage-processed antigen (P), act as helper cells for αAg bearing T-dependent B cells. The Lyt 1 αAg T cells also act in feedback suppression. Lyt 23 αAg and Lyt 23 αId T cells act in the suppressor circuit so as to induce antigen nonspecific suppressor effector cells (TS). These interfere with the functions of Lyt 1 T cells and B cells.

Antibody also serves as an immunoregulatory agent. Anti-antigen (Ab_1) can interact with cells with αId receptors. The net effect is generally suppression; however, both suppressor and helper pathways may be activated and the net effect could be either, depending upon the relative strength of one pathway versus another. Finally, anti-Ag induces B2s (the whole population of B cells with receptors for Id) to produce Ab_2. This anti-idiotype antibody serves to further modulate the responses of cells with the appropriate receptors as shown. Whereas some of the B cells can respond to antigen (Ag) without the need for T cell help, it appears that Ab_2 requires both the appropriate B cells and T cell help.

factors, produced by different cells in the regulatory pathway, which may mediate the effects of particular cells. In addition, there appear to be distinct signals for differentiation and proliferation. Finally, the interference with suppression —fundamental to the development of an immune response—may involve multiple mechanisms. These are reflected in ontogeny by initial suppression at birth; interference with suppression and development of immune capacity; and ultimately new development of adult suppressor mechanisms to regulate immune responsiveness.

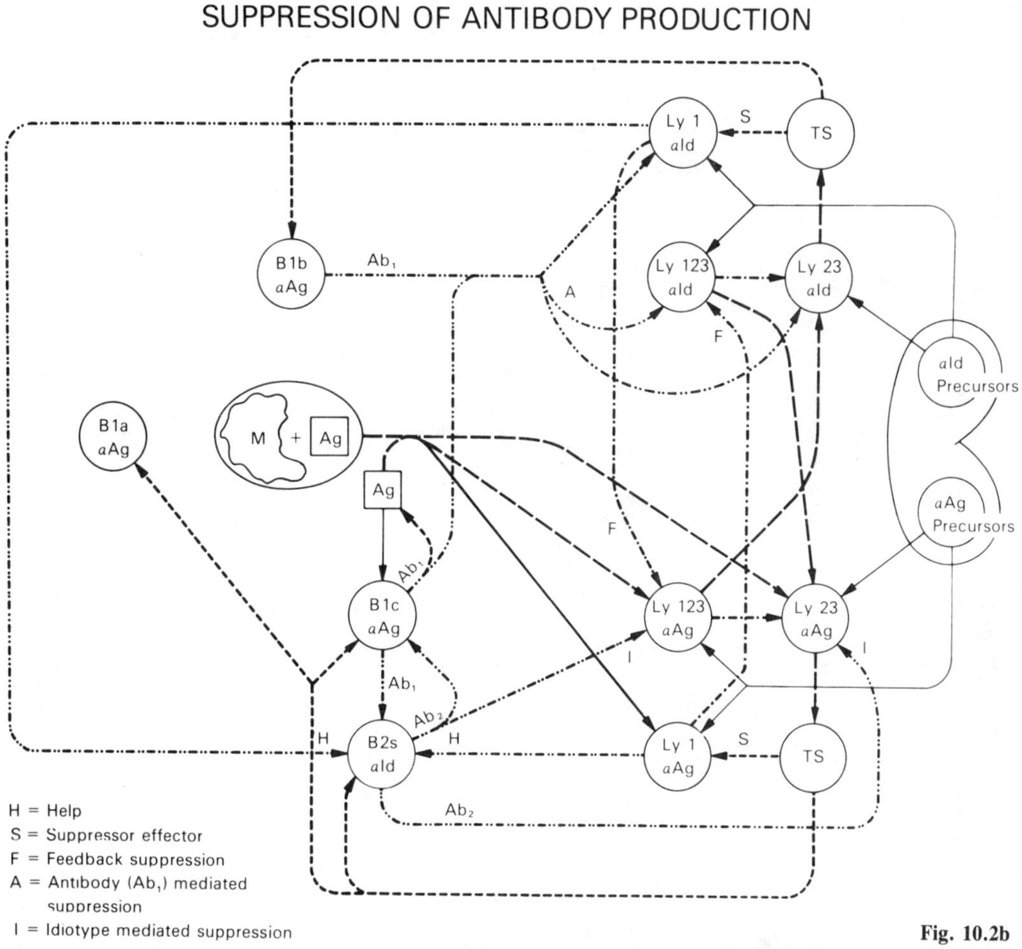

Fig. 10.2b

The Human Immune System

The functional characteristics of the human immune responses are analogous to those of the mouse. They involve antigen-presenting cells, B cells and helper, suppressor and cytotoxic T cells. However, until recently, physical characterization of subsets of the three immunocompetent cell lineages has not been possible. The demonstration that T cells with receptors for the Fc fragment of IgM (T_{μ}) subserve helper effects, whereas T cells with receptors for Fc-IgG (T_{γ}) subserve suppression (Moretta et al., 1977), has enabled some advances in our understanding of autoimmune diseases. Futhermore, it has led to the demonstration of human feedback inhibition (Heijnen et al., 1979, see Fig. 10.3). However, these surface markers are not necessarily stable (Pichler et al., 1978) and the presence of Fc IgG-receptors on non-T cells has led to some confusion about the nature of T_{γ} cells (Reinherz et al., 1980; Pichler and Broder, 1981). Both T_{γ} and T_{μ} cells are heterogenous with regard to expression of subset-specific differentiation antigens (Pichler and Broder, 1981). Also, suppression in some systems does not depend upon the presence of T_{γ} cells (Haynes and Fauci, 1978). Nevertheless, it appears that many T_{γ} cells do subserve suppression and that such cells are preferentially lost in systemic lupus erythematosus (SLE), a disease characterized by decreased suppressor function (Fauci et al., 1978).

Most recently, analysis of T cells, B cells and macrophages with the help of a myriad of monoclonal antibodies has not only enabled the

REGULATION OF ANTIBODY PRODUCTION — A SIMPLIFIED VIEW

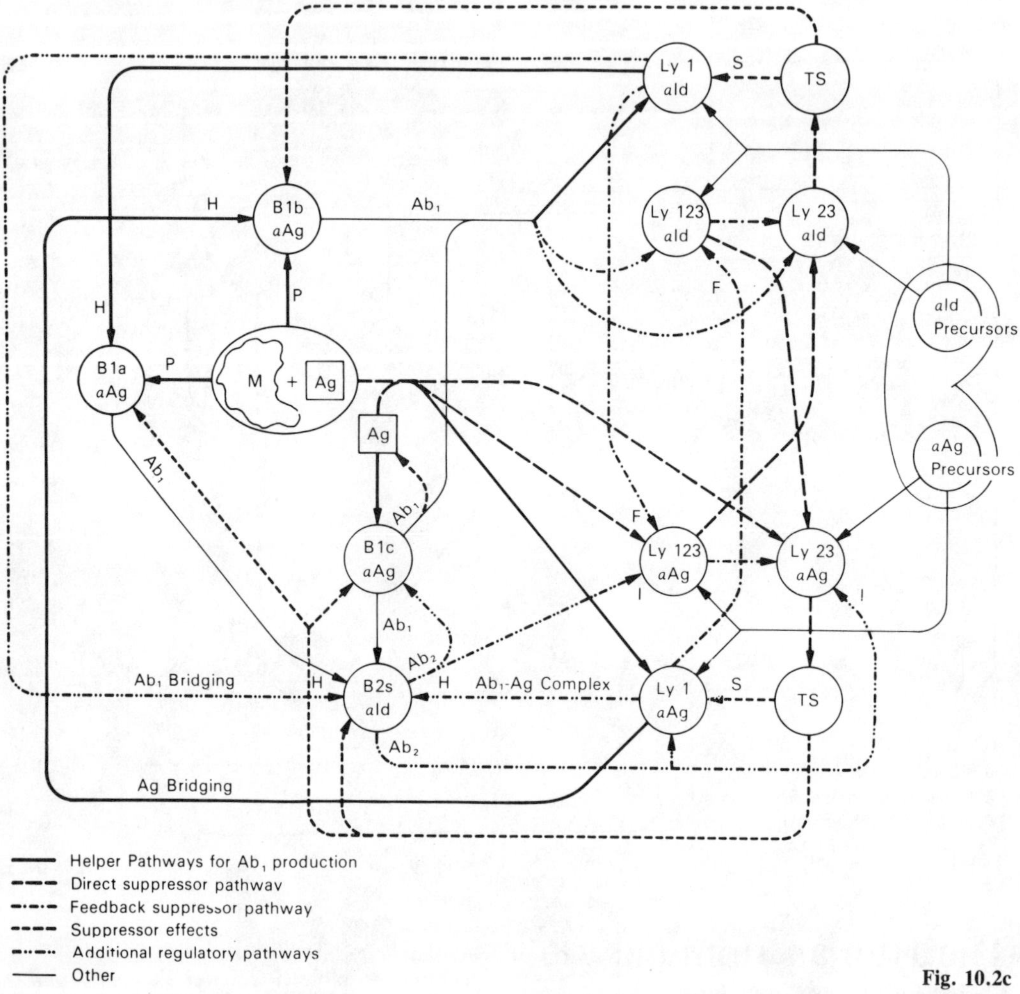

Fig. 10.2c

characterization of antigens on functionally distinct cell subsets, but also the characterizaton of differentiation antigens on these cells (Reinherz et al., 1979a; Reinherz et al., 1980a; Ledbetter et al., 1981; Raff et al., 1980; Abramson et al., 1981; Chapters 1 to 3). On the basis of analogies between the murine Lyt system and the human Leu antigen system (Ledbetter et al., 1981), a simplified view of the human immune system is presented in Figure 10.4. The figure has been generated using Figure 10.2, the analogies between mouse and human markers and the functional data available from human studies. Leu 1 (but also other antigens characterized by monoclonal antibodies, such as Leu 4, OKT 1, and OKT 3) is a general marker for T cells and thus equivalent to Lyt 1; Leu 2 (but also OKT 5 and OKT 8) is a marker for the suppressor/cytotoxic cell populations and its antigens Leu 2a and Leu 2b correspond to Lyt 2 and Lyt 3, respectively; finally, Leu 3 (but also OKT 4) is present on the inducer cell subset. Inducer populations include inducers of both helper and suppressor circuits (Reinherz et al., 1979; Thomas et al., 1980). Thus, an inducer cell may induce a B cell to become an antibody-producing cell or an inducer cell (perhaps a different inducer cell) may induce a suppressor cell precursor to become an effector suppressor cell.

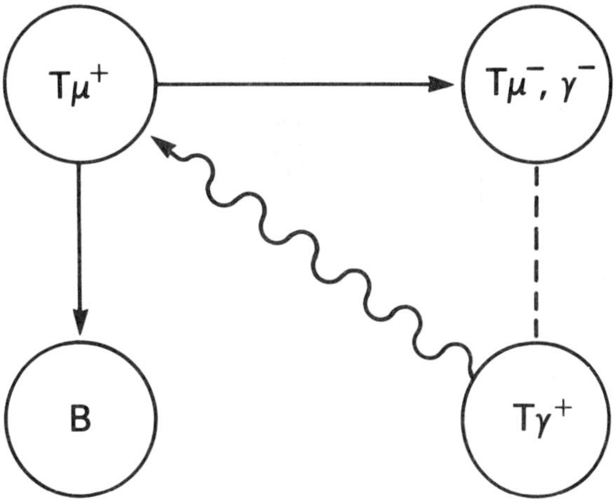

Fig. 10.3 Feedback inhibition by human T cells. A primed Tμ cell (a cell with a receptor for the Fc portion of IgM) induces a $T_{\mu-\gamma-}$ cell (a T cell lacking receptors for the Fc portion of IgM and IgG) to give rise to a Tγ suppressor effector cell. This Tγ cell has receptors for the Fc portion of IgG. In a manner analogous to the murine system shown in Figure 10.1 this suppressor cell interferes with B cell function by inhibiting the Tμ helper cell. It may also act directly on B cells to inhibit proliferation and/or differentiation. This type of feedback loop is only a portion of the immune network shown in Figure 10.4. In the latter, rather than using Tμ and Tγ cells, the more stable Leu markers are used.

The analogy of the human to the mouse system is not complete; we have ignored, in the diagram for the murine immune system (Fig. 10.2) the fact that all T cells, including the Lyt 2,3 cells, have at least small amounts of Lyt 1. In addition, the Leu 3 antigen, which is characteristic of human inducer cells, has no known analogue in the mouse. Finally, in contrast to experiments in murine models, there is no certanty about the role of human Leu 1,2,3-positive cells. Whereas murine Lyt 1,2,3 cells as determined by column adherence comprise up to 50% of the splenic T cell population (Cantor and Boyse, 1976), a maximum of 10% of human peripheral blood T cells have antigens characteristic of both the helper and the suppressor/cytotoxic cell subsets (Biddison and Sharrow, personal communication). However, human peripheral blood may be inadequate for comparative studies and Leu 1,2,3 cells comprise the majority of thymic lymphocytes (Reinherz et al., 1980).

Disorders of Immune Regulation—An Approach

The complex cellular interactions detailed in Figures 10.2 and 10.4 indicate that the utility of cell surface characteristics for the classification of inducer and suppressor cells is somewhat limited, especially with regard to their application to disease states. Phenotypic inducer cells may be necessary for the activation and/or function of suppressor cells or may even contain a subset of suppressor effectors, the effects of which are masked by the remaining inducer cells. Therefore, a functional defect in an inducer cell populaton may lead to defective suppressor function. Thus, a numerical and/or functional defect in an inducer subset could paradoxically increase antibody production, by failure to induce suppressor cells, rather than decrease antibody production on the basis of decreased helper cells. [This is analogous to the discovery many years ago that patients with hypogammaglobulinemia had relatives with a markedly increased incidence in abnormal serum immunoglobulin levels; unlike the patients, relatives not only had decreased immunoglobulins, but frequently had increased quantities (Waldenstrom, 1961; Fudenberg, 1971).] Therefore, a finding of a decrease in inducer cells by phenotyping points to a possible immune regulatory defect, but it does not necessarily point to the exact nature of that defect. Moreover even functional assays for helper or suppressor function may not pinpoint the precise defect. It may be necessary to analyze inducer cells, suppressor cell precursors, mature suppressor cells and feedback regulation, as well as the relevant macrophages and secreted molecular intermediaries, in order to fully assess even one limb of a regulatory loop.

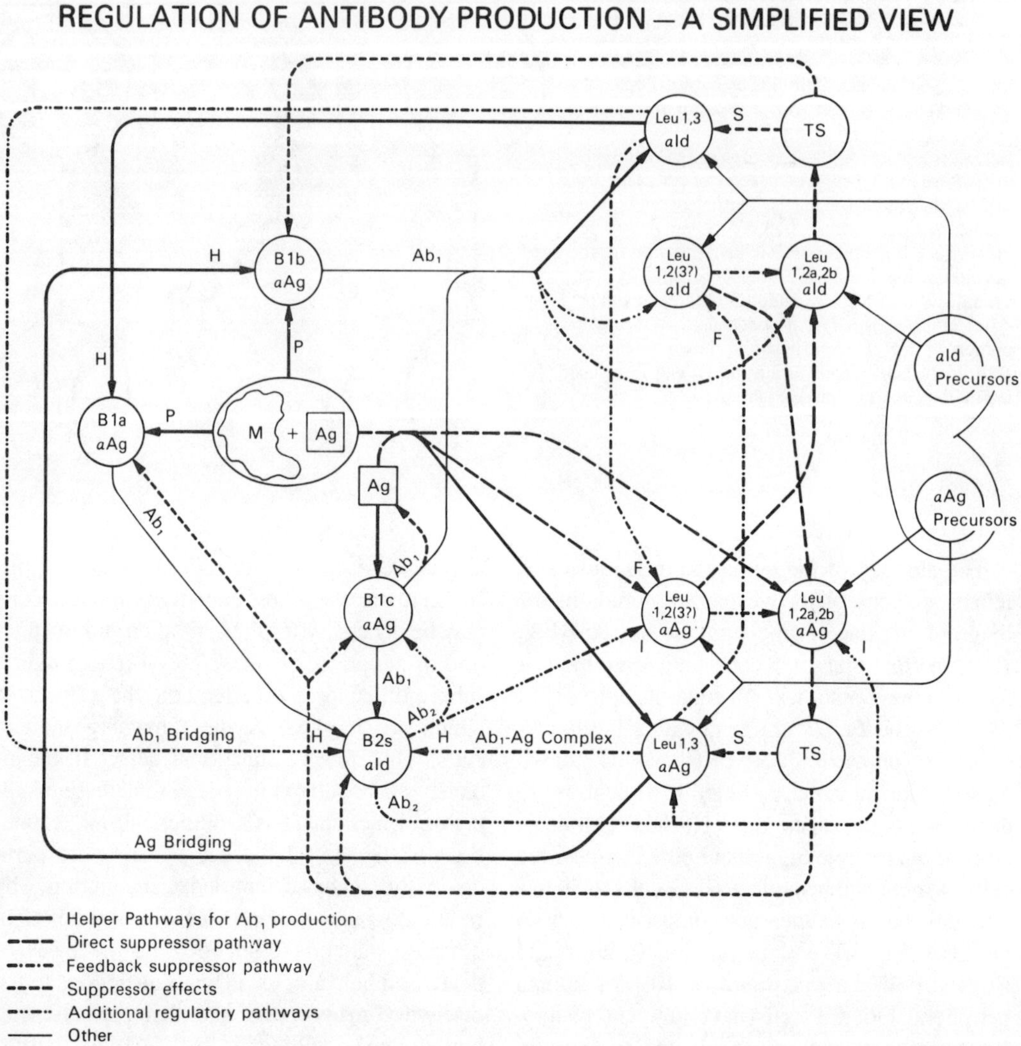

Fig. 10.4 A schematic for the human immune system showing a variety of cellular and humoral feedback loops. This diagram is an analogy from Figure 10.2, which shows the mouse system. The evidence available from the mouse is somewhat greater than that from man. As a result, this diagram is even more tenative than the mouse diagram. Nevertheless, the available human data are compatible with it. In this figure, Leu 1,3 cells represent "helper" cells, and Leu 1,2a,2b cells represent "suppressor" cells; however, because of the network nature of the immune system, such designations are inadequate. The Leu 1,3 cells are analogous to OKT-4 cells and the Leu 1,2a,2b cells are analogous to OKT-8 cells. The importance of Leu 1,2,3 cell is still uncertain. The network functions exactly as has been described in Figure 10.2

Many diseases may be characterized by primary B cell abnormalities, such as impaired or excessive B cell activation. Such events may be associated with abnormal responsiveness of such B cells to immune signals or abnormal regulatory cell function(s). The possibility of analyzing individuals with regard to their T cell subsets allows for the differentiation between primary B cell disorders and secondary B cell disorders. Moreover, understanding the different cellular interactions, and especially the sequential steps of regulation, ultimately should lead to clarification of pathogenetic mechanisms in diseases involving abnormalities of the immune system. Below we will illustrate these points with several human diseases of immune regulation.

A very large number of human diseases are characterized by immune abnormalities. It is often difficult to know whether the immune abnormality is the cause or the result of the disease process. Nevertheless, for many of the diseases, the immune defect appears to be a major feature of the disease. Moreover, one causative abnormality may induce various secondary ones due to the network nature of the immune system. Diseases of man include those characterized by abnormalities in the number or function of T cells, B cells or macrophages. Obviously, any of these defects would represent an abnormality of immune regulation. In the present chapter we will emphasize diseases characterized by abnormalities in regulatory T cell populations and only touch upon the others, which will be dealt with in greater detail in other chapters. A summary of some of the disorders associated with T cell abnormalities is given in Table 10.1.

Before discussing disorders of human immune regulation in detail, it would be helpful to explore how the cellular basis of a disease in the mouse system may be viewed in the diagram presented as Figure 10.2.

Athymic (nude) mice lack mature T cells. These mice can respond efficiently to antigen only with B cells that do not require T cell help. In addition, with inadequate T cells, they cannot produce anti-idiotypic antibody. Finally, they do not have mature T cells to give rise rapidly to effector suppressor cells (Ts). Therefore, these mice fail to respond very well to thymic-dependent antigens. They can respond to antigens which do not require T cell help; however the response is somewhat prolonged in the absence of the usual suppressor circuits. Nude mice fail to reject tumor grafts, succumb to viral infections and may develop autoantibodies (Gershwin et al., 1975; Morse et al., 1974). A more complex disease is murine lupus (Steinberg et al., 1981; Theofilopoulos and Dixon, 1981; Datta and Schwartz, 1978). In this disease, there is an increase in B cell activity prior to deliberate antigenic stimulation; however, there is an associated impaired response to primary immunization. From the diagram, it can be seen that excessive activity of helper circuits or decreased activity of suppressor circuits could be responsible for production of autoantibodies. Moreover, defects in the suppressor circuits could occur at several points. Finally, the excessive B cell activity would be expected to result in a marked increase in suppressor effector cells which would interfere with primary immune responses, but which might not interfere with secondary immune responses (Ranney and Steinberg, 1976). Thus, murine lupus could arise from a defect in anti-Id cells (or a subset of

Table 10.1 Disorders of Immune Regulations—T Cell Abnormalities

Maturation arrest of thymocytes	Severe combined immune deficiency disease
Impaired numbers or functions of inducer T cells for B cells	Common variable hypogammaglobulinemia with B cells; acquired hypogammaglobulinemia
Excess activated suppressor cells	Common variable hypogammaglobulinemia; infectious mononucleosis; lepromatous leprosy; chronic graft vs. host disease; certain viral diseases; certain normals
Reduced R_T (inducer/suppressor ratio)[a]	Common variable hypogammaglobulinemia; certain normals; some patients with autoimmune diseases including Sjogren's syndrome, juvenile rheumatoid arthritis and systemic lupus
Increased R_T	Many patients with autoimmune diseases including systemic lupus, multiple sclerosis, biliary cirrhosis, Sjogren's syndrome, severe atopic eczema, syndroms of excess IgE, graft vs. host disease, kidney allograft rejection

[a]It should be noted that, although the ratio appears to be important, an abnormal ratio (R_T) could be caused by a marked increase in one population or a marked decrease in another, with different causes and consequences; in addition, an abnormality in one subpopulation of either the inducer or suppressor phenotype may or may not be identifiable as an abnormal ratio. For example, a marked decrease in inducers of suppressors might not be revealed in an abnormal ratio if there are adequate numbers of inducers of B cells. This is seen in some patients with autoimmune diseases.

anti-Id cells), anti-Ag cells (or a subset of anti-Ag cells), Lyt 1,2,3 cells, Lyt 1 cells, Lyt 2,3 cells or a defect in the macrophages necessary for the function of these different lymphocytes. Moreover, anti-T cell antibodies and immune complexes may further interfere in the context of already deranged immune regulation. Viral infections as subclinical disease or via polyclonal activation or formation of immune complexes may interfere with normal immune regulation. The multiple potential defects are well reflected in the present knowledge of murine SLE.

Autologous Mixed Lymphocyte Reaction

The in vitro proliferation of T cells to autologous non-T cells has been termed the autologous mixed lymphocyte reaction (AMLR). In man, B cells, ''null'' cells and macrophages appear to stimulate the AMLR. The involvement of Ia or DR determinants on stimulating cells (Yamashita and Shevach, 1980; Weksler et al., 1978) is of great interest. Such a requirement points to Ia as the self-recognition structure necessary for the autologous non-T cell-T cell interaction. This may well be the structure necessary for antigen presentation when non-T cells present antigens to T cells. However, Ia antigens may not be the only ones responsible for stimulation of autologous T cells, since ''null'' cells, which are effective AMLR stimulators, have not been found to bear DR antigens (Kay and Horwitz, 1980). Thus, aside from Ia antigens, T cell stimulation in the AMLR could involve non-Ia antigens encoded by the major histocompatibility complex. Different stimulator populations may act upon different responder cell populations. A subset of macrophages induces proliferation of a defined T cell subset that is involved in antigen recognition (Raff et al., 1980); another macrophage subpopulaton may be responsible for macrophage-induced suppression of the AMLR (Smolen et al., 1981a). An additional indication for cell-cell communication during the AMLR is the generation of helper, suppressor and cytotoxic functions of AMLR-primed T cells in secondary test systems priming (Hausmann and Stobo, 1979; Sakane and Green, 1979; Van de Stouwe et al., 1978). Recent studies indicate that regulation occurs even during a primary AMLR; suppressor T cells act to decrease the proliferative response (Smolen et al., 1981a). It is conceivable that AMLR-activated T cells are involved in the regulation of the function of the non-T cells stimulating the reaction. Thus, in Figure 10.4, a Leu 3 αAg cell may proliferate and induce B cell activation and differentiation; a Leu 3αId cell induces either Leu 2 suppressor or cytotoxic cells to become activated. An entire circuit appears to be operative in the AMLR (Smolen, et al., J. Immunol. Sept. 1982 in press).

Patients with a variety of diseases associated with abnormal immune regulation have been found to be deficient in the so-called autologous mixed lymphocyte reaction (AMLR). What are the common features of diseases such as SLE, primary biliary cirrhosis, Sjögren's syndrome and Hodgkin's disease, in which the AMLR has been reported deficient (Sakane et al., 1978b; James et al., 1980; Miyasaka et al., 1980; Engleman et al., 1980)? A general common feature is the derangement of the immune system. Another common feature is deficient mitogen responsiveness; often there is also deficiency of Con A-induced suppressor cell activity. These patients also have increased numbers of macrophage-like cells in the circulation which may be responsible for macrophage-mediated suppressor effects (Rice et al., 1979). Finally, at least in some of these diseases highly activated B cells and T cells may be found, the latter exemplified by the presence of Ia-positive T cells in the circulation (Yu et al., 1980). Thus, a possible explanation for the deficiency of the AMLR in so many diseases with different regulatory abnormalities may simply be a refractoriness of activated lymphocytes to new stimulatory signals in vitro. Such in vivo activation of T cells, theoretically, may be due to an ongoing AMLR. Not only have activated B cells been shown to be very potent stimulators of the AMLR (James and Strober, 1981), but an in vivo AMLR response would also be consistent with the loss of self-tolerance often observed in these diseases, here involving stimulating B cell antigens. Then, the

AMLR response of healthy individuals, as it is observed in vitro, would reflect a loss of self-tolerance. When this has occurred in vivo, compensatory suppressive factors already may have been released.

The deficient AMLR in disease states may have another basis than in vivo activation involving different points in the regulatory circuit. Any of the following could cause a reduced AMLR: insufficient stimulation by one stimulator cell population or more, numerical or functional deficiency of one responder T cell subset or more to one stimulator cell population or more, increased suppression or decreased induction of the AMLR or a combination of such defects. The apparent importance of the AMLR in immunoregulatory circuits and its derangement in association with a variety of immune diseases suggests that dissection of this phenomenon will lead to greater understanding of the regulatory abnormalities in the individual diseases.

Systemic Lupus Erythematosus as a Model for Autoimmunity

Murine SLE

Mice of the strains MRL/1, BXSB, NZB and (NZB × NZW)F_1 illustrate both the complexity and the variety of immune regulatory abnormalities found in humans with SLE (Steinberg et al., 1981; Theofilopoulos and Dixon, 1981; Datta and Schwartz, 1978; Gershon et al., 1978; Cantor et al., 1978). All manifest B cell hyperactivity, defects in tolerance induction, autoantibody production and immune complex renal disease. Despite the marked immune activity, they have reduced primary immune responses to test antigens. All die prematurely; however, the pace and details of their illnesses vary.

MRL/1 mice have marked proliferation of T cells with a helper phenotype. They produce moderate amounts of antibodies to native DNA and large amounts of anti-single stranded DNA. MRL/1 mice also produce antiglobulins and anti-Sm. Females have somewhat more rapidly progressing disease than do males; however, both sexes die quite prematurely with marked immune complex glomerulonephritis. The disease is ameliorated by neonatal thymectomy (Steinberg et al., 1980). One of the immunoregulatory problems thought to be important in disease development is failure of Lyt 1 cells to be suppresed by Lyt 2,3 suppressor cells. Such a failure could result from a defect in the responses of Lyt 1 cells to suppressive signals. Alternatively, the Lyt 1 cells may be unable to effectively interact with Lyt 1,2,3 cells to induce adequate suppressor function (See Fig. 10.2). The MRL/1 mouse is characterized by B cell hyperactivity unresponsive to normal immune regulatory signals. However, these MRL/1 mice have marked proliferation of a T cell subset which usually subserves inducer function (Theofilopoulos and Dixon, 1981; Warner, 1980). The autoimmune phenomena in these mice may be induced by such Lyt 1 cells which drive B cells, but which fail to function normally in response to suppressor signals (Gershon et al., 1978). The resulting proliferation of Lyt 1 cells leads to marked lymph node enlargement. Androgen administration has a beneficial effect upon the autoimmune process of these mice. Whether or not the androgens act on regulatory pathways has not been determined; however, we believe that it is likely that the androgens act to alter maturation of cells in the pathway from marrow pre-T cells to mature thymocytes in such a manner that suppressor function is augmented and helper function is reduced.

Mice of the (NZB × NZW) F_1 cross show an even more marked amelioration of disease with androgen therapy. These mice develop immune complex glomerulonephritis and large amounts of antibodies to double- and single-stranded DNA. These features of illness can be almost completely suppressed by administration of androgens from very early in life. However, whereas thymectomy essentially prevents disease in MRL/1 mice, it accelerates the disease of (NZB × NZW) F_1 mice, suggesting that the latter have a deficiency of suppressor function (Steinberg et al., 1970, 1980). Thus, the role of the thymus in disease production may be different in the two SLE models and yet the beneficial effects of androgens may be very similar. It is likely that androgens can act at several steps in the immune system. Thus, they might be capable of effectively altering more than one type of immunoregulatory abnormality. (NZB × NZW) F_1 mice have been shown to lose T-dependent suppression with age (Steinberg and Klassen, 1977), although non-T cell suppressor mechanisms may increase with age (Roder et al., 1975). This former defect may stem from an inability to activate Lyt 1,2,3 suppressor cell precursors by signals from Lyt 1 inducers (Cantor et al., 1978). The latter appears to result from marked immune hyperactivity which characterizes the autoimmune state. Although both MRL/1 and (NZB × NZW) F_1 mice have B cell hyperactivity, the T cell abnormalities appear to be important to the ultimate clinical illness. This is especially true of MRL/1 mice, which do not get very ill if they are thymectomized.

BXSB mice manifest much less in the way of antibodies to DNA than do MRL/1 or (NZB × NZW) F_1 mice. The BSXB females do not get sick early in life, whereas the males die quite prematurely. The sex difference appears unrelated to sex hormones; it is attributed rather to some factor on the Y chromosome which accelerates disease in an autoimmune susceptible strain. The factor is expressed in the stem cells of the male as demonstrated by adoptive transfer experiments. Theofilopoulos and Dixon, (1981).

NZB mice, which are the most studied of all strains, develop disease rather late in life. These mice make only small amounts of anti-DNA; they produce large amounts of antibodies to T cells and erythrocytes. They manifest marked B cell hyperactivity which terminates in splenic hyperdiploidy and a poorly differentiated malignancy in many mice. Others die with severe hemolytic anemia or immune complex renal disease. The full expression of disease in NZB mice requires a number of genes (estimated to be at least six), although individual traits may be controlled by fewer genes (Raveche et al., 1981). For example, anti-DNA and anti-T cell antibodies are largely regulated by independent single genes. Similar studies on background genes for BXSB and MRL/1 mice are not yet available; however; the 1pr/1pr gene can impose upon other strains both lymphoproliferation and autoantibody production, suggesting that this single gene is very important in the development of autoimmunity in association with the appropriate ''background'' genes of several strains.

The marked B cell hyperactivity in NZB mice begins before birth. Nevertheless, an immune regulatory defect may be very important for disease expression. A defect in numbers of Lyt 1,2,3 cells has been described for these mice. As a result, they may be unable to manifest feedback suppression (see Fig. 10.2). According to this concept, Lyt 1 cells do not find adequate numbers of Lyt 1,2,3 cells to act as intermediaries on the way to Lyt 2,3 cells and ultimately the TS effector. Moreover, NZB thymocytes interfere with the development of tolerance and contribute to autoantibody production. Recent studies indicate that NZB thymocytes are sufficient to interfere with tolerance induction in females, whereas in males NZB thymocytes are not sufficient to prevent tolerance; an abnormal B cell is also necessary (Laskin et al., 1981). Thus, androgens apparently can allow the immune system of the organism to be more grossly deranged before autoimmunity is fully expressed.

Despite the marked immune hyperactivity of young SLE-prone mice, older mice actively exhibiting autoimmunity are hyporesponsive to primary immunization. They have marked impairment in responses to mitogens, cell mediated immunity and humoral immunity. Some of these defects relate to suppressive factors released by monocytes as a result of the marked spontaneous immune hyperactivity associated with the autoimmune state.

What do the various mice tell us about the pathogenesis of SLE? First, they indicate that the genetic basis of the illness may be different and yet still be called lupus. Secondly, murine lupus may have different cellular bases. Moreover, the details of the immunoregulatory defects may be different in different strains. Even studies of mice not prone to develop autoimmunity have shed light upon the development of SLE. For example, administration of polyclonal activators, which accelerate disease in autoimmune mice (Steinberg et al., 1969), induce anti-DNA and other autoantibodies in nonautoimmune mice (Louis and Lambert, 1979). Moreover, thymectomy may be associated with autoimmune features, presumably because of removal of cells necessary for suppressor circuits (Steinberg et al., 1970; Yunis et al., 1967. A combination of these two procedures, thymectomy plus administration of polyclonal B cell activators, has led to the rapid development of autoimmunity. Moreover, anti-DNA production was markedly inhibited by the presence of a thymus (Smith et al., 1981). Thus, at least two factors appear to be important to the development of autoimmunity; these are impaired T cell regulation and polyclonal B cell activation.

Human SLE

From the animal studies, it might be expected that analysis of human SLE might be hopelessly complex. We do not have highly inbred human populations, we cannot do thymectomy or cell transfer studies and we cannot alter sexually before puberty. Perhaps most importantly, we cannot study humans with SLE prior to the development of illness. Thus, the defects observed during active disease may result from, rather than cause, the illness. From a practical point of view, we usually have to settle for peripheral blood for most studies and use marrow, spleen and lymph nodes much less often. Moreover, in the overwhelming majority of instances we can only get the blood after the disease process is already in progress and often only after some treatment has been instituted. Despite these tremendous disadvantages, the picture of human SLE is becoming clearer. Most of the human studies are based upon concepts developed in mice. Humans with active SLE, like mice, have markedly increased B cell activity manifested by hypergammaglobulinemia, autoantibody production, Ig production in vitro (reverse plague assay) and circulating activated B-cells. In contrast, T cell functions are generally reduced. There is impaired skin reactivity to test antigens and decreased in vitro responses. They also have immune regulatory abnormalities. These are common but not universal. In fact, we should expect that there might be people with immune abnormalities rather like the various mice with SLE-like illnesses. However, to date, most of the studies have emphasized defects in suppressor cell generation (Abdou et al., 1976; Fauci et al., 1978; Sakane et al., 1978a). Many investigators have found that patients with active SLE have defective suppressor cell function. This has been found for systems involving and not involving mitogen-activated cells. It appears that the defect in suppressor function is one of failure to produce adequate suppressor signals for the responding population rather than a defect in receiving suppressor signals. Whether this represents a defect in or deficit of suppressor cell precursors or their differentiation has not yet been elucidated. However, some patients with SLE have normal suppressor function (Sakane, et al. 1978a). Moreover, some patients produce antibodies which preferentially interact with suppressor cells or cells necessary for suppression (Sakane et al., 1979). As a result, it is very difficult to determine whether the antibodies or the cellular abnormalities came first.

Furthermore, many of the T cell deficiencies of active SLE patients may result from the disease process, as appears to be the case in mice with active disease. Thus, impaired responses to skin testing and other defects may result from the autoimmune activity rather than be a clue to its pathogenesis.

Family studies suggest that defective suppressor cell activity may be a genetic trait (Miller and Schwartz, 1979) and may require additional abnormalities to become a pathogenic factor. In addition, a defect in inducer cell activity may be present in SLE patients, concomitant with or independent of suppressor cell abnormalities (Delfraissey et al., 1980). A combination of such defects may result from a failure of feedback-inhibitory circuits (Heijnen et al., 1980). As human T cells become better defined, it may be possible to examine in detail various regulatory circuits suggested in Figure 10.4 and define patients with abnormalities at different points, all with the same symptom complex we call SLE. Thus, many patients with SLE have a defect in T cells with the suppressor phenotype (Morimoto et al., 1980). However, a study in additional patients of ratios of helper cell phenotype to suppressor cell phenotype (R_T = % helper/% suppressor) suggests a correlation with certain clinical features. Patients without renal disease appear to be more likely to have high R_T (Smolen et al., 1982a). These studies suggest that there are subtypes of human SLE analogous to subtypes of mouse SLE. This is reflected by differences in clinical features, T cell subsets and immunoregulatory pathways and genetic differences. The genetic heterogeneity of non-inbred humans may be responsible for a much more diverse group of defects than is found in inbred mice. Nevertheless, the same principles appear to apply to humans as had been found for mice.

Immunoregulatory Abnormalities in Rheumatoid Arthritis Syndromes

Adult Rheumatoid Arthritis (RA)

Several recent investigations in human RA have revealed a derangement of immunoregulatory processes. For example, a deficiency of Con A-inducible suppressor cells has been found in patients with RA. This deficiency is most pronounced in active early RA and may be accompanied by anti-T cell antibodies (Abdou et al., 1979). In later stages, the suppressor cell deficiency is only minimal and involves primarily patients who are not treated with remission-inducing drugs (Smolen et al., 1981c). Synovial lymphocytes, however, may lack spontaneous and Con A-inducible suppressors at all stages (Chattopadhyay et al., 1979).

A more specific regulatory deficiency has been suggested by investigations of the association of RA with Epstein-Barr virus (EBV) infection. RA patients have circulating antibodies to a nuclear antigen of EBV-infected cells (RANA) (Alspaugh et al., 1978). In addition, their lymphocytes undergo enhanced transformation into lymphoblastoid cell lines after EBV inoculation (Bardwick et al., 1980). In fact, RA lymphocytes tend to transform spontaneously into cell lines much more often than do normal lymphocytes (Vaughan, 1979). Taken together, these data hint at a possible defect in EBV-specific suppressor cells. Such a defect has recently been demonstrated. EBV-induced immunoglobulin secretion by RA B lymphocytes is not suppressed in vitro by RA T cells (Tosato et al., 1981). This is in contrast to EBV-stimulated lymphocytes from normal patients and even patients with SLE, in whom suppression of EBV-induced Ig synthesis is normal. It is also in contrast to suppression of mitogen-induced immunoglobulin production which is normal in the same RA patients. These results suggest that EBV might be an important pathogenetic factor in the induction or perpetuation of RA. They also indicate that a specific suppressor T cell defect could be responsible for uncontrolled autoantibody production by B cells following stimulation with EBV virus. The polyclonal B cell activation and the resulting inflammatory processes could lead to production of antibodies to collagen (Steffen, 1970; Menzel et al., 1978) and the production of anti-immunoglobulins (Steffen, 1970; Johnson and Faulk, 1976). In addition, a suppressor cell defect predisposes to autoreactivity against collagen (Smolen et al., 1981c; Solinger and Stobo, 1981). Finally, RA patients may also manifest excessive secretion by lymphocytes of soluble products, which enhance fibroblast proliferation and collagen synthesis (Johnson and Ziff, 1976).

Although the in vitro studies of immune regulation in RA are preliminary, the abnormalities are consistent with recent studies of T cell phenotypes. Increased R_T has been found in peripheral blood from RA patients and increased as well as decreased R_T was observed using synovial lymphocytes (Fox and Vaughan, 1981). Thus, as in SLE, the symptom complex of RA may be common to a variety of regulatory abnormalities. This assumption is in accordance with the differences in disease courses and manifestations of RA in individual patients, as well as with the demonstration of differences in disease features in patients with different genetic backgrounds (Scherak et al., 1981).

Juvenile Rheumatoid Arthritis (JRA)

The clinical heterogeneity of JRA, which can be a pauci-articular, a polyarticular or a systemic disease, makes different regulatory abnormalities in its pathogenesis at least as plausible as in SLE or RA. Recent studies have revealed that patients with active JRA lack a subset of inducer T cells which are necessary for the induction of mature suppressor cells from presuppressor cells (Morimoto et al., 1981). In the absence of adequate inducer function, there is markedly impaired suppression of in vitro immunoglobulin synthesis. The same patients had circulating antibodies which bound to a normal T cell subset which participated in suppression. These antibodies could bring about reduced suppression by interfering with the function of a suppressor cell and/or an inducer cell for suppressor cells possibly participating in feedback inhibitory circuits. These data would suggest that, according to Figure 10.4, a Leu 3 inducer cell failed (because of inadequate numbers or functional defects) to induce a Leu 1,2,3 precursor cell to signal or differentiate into a Leu 2 suppressor cell. Consistent with this formulation, analysis of T cell subsets has revealed a decrease in active JRA of the phenotypical inducer cell population, thereby yielding a low R_T (Morimoto et al., 1981).

The immunoregulatory effects of JRA antilymphocyte antibody are reported to be mimicked by immune complexes or even monomeric IgG (Froelich et al., 1981). Thus, it may be anticipated that further studies of JRA T cell populations by phenotyping and functional analyses may reveal a variety of regulatory abnormalities. Such a heterogeneity would not only be in accordance with the different clinical subsets, but also with differences between these subsets in the expression of autoantibodies to collagen (Steffen et al., 1980) and in MHC-coded antigens (Stastny and Fink, 1979).

"Organ-specific" Autoimmune Diseases

"Organ-specific" autoimmune diseases are characterized by the occurrence of humoral and cellular immune reactivity to organ-specific autoantigens, in conrast to nonspecific ones such as DNA, immunoglobulin and collagen. Organ-specific autoimmune diseases include juvenile onset, insulin-dependent diabetes (IDD), Graves' disease, chronic thyroiditis (Hashimoto), idiopathic Addison's disease, pernicious anemia and myasthenia gravis.

Juvenile Onset Insulin-dependent Diabetes Mellitus (IDD)

In IDD (type I diabetes), a viral infection (Coxsackie B, mumps) causing pancreatic insulitis may trigger the disease (Craighead, 1981; Nerup and Lernmark, 1981). The participation of immunologic mechanisms in the pathogenesis is indicated by the presence of autoantibodies, as well as by the association with certain HLA antigens. Differences in the expression of autoantibodies and HLA antigens in groups of patients with IDD have indicated a heterogeneity of this disease. IDD patients with HLA B8/DR 3 are more often female, have persistence of anti-islet cell antibodies beyond the period of early disease and autoantibodies to other organ-specific antigens and tend to develop polyendocrine disease. These features are uncommon in IDD patients bearing HLA B15/DR4, who tend to have an early onset of the disease and often develop antibodies to exogenously administered insulin (Rotter and Rimoin, 1981). Such differences have prompted the postulate of three groups of IDD; these are viral induced IDD, autoimmune IDD and an overlapping group (Irvine, 1977). Thus, one subtype of IDD could be associated with an abnormal immune response to viral antigens. Studies in mice infected with diabetogenic virus have indicated that T cells are necessary for the genesis of this disease, since athymic (nude) mice, but not their crosses, are resistant to the development of diabetes. Furthermore, androgens which normally act to increase suppressor cell activity enhance the development of virally induced diabetes mellitus (Craighead, 1981). Thus, in the context of our diagram, one could envisage a (virus-specific) increased TS activity (Leu 2αAg) impairing rapid elimination of the virus. The other subtype of IDD, possibly also triggered by environmental agents, has an islet cell-specific B cell hyperactivity as its major pathogenic principle. A TS deficiency may be associated, and accompanied polyclonal B cell activation leading to a variety of autoantibody responses in a genetically predisposed individual may ultimately result in polyendocrine disease. (A similiar genetic and immunologic heterogeneity is found in chronic active hepatitis.) In contrast to IDD, immunoregulatory abnormalities do not account for non-insulin-dependent diabetes mellitus (type II). These patients, in contrast to IDD patients, have no indication of insulitis and no marked decrease in pancreatic islet cells and are very often hyperinsulinemic and obese. Abnormalities in responsiveness to insulin and/or the release of insulin are the cause of the disease. Although genetic predisposition is clearly involved, it is not associated with the HLA complex in type II diabetes. Finally, in some patients, diabetes is due to the blocking activity of autoantibodies to the insulin receptor. Patients with these antibodies often have acathosis nigricans and/or SLE or Sjoegren's syndrome (Kahn, 1980). The antireceptor antibodies may be due to an immunologic reaction against receptor molecules. Alternatively, they can be regarded as anti-idiotype antibodies to anti-insulin antibodies (Sege and Peterson, 1978) (Ab2 in Fig. 10.4).

Thyroid Disorders, Addison's Disease and Pernicious Anemia

Circulating stimulating antibodies to the TSH receptor are a hallmark of Graves' disease (Adams et al., 1974). In contrast, chronic thyroiditis may be accompanied by blocking antibodies to the TSH receptor which prevent the regeneration of thyroid cells (Drexhage et al., 1981). Autoantibodies to thyroglobulin and thyroid microsomes are commonly observed in thyroiditis and are less often found in Graves' disease. The induction of an experimental Hashimoto-like thyroiditis by injection of thyroglobulin makes this antigen attractive as a pathogenetic agent. A combination of genetic predisposition, insufficient tolerance to thyroglobulin and triggering environmental agents may be responsible for the development of the disease. However, other thyroid antigens may also induce disease. Moreover, spontaneous thyroiditis in animals is regulated by multiple genes and by thymic function. Neonatally thymectomized buffalo rats have a marked acceleration of thyroiditis. In man, viral induced thyroiditis may cause an inflammatory response sufficient to allow release of thyroid antigens into the circulation so as to lead to immunization. Genetic susceptibility to such immunization may be critical. Two genes may be necessary, one for generalized immune hyperactivity or defective regulation and one for response to thyroid antigens. The antibody response appears to be critical to disease development. Subsequently, lymphocytes infiltrate the gland. We believe that ADCC is an important mechanism of thyroid destruction.

Very similar causes may lead to idiopathic Addison's disease, which is characterized by autoantibodies to adrenal cell antigens and cellular abnormalities in response to such antigens (Irvine, 1978a).

Patients with autoimmune pernicious anemia and the associated atrophic gastritis develop antibodies to gastric parietal cells and to intrinsic factor; the latter may be regarded as antireceptor antibodies, since they very commonly block the formation of the intrinsic factor–Vitamin B12 complex. The high incidence of pernicious anemia in patients with hypogammaglobulinemia suggests that additional mechanisms such as bacterial overgrowth of the stomach may contribute to disease expression.

Myasthenia Gravis

In myasthenia gravis, autoantibodies to the acetylcholine receptor of striated muscle may be responsible for receptor destruction and disease manifestations (Drachman, 1978). The associated thymic hyperplasia or thymoma in the majority of the cases, as well as the beneficial effects of thymectomy in this disease, suggests participation of regulatory abnormalities, probably excessive helper function relative to suppressor function. This could be excessive activity of a subset of cells subserving anti-Id helper function without adequate counterbalancing suppressor function. The acetylcholine receptor of thymic myoid cells may be the initial target of the abnormal immune response. Alternatively, or in addition, thymic hormones may play an important role since thymectomy does not improve myasthenia gravis if (ectopic?) thymic hormone production is sustained (Twomey et al., 1979).

General Considerations

The organ-specific autoimmune diseases discussed here have much more in common than organ specificity. Additionally, a variety of organ-specific autoantibodies may be found in relatives of patients with such diseases; patients with organ-specific autoimmunity tend to have autoantibodies against antigens of uninvolved organs (Irvine, 1978b); anti-receptor autoantibodies are observed or even pathogenetic; some patients have polyendocrine autoimmune disease, often associated with myasthenia gravis (Rose, 1980); and, with the exception of subacute thyroiditis and a subtype of IDD, all diseases are associated with HLA DR3 (Bernoco and Terasaki, 1978). These common denominators are a very strong argument for a common immunoregulatory aberration in the majority of organ-specific autoimmune diseases. Minute differences in genetic predisposition, abnormal handling of environmental agents or loss of tolerance to specific antigens, alone or in combination, may be responsible for the selection of the target organ. The common abnormality may lie primarily in an immunoregulatory defect. For example, such a defect might be hyperactivity of antigen-specific T helper cells or one which predisposes to the production of anti-idiotype antibodies since such antibodies may react with receptor molecules. Such a formulation would suggest that these diseases result from excessive immune regulation. This would contrast with the organ nonspecific diseases, in which immune regulation appears to be inadequate rather than excessive. However, both kinds of diseases could be initiated by excessive responsiveness. What is observed in the organ-specific disease is a reaction of activation of a specific regulatory pathway which is especially active. In contrast, in the nonspecific diseases, the major attempts at control are toward TS production and those are inadequate to control the initiating processes.

Other Disorders of Immunoregulation

Celiac Disease and Dermatitis Herpetiformis

In celiac disease, the wheat protein gliadin induces antibodies and cellular reactions in susceptible individuals (Strober et al., 1975). An immune complex type of inflammatory reaction occurs at the site of gliadin absorption in the jejunum. A gliadin-free diet leads to complete remission of the disease. Thus, a genetically determined abnormality in the handling of gliadin leads to an immune-mediated disease. Moreover, the same antigen seems to be of major importance in the pathogenesis of dermatitis herpetiformis (DH), in which gliadin-antigliadin complexes may play a pathogenetic role and which is ameliorated by cessation of gliadin intake (Katz et al., 1981). The association with HLA DR3 is similar to that of celiac disease (Bernoco and Terasaki, 1978) and some patients with DH may have asymptomatic bowel involvement. The similarities between DH and CD are astounding. One may assume that the different diseases result from minimal differences in the regulation of the immune response to gliadin leading to circulating IgA-antigliadin-gliadin immune complexes in one and fixation of antigliadin antibodies in the gut in the other. These diseases are related to many of the preceding diseases, especially in the HLA DR3 association; however, here an initiating antigen has been identified.

Hepatitis B Virus-associated Diseases

Hepatitis B virus (HBV) is associated with chronic active hepatitis (CAH), polyarteritis nodosa (PAN) and essential mixed cryoglobulinemia (EMC). Although patients with PAN and EMC may also suffer from subclinical to severe liver disease, the differences in clinical and serological features between these diseases are consistent with different responses to HBV infection. An abnormal immune response to the virus itself may secondarily initiate autoimmune responses to liver proteins (Vyas et al., 1978).

The immune complexes in EMC are different from those in PAN; in the former rheumatoid factor production and monoclonal antibodies are often observed (Gorevic et al., 1980). Moreover, some immunoglobulins present in the cryoprecipitate have anti-idiotype specificity (Geltner et al., 1980). Most patients with these HBV-associated diseases are male. In contrast, females with similar diseases tend not to have evidence of HBV infection. The CAH found in women is associated with HLA DR3 and responds better to corticosteroid therapy. The male predominance in HBV-associated chronic diseases may be related to a relative deficiency of the male immune system, as compared to the female one, in mounting a sufficient immune response to the virus (Drews et al., 1978). This results in circulating immune complexes and organ-localized immune disease. Similar pathogenic effects of chronic viral infection with virus-anti-virus complexes are observed in many animal species. Ironically, treatment with immunosuppressive drugs may reduce antibody production and improve the disease process without altering the underlying viral infection.

Epstein-Barr Virus-associated Diseases

Epstein-Barr virus (EBV) infections have received major attention in connection with immune regulation in recent years. It has been known for more than a decade that EBV is the cause of a benign lymphoid disease [infectious mononucleosis (IM)], a malignant lymphoid disease (Burkitt's lymphoma) and an epithelial malignancy (nasopharyngeal carcinoma).

B lymphocytes are the target lymphoid cells for infection by this herpes virus. The result is marked B cell stimulation and proliferation. In infectious mononucleosis, this event is followed by benign T cell proliferation. The T cells bear surface antigens characteristic of the suppressor/cytotoxic cell subset (DeWaele et al., 1981) and exert vigorous suppressor cell activity (Tosato et al., 1981). There is an associated loss of responsiveness (anergy) to other antigens. In addition, antilymphocyte antibodies are produced. Only rarely is IM a lethal disease in man. In certain regions, especially in Africa, EBV infection leads to the development of Burkitt's lymphoma in children. Whether the lymphomagenesis is due to infection with EBV early in life or to additional environmental factors, such as chronic infections, is not known. The EBV-infected cells exhibit a surface antigen which is a specific target for cytotoxic T cells of IM patients (Svedmyr and Jondal, 1975). It appears that defects in the regulation of the immune response to EBV are essential in the development of this malignancy. Thus, an EBV-specific suppressor cell defect may turn a benign EBV-induced illness into a malignancy. The possible association between EBV infection and rheumatoid arthritis discussed above points to the further heterogeneity of abnormal responses to infection with this virus.

Graft Versus Host Disease

Patients receiving bone marrow transplants frequently have developed graft versus host disease (GVHD). This result has allowed investigators to better understand human immune regulation and its relationship to studies in experimental animals. Patients with acute graft versus host disease were found to lack a subset of T cells which functionally subserved suppression. Patients with chronic graft versus host disease were heterogeneous; some had decreased suppressor cells and others had increased numbers of suppressor cells. Both acute and chronic diseases were characterized by T cells bearing Ia antigens, indicating activation (Reinherz et al.,

1979b). These studies indicate that immune regulatory abnormalities are associated with human graft versus host disease. By themselves, the results might not be either very interesting or very surprising. However, graft versus host disease has been associated with the development of autoimmune disease in humans and in experimental animals. In experimental animals, in addition to the development of an illness resembling systemic lupus erythematosus, graft versus host disease may result in the development of lymphoid malignancy (Gleichmann et al., 1978). Thus, an abnormality of immune regulation associated with autoimmunity may be characterized by a loss of suppressor cells. The loss of suppressor cells and the profound immune stimulation characterizing GVHD may be sufficient to cause autoimmunity. However, in some affected individuals it may be possible for the previously intact immune system to activate feedback regulatory circuits resulting in the supply of large numbers of suppressor cells. Whether or not such cells might be capable of retarding or preventing subsequent autoimmune disease is unknown. However, an autoimmune process may be associated initially with reduced suppressor function and later, during the full-blown illness, increased suppressor function (Ranney and Steinberg, 1976). Thus analysis late in the illness may not be adequate to point to pathogenetic factors.

Additional Factors Affecting Disorders of Immune Regulation

Having defined and discussed some aspects of normal immune regulation and some immunologic sequelae of its dysfunction, we will focus upon additional factors that influence the balance of the immune system in health and disease. Although the *genetics* of immunologically mediated diseases have not yet been resolved, the association of many of these diseases with genes coding for specific HLA antigens implies that these individuals are more prone to develop abnormalities within the immunoregulatory circuits than are others. Details of these associations and of the importance of genes within the major histocompatibility complex have been outlined in Chapter 4. However, it is obvious that the specific defects that lead to the expression of a specific disease may be governed by different genes in different diseases, even though they may be linked to the same major histocompatibility gene. Thus, HLA DR3 has been found associated with IDD, celiac disease, Graves' disease, Addison's disease, chronic active hepatitis, pernicious anemia, Sjogren's syndrome and systemic lupus erythematosus; HLA DR4 is highly increased in rheumatoid arthritis, IDD and chronic active hepatitis (Bernoco and Terasaki, 1978). Obviously a single gene defect cannot explain all of the diseases linked to one HLA antigen. Either additional genes or important environmental differences (or both) must account for differences in disease expression. Moreover, a genetic disease predisposition may be primarily nonspecific and its evolution into a specific disease be dependent upon the environmental agent triggering the process and the immunoregulatory balance at that time or thereafter. However, the multifactorial and multigenic nature of SLE in mice (Steinberg et al., 1981; Raveche et al., 1981) suggests that human diseases may also be multifactorial in pathogenesis.

Nutritional factors can influence the immune status importantly. Simple dietary manipulations have been shown to influence the prognosis of murine SLE and also of human "degenerative" cardiovascular diseases. Since the latter may have some immunologic basis (Mathews et al., 1971; Smolen et al., 1978), this aspect should not be neglected with regard to its possible effects upon immune regulation. Moreover, recent studies of the effects of lipoproteins upon immune regulation indicate substantial interrelationships with the immune system (Curtiss and Edgington, 1981; Prickett, et al 1981).

Related to the nutritional aspects are the *sex hormone effects* upon the immune system. Estrogens tend to increase the ratio of helper to suppressor function, whereas androgens tend to reduce that ratio. In nonautoimmune mice, androgens reduce most immune responses. Thus, the increased incidence of autoimmune disease in (NZB × NZW)F_1 females, and in human females, fits with the basic suppressive effects of androgens on immunity and stimulatory effects of estrogens. However the details of the cellular mechanisms involved in sex hormone-mediated effects are not yet elucidated. In fact, there may be effects at multiple steps in maturation, as well as on different cell types. Androgens may increase suppressor effects by acting upon bone marrow precursors. These cells are characterized by the enzyme 20-hydroxysteroid dehydrogenase, the expression of which is influenced by androgens (Fuks and Weinstein, 1979). Furthermore, effects of sex hormones upon the maturation of T cells in the thymus are also likely, since thymic epithelium contains receptors for both androgens and estrogens (Raveche et al., 1980; Siiteri et al., 1980). Androgens may also indirectly affect T cell function, since the production of anti-T cell antibodies in mice can be abrogated by androgens (Raveche et al., 1976). These theoretical effects of sex hormones may have profound effects in practice; androgens markedly retard disease of (NZB × NZW)F_1 and MRL/1 mice (Steinberg et al., 1981).

The occurrence of *autoantibodies to lymphocytes* in a varity of autoimmune and lymphoproliferative diseases is a potential explanation for some functional defects. Some antibodies from patients with SLE and JRA may specifically react with T cell subsets involved in suppressor functions (Sakane et al., 1979; Morimoto et al., 1981). These antibodies can eliminate regulatory T cells by complement-mediated killing, ADCC and opsonization and uptake by the reticuloendothelial system (Kumagai et al., 1981). However, such anti-T cell antibodies tend to occur in active disease rather than during inactive phases and thus they may result from the immune stimulation associated with the disease itself. Moreover, some of the observed effects with autoimmune sera may be due to immune complexes. However, the mere binding to cell surface antigens of either antibodies or immune complexes may perturb the normal function or traffic of the cell. This perturbation need not be uniform, since we know from studies on B cell activation that in vitro treatment with anti-immunoglobulin may polyclonally activate these cells, whereas administration of anti-immunoglobulins to cells from newborn animals suppresses B cells (Lawton and Cooper, 1974; Gausset et al., 1976).

Regulatory effects of *immune complexes* have been much less appreciated than their effects in eliciting inflammatory responses. However, the presence of Fc receptors on a variety of cell populations makes the Fc part of the immune complex an attractive modulatory molecule. Not only can such complexes activate macrophages and thereby enhance macrophage associated immunoregulatory processes, but fragments derived from the Fc part of the immunoglobulin molecule can induce suppression of antibody responses to the complex-bound antigen via activation of the feedback-inhibitory loop (Rao et al., 1980).

Summary

A number of diseases are characterized by immune abnormalities. It is clear that at least some of these diseases have at their bases a fundamental derangement of the immune system. These may be reflected in immune deficiencies and secondary immunoregulatory problems. An additional group of diseases with immune abnormalities appears to be more complex in terms of pathogenesis. Many of these are multifactorial; that is, multiple factors combine to bring about the illness. For example, a disease may result from genetic factors, an environmental trigger, an immune defect and the absence or presence of androgens. Many such diseases are properly viewed as diseases of immune regulation; however, it must be recognized that additional factors may be critical to disease development. Moreover, for certain of these diseases, defects in different parts of the immunoregulatory circuit may each be capable of bringing about the same clinical syndrome. Finally, the secondary immunoregulatory abnormalities may be very important clinically. In other words, although one immunoregulatory problem may be responsible for disease initiation, other immunoregulatory defects may be most prominent during the active illness. The latter may require even more attention, with regard to therapy, than the former.

Our current ability to define subsets of cells which participate in human immune regulation is still quite limited. We are able to appreciate subsets of T cells, B cells and macrophages; however, precise functional subsets have not been fully defined. We are limited to only the crudest separation by the available monoclonal antibodies to lymphocyte subsets. Moreover, the immunoregulatory circuits presented herein are only tentative; they may evolve as our information about the immune system becomes more precise. As a result, we have only been able to hint at diseases with particular immunoregulatory abnormalities. These are based upon carefully performed studies. Nevertheless, we anticipate that as more data become available, the defects will be better defined. In addition, we have included discussions of environmental agents such as dietary substances and viruses. Such agents are critical as triggers for many diseases. By themselves, they may be incapable of inducing the pathologic changes we recognize as an illness. However, without them the same underlying abnormalities of the host may also not yield the illness. It is becoming clearer that one must understand not only host abnormalities, but also the factors which serve to trigger an illness.

We conclude that many human illnesses are caused by and/or result in diseases of immune regulation. A fuller understanding of these diseases will result in better knowledge of the immune system in general and should provide a basis for intelligent approaches to therapy of these disorders.

References

Abdou, N.I., Pascual, F., and Pacela, L.S. 1979. Suppressor T cell dysfunction and anti suppressor T cell antibody in active early rheumatoid arthritis. Arthritis Rheum 22:486.

Abdou, N.I., Sagawa, A., Pascual, E., Herbert, J., and Sadhegee, S. 1976. Suppressor T cell abnormality in idiopathic system lupus erythematosus. Clin Immunol Immunopathol 6:192–199.

Abramson, C.S., Kersey, J.H., and LeBien, T.W. 1981. A monoclonal antibody (BA-1) reactive with cells of human B lymphocyte lineage. J Immunol 126:83–88.

Adams, D.D., Kennedy, T.H., and Stewart, R.D. 1974. Correlation between long-acting thyroid stimulator protector levels and thyroid ^{131}I uptake. Brit Med J 2:199.

Ahmed, A., Scher, I., Sharrow, S.O., Smith, A.H., Paul, W.E., Sachs, D.H., and Sell, K.W. 1977. B lymphocyte heterogeneity development of an alloantiserum which distinguishes B lymphocyte differentiation alloantigens. J Exp Med 145:101.

Alspaugh, M.A., Jensen, F.C., Robin, H., and Tan, E.M. 1978. Lymphocytes transformed by Epstein-Barr virus: Induction of nuclear antigen reactive with antibody in rheumatoid arthritis. J Exp Med 147:1018–1027.

Bardwick, P.A., Bluestein, H.G., Zvaifler, N.J., Depper, J.M., and Seegmiller, J.E. 1980. Altered regulation of Epstein-Barr virus induced lymphoblast proliferation in rheumatoid arthritis lymphoid cells. Arthritis Rheum 23:626–632.

Bernoco, D., and Terasaki, P.I. 1978. HLA-D and disease. In: Genetic Control of Autoimmune Disease, eds. N.R. Rose, P.E. Bigazzi, and N.L. Warner, pp. 3–11. Elsevier-North Holland; New York.

Cantor, H., and Boyse, E.A. 1976. Regulation of cellular and humoral immune responses by T-cell subclasses. Cold Spring Harbor Symp Quant Biol 41:23.

Cantor, H., McVay-Bourdreau, L., Hugenberger, J., Naidorf, F., Shen, F.W., and Gershon, R.K. 1978. Immunoregulatory circuits among T-cell sets. II. Physiologic role of feedback inhibition in vivo: Absence in NZB mice. J Exp Med 147:1116.

Chattopadhyay, C., Chattopadhyay, H., Natvig, J.B., and Mellbye, O.J. 1979. Rheumatoid synovial lymphocytes lack concanavalin-A-activated suppressor cell activity. Scand J Immunol 10:479–486.

Claman, H.N., Chaperon, E.A., and Triplett, R.F. 1966. Immunocompetence of transferred thymus marrow combinations. J Immunol 97:928.

Cohen, S., Pick, E., and Oppenheim, J.J., eds. 1978. Biology of the Lymphokines. Academic Press; New York.

Cowing, C., Schwartz, B.D., and Dickler, H.B. 1978. Macrophage Ia antigens. I. Macrophage populations differ in their expression of Ia antigens. J Immunol 119:1584.

Craighead, J.E. 1981. Viral diabetes mellitus in man and experimental animal. Am J Med 70:127–134.

Curtiss, L.A., and Edgington, T.S. 1981. Immunoregulatory plasma low density lipoprotein: The biologic activity and receptor-binding specificity is independent of neutral lipids. J Immunol 126:1008–1012.

Danon, F., and Seligman, M. 1973. Serum monoclonal immunoglobulins in childhood. Arch Dis Childhood 48:102.

Datta, S.K., and Schwartz, R.S. 1978. Genetic, viral, and immunological aspects of autoimmune disease in NZB mice. In: Genetic Control of Autoimmune Disease, eds. N.R. Rose, P.E. Bigazzi, and N.L. Warner, pp. 193. Elsevier-North Holland; New York.

Delfraissy, J.F., Segand, P., Gelanand, P., Wollond, C., Massias, P., and Dormont, J. 1980. Deprived primary in vitro antibody response in untreated systemic lupus erythematosus. T helper cell defect and lack of defective suppressor cell function. J Clin Invest 66:141–148.

DeWaele, M., Thielemans, C., and Van Camp, B.K.G. 1981. Characterization of immunoregulatory T cells in EBV-induced infectious mononucleosis by monoclonal antibodies. N Engl J Med 304:460–462.

Drachman, D.B. 1978. Myasthenia gravis. N Engl J Med 298:136.

Drews, J.S., London, W.T., Lustbader, E.D., Hessler, J.E., and Blumberg, J.S. 1978. Hepatitis B virus and sex ratio of offspring. Science 201:687.

Drexhage, H.A., Bottazo, G.F., Bitensky, L., Chayen, J., and Doniach, D. 1981. Thyroid growth-blocking antibodies in primary myxoedema. Nature 289:594–596.

Eardley, D.D., Hugenberger, J., McVay-Boudreau, L., Shen, F.W., Gershon, R.K., and Cantor, H. 1978. Immunoregulatory circuits among T-cell sets. I. T-helper cells induce other T cells to exert feedback inhibition. J Exp Med 147:1106.

Eichmann, K. 1978. Expression and Function of idiotypes on lymphocytes. Adv Immunol 26:195–254.

Engleman, E.G., Benike, C.J., Hoppe, R.T., Kaplan, H.S., and Berberich, F.R. 1980. Autologous mixed lymphocyte reaction in patients with Hodgkin's disease. Evidence for a T cell defect. J Clin Invest 66:149–158.

Fauci, A.S., Steinberg, A.D., Haynes, B.F., and Whalen, G. 1978. Immunoregulatory aberrations in systemic lupus erythematosus. J Immunol 121:1473–1479.

Fox, R.I., and Vaughan, J.H. 1981. Lymphocyte subsets in rheumatoid arthritis. Clin Res 29:102A.

Froelich, C.J., Bankhurst, A.D., Crowe, W.E., Williams, R.C., Warner, N.L., and Levinson, J.E. 1981. Flow cytometry and cytoadherence studies of sera from children with juvenile rheumatoid arthritis and normal controls. Arthritis Rheum 24:457–463.

Fuks, A.S., and Weinstein, Y. 1979. 20α hydroxysteroid dehydrogenase (20αSDH) activity in New Zealand mice T lymphocytes and bone marrow cells: Effect of age, sex, and castration. J Immunol 123:1266–1271.

Gausset, P., Delepesse, G., and Hubert, C. 1976. In vitro response of subpopulations of human lymphocytes. II. DNA synthesis induced by anti-immunoglobulin antibodies. J Immunol 116:446.

Geltner, D., Franklin, E.C., and Fragione, B. 1980. Anti-idiotypic activity in the IgM fractions of mixed cryoglobulins. J Immunol 125:1530–1535.

Germain, R.N., and Benacerraf, B. 1980. A single major pathway of T-lymphocyte interactions in antigen-specific immune suppression. Scand J Immunol 13:1–10.

Gershon, R.K. 1974. T cell control of antibody production. Contemp Top Immunogiol 3:1.

Gershon, R.K., Horowitz, M., Kemp, J.D., Murphy, D.B., and Murphy, E.D. 1978. The cellular site of immunoregulatory breakdown in the 1pr mutant mouse. In: Genetic Control of Autoimmune Disease, eds. N.R. Rose, P.E. Bigazzi, and N.L. Warner, pp. 223–227. Elsevier North Holland; New York.

Gershwin, M.E., Merchant, B., Gelfand, M.C., Vickers, J., Steinberg, A.D., and Hansen, C.T. 1975. The natural history and immunopathology of outbred athymic (nude) mice. Clin Immunol Immunopathol 4:324–340.

Gleichmann, E., Issa, P., Van Elven, E.H., and Lamers, M.C. 1978. The chronic graft-versus-host reaction: A lupus erythematosus-like syndrome caused by abnormal T-B cell interaction. Clin Rheum Dis 4:587–602.

Good, R.A., Fernandes, G., and West, A. 1979. Nutrition, immunologic aging, and disease. In: Aging and immunity, eds. Singhal, Sinclair, and Stiller, pp. 141–163. Elsevier-North Holland; New York.

Gorevic, P.D., Kassab, H.J., Levo, Y., Kohn, R., Meltzer, M., Rose, P., and Franklin, E.C. 1980. Mixed cryoglobulinemia: Clinical aspects and long-term follow-up of 40 patients. Am J Med 69:287–308.

Hausmann, P.B., and Stobo, J.D. 1979. Specificity and function of a human autologous reactive T cell. J Exp Med 149:1537–1542.

Haynes, B.F., and Fauci, A.S. 1978. Activation of human B lymphocytes. X. Heterogeneity of concanavalin A-generated suppressor cells of the pokeweed mitogen-induced plaque-forming cell response of human peripheral lymphocytes. J Immunol 121:559–565.

Heijnen, C.J., Uytedehaag, F., and Ballieux, R.E. 1980. In vitro antibody response of human lymphocytes. Springer Sem Immunopathol 3:63–92.

Heijnen, C.J., Uytedehaag, F., Pot, C.H., and Ballieux, R.E. 1979. Feedback inhibition of human primed T-helper cells. Nature 280:589–591.

Hoffmann, M.K., 1980. Antibody regulates the cooperation of B cells with helper cells. Immunol Rev 49:79–91.

Huber, B.T., Gershon, R.K., and Cantor, H. 1977. Identification of a B-cell surface structure involved in antigen dependent triggering: Absence of the structure on B cells from CBA/N mice. J Exp Med 145:10.

Irvine, W.J. 1977. Classification of idiopathic diabetes. Lancet 1:638–642.

Irvine, W.J. 1978a. Adrenalitis, hypoparathyroidism, and associated diseases. In: Immunological Diseases, ed. M. Santer, vol. 2, pp. 1278–1295. Little, Brown and Co.; New York.

Irvine, W.J. 1978b. The immunology and genetics of autoimmune disease. In: Genetic Control of Autoimmune Disease, eds. N.R. Rose, P.E. Bigazzi, and N.L. Warner, pp. 77–100. Elsevier-North Holland; New York.

James, S.P., Elson, C.O., Waggoner, J.G., Jones, E.A., and Strober, W. 1980. Deficiency of the autologous mixed lymphocyte reaction in patients with primary biliary cirrhosis. J Clin Invest 66:1305–1310.

Janeway, C.A. 1980. Idiotypic control: The expression of idiotypes and its regulation. In: Strategies of Immune Regulation, ed. E. Sercarz, pp. 179–198. Academic Press; New York.

Johnson, P.M., and Faulk, W.P. 1976. Rheumatoid factor: Its nature, specificity, and production in rheumatoid arthritis. Clin Immunol Immunopathol 7:414–430.

Johnson, R.L., and Ziff, M. 1976. Lymphokine stimulation of collagen accumulation. J Clin Invest 58:240–252.

Kahn, C.R. 1980. Role of insulin receptors in insulin-resistant states. Metabolism 29:455–466.

Katz, S.I., Hall, R.P. Lawley, T.J., and Strober, W. 1980. Dermatitis herpetiformis: The skin and the gut. Annals Int Med 93:857–874.

Kay, H.D., and Horwitz, D.A. 1980. Evidence by reactivity with hybridoma antibodies for a probably myeloid origin of peripheral blood cells active in natural cytotoxicity and antibody-dependent cell-mediated cytotoxicity. J Clin Invest 66:847.

Kumagai, S., Steinberg, A.D., and Green, I. 1981. Antibodies to T cells in patients with SLE mediated ADCC against human T cells. J Clin Invest 67:605–614.

Laskin, C.A., Taurog, J.D., Smathers, P.A., and Steinberg, A.D. 1981. Studies of defective tolerance in murine lupus. J Immunol 127:1743–1747.

Lawton, A.R., and Cooper, M.D. 1974. Modification of B lymphocyte differentiation by anti-immunoglobulins. Contemp Topics Immunobiol 3: 193.

Ledbetter, J.A., Evans, R.L., Lipinski, M., Cunningham-Rundles, C., Good, R.A., and Herzenberg, L.A. 1981. Evolutionary conservation of surface molecules that distinguish T lymphocyte helper/inducer and T cytotoxic/suppressor subpopulations in mouse and man. J Exp Med 153:310–323.

Louis, J.A., and Lambert, P.H. 1979. Lipopolysaccharides: From immune stimulation to autoimmunity. Springer Sem Immunopathol 2:215–228.

MacDermott, R.P., and Stacey, M.C. 1981. Further characterization of the human autologous mixed leukocyte reaction (MLR). J Immunol 126:729–734.

Mathews, J.D., Whittingham, S., and Mackay, I.R. 1974. Lancet ii:1423.

Menzel, E.J., Steffen, C., Kolarz, G., Kojer, M., and Smolen, J.S. 1978. Demonstration of anti-collagen antibodies in rheumatoid arthritis synovial fluids by ^{14}C-radioimmunoassay. Arthritis Rheum 21:243–248.

Miller, J.F.A.P., and Mitchell, G.F. 1968. Cell to cell interaction in the immune response. I. Haemolysin forming cells in neonatally thymectomized mice reconstituted with thymus or thoracic duct lymphocytes. J Exp Med 128:801.

Miller, K.F., and Schwartz, R.S. 1979. Familian abnormalities of suppressor function in systemic lupus erythematosus. N Engl J Med 301:803–809.

Miyasaka, M., Sauvezie, B., Pierce, D.A., Daniels, T.E., and Talal, N. 1980. Decreased autologous mixed lymphocyte reaction in Sjogren's syndrome. J Clin Invest 66:928–933.

Moller, G. 1975. Subpopulations of B lymphocytes. Transpl Rev 23:1–174.

Moretta, L., Webb, S.R., Grossi, C.E., Lydyard, P.M., and Cooper, M.D. 1977. Functional analysis of two human T-cell subpopulations: Help and suppression of B cell responses by T cells bearing receptors for IgM (T_M) or IgG (T_G). J Exp Med 146:184.

Morimoto, C., Reinherz, E.L., Borel, Y., Mangzourais, E., Steinberg, A.D., and Schlossman, S.F. 1981. An autoantibody to an immunoregultory inducer population in patients with juvenile rheumatoid arthritis (JRA). J Clin Invest. 67:753–761.

Morimoto, C., Reinherz, E.L., Schlossman, S.F., Schur, P.H., Mills, J.A., and Steinberg, A.D. 1980. Alterations of immunoregulatory T cell subsets in active systemic lupus erythematosus. J Clin Invest 66:1171–1174.

Morse, H.C., III, Steinberg, A.D., Schur, P.H., and Reed, N.D. 1974. Spontaneous "autoimmune disease" in nude mice. J Immunol 113:688–697.

Mosier, D.E., and Coppleson, L.W. 1968. A three-cell interaction required for the induction of the primary immune response in vitro. Proc Natl Acad Sci 61:542.

Nerup, J., and Lernmark, A. 1981. Autoimmunity in insulin-dependent diabetes mellitus. Am J Med 70:135–141.

Novotny, E.A., Raveche, E.S., Sharrow, S.O., and

Steinberg, A.D. 1981. Effect of sex hormones on thymocyte subpopulations. Arthritis Rheum 24:S85.

Pichler, W.J., and Broder, S. 1981. In vitro functions of human T cells expressing Fc-IgG or Fc-IgM receptors. Immunol Rev 56, In press.

Pichler, W.J., Lum, L., and Broder, S. 1978. Fc-receptors on human T lymphocytes. I. Transition of T_γ to T_μ cells. J Immunol 121:1540–1548.

Prickett, J.D., Robinson, D.R., and Steinberg, A.D. Dietary enrichment with the polyunsaturated fatty acid eicosapentaenoic acid prevents proteinuria and prolongs survival in NZB × NZW F, mice. 1981. J Clin Invest 68:556–559.

Radl, J. 1980. Idiopathic paraproteinemia—a consequence of an age-related deficiency in the T immune system. Clin Immunol Immunopathol 14:251–254.

Raff, H.V., Picker, L.J., and Stobo, J.D. 1980. Macrophage heterogeneity in man: A subpopulation of HLA-DR-bearing macrophages required for antigen-induced T cell activation also contains stimulators for autologous-reactive T cells. J Exp Med 152–581.

Ranney, D.F., and Steinberg, A.D. 1976. Differences in the age-dependent release of a low molecular weight suppressor (LMWS) and stimulators by normal and NZB/W lymphoid organs. J Immunol 117:1219–1225.

Rao, V.S., Bennett, J.A., Shen, F.W., Gershon, R.K., and Mitchell, M.S. 1980. Antigen-antibody complexes generate Lyt 1 inducers to suppressor cells. J Immunol 125:63–67.

Raveche, E.S., Klassen, L.W., and Steinberg, A.D. 1976. Sex differences in the formation of anti-T cell antibodies. Nature 263:415–416.

Raveche, E.S., Novotny, E.A., Hansen, C.T., Tjio, J.H., and Steinberg, A.D. 1981. Genetic studies in NZB mice. V. Recombinant inbred lines demonstrate that separate genes control autoimmune phenotype. J Exp Med 153:1187–1197.

Raveche, E.S., Vigerski, R., Rice, M.K., and Steinberg, A.D. 1980. Murine thymic androgen receptors. J Immunopharmacol 2:425–434.

Reinherz, E.L., Kung, P.C., Goldstein, G., and Schlossman, S.F. 1979a. Separation of functional subsets of human T cells by a monoclonal antibody. Proc Natl Acad Sci USA 76:4061–4065.

Reinherz, E.L., Parkman, R., Rappeport, J., Rose, F.S., and Schlossman, S.F. 1979b. Aberrations of suppressor T cells in human graft-versus-host disease. N Engl J Med 300:1061–1068.

Reinherz, E.L., Moretta, L., Roper, M., Breard, J.M., Mingari, M.C., Cooper, M.D., and Schlossman, S.F. 1980a. Human T lymphocyte subpopulations defined by Fc receptors and monoclonal antibodies. A comparison. J Exp Med 151:969–974.

Reinherz, E.L., Kung, P.C., Goldstein, G., Levy, R.H., and Schlossman, S.F. 1980b. Discrete stages of intrathymic differentiation: Analysis of normal thymocytes and leukemic lymphoblasts of T-cell lineage. Proc Natl Acad Sci USA 77:1588–1592.

Rice, L., Laughter, A.H., and Twomey, J.J. 1979. Three suppressor systems in human blood that modulate lymphoproliferation. J Immunol 122:991–996.

Roder, J.C., Bell, D.A., and Singhal, S.F. 1975. Suppressor cells in New Zealand mice: possible role in the generation of autoimmunity. In: Suppressor Cells in Immunity, eds. S.K. Singhal and N.R. St. C. Sinclair, pp. 164–173. The University of Western Ontario; London, Ontario.

Rose, N.R. 1980. Endocrine diseases. In: Basic and Clinical Immunology, eds. H.H. Fudenberg, D.P. Stites, J.L. Caldwell, and J.V. Wells, pp. 644. Lange; Los Altos.

Rosenthal, A.S., and Shevach, E.M. 1973. The function of macrophages in antigen recognition by guinea pig T lymphocytes. I. Requirement for histocompatible macrophages and lymphocytes. J Exp Med 138:1194.

Rotter, J.I., and Rimoin, D.L. 1981. The genetics of the glucose intolerance disorders. Am J Med 70:116–126.

Rozing, J., Brons, N.H.C., and Benner, R. 1977. B-lymphocyte differentiation in lethally irradiated and reconstituted mice. II. Recovery of humoral immune responsiveness. Cell Immunol 29:37.

Sakane, T., and Green, I. 1979. Specificity and suppressor function of human T cells responsive to autologous non-T cells. J Immunol 123:584–589.

Sakane, T., Steinberg, A.D., and Green, I. 1978a. Failure of autologous mixed lymphocyte reactions between T and non-T cells in patients with systemic lupus erythematosus. Proc Nat Acad Sci USA 75:3464–3468.

Sakane, T., Steinberg, A.D., and Green, I. 1978b. Studies of immune functions of patients with systemic lupus erythematosus. I. Dysfunction of suppressor T cell activity related to impaired generation of, rather than response to, suppressor cells. Arthritis Rheum 21:657–664.

Sakane, T., Steinberg, A.D., Reeves, J.P., and Green, I. 1979. Studies of immune functions of patients with systemic lupus erythematosus. Complement dependent immunoglobulin M anti-thymus derived cell antibodies preferentially inactivate suppressor cells. J Clin Invest 63:954–965.

Scherak, O., Smolen, J.S., and Mayr, W.R. 1981. HLA-DR antigens and disease patterns of rheumatoid arthritis. In press.

Schwartz, M., Novivk, D., Givol, D., and Fuchs, S. 1978. Induction of anti-idiotypic antibodies by immunization with syngeneic spleen cells educated with acetylcholine receptor. Nature 273:543.

Sege, K., and Peterson, P. 1978. Use of anti-idiotype antibodies as cell surface receptor probes. Proc Natl Acad Sci USA 75:2433.

Siiteri, P.K., Jones, L.A., Roubinian, J., and Talal, N. 1980. Sex steroids and the immune system. Sex differences in autoimmune disease in NZB/NZW hybrid mice. J Steroid Biochem 12:425.

Smith, H.R., Smathers, P.A., Raveche, E.S., and Steinberg, A.D. 1981. Induction and thymic inhibition of anti-ssDNA with polyclonal B cell activators (PCBCA). Arthritis Rheum 24:S63.

Smolen, J.S., Chused, T.M., Leiserson, W., Reeves, J.P., and Steinberg, A.D. 1982a. Heterogeneity of immunoregulatory T cell subsets in systemic lupus erythematosus. Correlation with clinical features. Amer. J. Med. 72:783–790.

Smolen, J.S., Lanzer, G., Scherak, O., Menzel, E.J., Mayr, W.R., Steffen, C., and Knapp, W. 1981c. Concanavalin A induced suppressor cell activity and in vitro immunoglobulin secretion in rheumatoid arthritis: Correlation with clinical and immunological parameters. Rheumatol Internat. In press.

Smolen, J.S., Sharrow, S.O., Reeves, J.P., Boegel, W.A., and Steinberg, A.D. 1981. The human antalogous mixed lymphocyte reaction. Suppression by macrophages and T cells 1981b. J Immunol 127:1987–1993.

Smolen, J.S., Youngchaiyud, U., Weidinger, P., Kojer, M., Endler, A.T., Mayr, W.R., and Menzel, E.J. 1978. Autoimmunological aspects of thromboangiitis obliterans (Buerger's Disease). Clin Immunol Immunopathol 11:168–177.

Stastny, P., and Fink, C.W. 1979. Different HLA-D associations in adult and juvenile rheumatoid arthritis. J Clin Invest 63:124–130.

Steffen, C., Saenger, L., and Menzel, E.J. 1980. Demonstration of antibodies to denatured type I and type II collagen in juvenile rheumatoid arthritis, Still's syndrome, and controls by (^{14}C)-collagen radioimmunoassay. Scand J Rheumatol 9:69–76.

Steffen, C. 1970. Considerations of pathogenesis of rheumatoid arthritis as collagen autoimmunity. Z Immunforsch (Immunobiol) 139:219–227.

Steinberg, A.D., Baron, S., and Talal, N. 1969. The pathogenesis of autoimmunity in New Zealand Mice. I. Induction of anti-nucleic acid antibodies by polyinosinic, polycytidylic acid. Proc Natl Acad Sci USA 63:1102–1107.

Steinberg, A.D., Huston, D.P., Taurog, J.D., Cowdery, J.S., and Raveche, E.S. 1981. The cellular and genetic basis of murine lupus. Immunol Rev 55:121–154.

Steinberg, A.D., and Klassen, L.W. 1977. Role of suppressor T cells in lymphopoietic disorders. Clin Haematol 6:439–478.

Steinberg, A.D., Law, L.W., and Talal, N. 1970. The role of the NZB/NZW F_1 thymus in experimental tolerance and autoimmunity. Arthrits Rheum 13:369–377.

Steinberg, A.D., Roths, J.B., Murphy, E.D., Steinberg, R.T., and Raveche, E.S. 1980. Effects of thymectomy or androgen administration upon the autoimmune disease of MRL/Mp-1pr/1pr mice. J Immunol 125:871–873.

Strober, W.R., Falchuk, Z.M., Rogentine, G.N., Nelson, D.L., and Klaeveman, H.L. 1975. The pathogenesis of gluten-sensitive enteropathy. Annals Int Med 83:242–256.

Svedmyr, E., and Jondal, M. 1975. Cytotoxic effector cells specific for B cell lines transformed by Epstein-Barr virus are present in patients with infectious mononucleosis. Proc Natl Acad Sci USA 72:1622–1626.

Theofilopoulos, A.N., and Dixon, F.J. 1981. Etiopathogenesis of murine SLE. Immunol Rev 55:179–216.

Thomas, Y., Sosman, J., Irigoyen, O., Friedman, S.M., Kung, P.C., Goldstein, G., and Chess, L. 1980. Functional analysis of human T cell subsets defined by monoclonal antibodies. J Immunol 125:2402–2408.

Tosato, G., Steinberg, A.D., and Blaese, R.M. 1981. Defective Epstein Barr virus (EBV) specific suppressor T cell function in rheumatoid arthritis. New England J. Med. 305:1238–1243.

Twomey, J.J., Lewis, V.M., Patten, B.M., Goldstein, G., and Good, R.A. 1979. Myasthenia gravis, thymectomy and serum thymic hormone activity. Am J Med 66:639–643.

Uhr, J.W., and Moller, G. 1968. Regulatory effects of antibody on the immune response. Advan Immunology 8:81.

Van de Stouwe, R.A., Kunkel, H.G., Halper, J.P., and Weksler, M.E. 1977. Autologous mixed lymphocyte culture reactions and generation of cytotoxic cells. J Exp Med 146:1809–1814.

Vaughan, J.H. 1979. Rheumatoid arthritis, rheumatoid factor and the Epstein-Barr virus. J Rheumatol 6:381.

Vyas, G.N., Cohen, S.N., and Schmid, R., eds. 1978. Viral Hepatitis. Franklin Institute Press.

Waldenstrom, J. 1961. Studies on conditions associated with disturbed gamma globulin formation (gammopathies). Harvey Lect 56:211–231.

Weksler, M.E., Kuntz, M.M., Birnbaum, G., and Innes, J.B. 1978. Lymphocyte transformation induced by autologous cells. Fed Proc 37:2370–2373.

Yamashita, U., and Shevach, E.M. 1980. The syngeneic mixed leukocyte reaction: The genetic requirements for the recognition of self resemble the requirements for the recognition of antigen in association with self. J Immunol 124:1773–1778.

Yu, D.T.Y., Winchester, R.J., Fu, S.M., Gibofsky, A., Ko, H.S., and Kunkel, H.G. 1980. Peripheral blood Ia positive T cells—Increases in certain diseases and after immunization. J Exp Med 151:91–100.

Yunis, E.J., Hong, R., Grewe, M.A., Martinez, C., Cornelius, E., and Good, R.A. 1967. Postthymectomy wasting associated with autoimmune phenomena. I. Antiglobulin positive anemia in A and C57BL/6 KS mice. J Exp Med 947–966.

Chapter 11

Immunobiology of Lymphoreticular Neoplasms

Richard J. Ford and Abby L. Maizel

Introduction

The human immune system consists of multiple populations of lymphoid and accessory cells that are generated from committed precursors in the bone marrow (Quesenbery and Levitt, 1979). These cells migrate from the primary lymphoid organ (the bone marrow) to peripheral secondary lymphoid organs and sites throughout the body forming the immune system (Ford, 1975). At these sites, cells of the T, B and monocyte/macrophage lineages undergo differentiation in their morphologic compartments (Sprent et al., 1971), achieving functional maturation and acquiring their genetically programmed effector function(s). Lymphocyte differentiation is normally a tightly regulated process that allows for the generation of genetically preprogrammed populations of immature and mature cells which interact to yield an immune response (Katz, 1977). Occasionally, however, due to unknown precipitating factors, a neoplastic transformation occurs in one of the clones comprising the T or B cell repertoire of the individual. This neoplastic clone then expands in an apparently unchecked and unregulated manner. The malignantly transformed clone usually appears to be "frozen" at a particular stage of maturation and proliferates continually without concomitant differentiation (Salmon and Seligmann, 1974). Lymphoid neoplasias in the human are referred to as malignant (non-Hodgkin's) lymphomas and lymphocytic leukemias; they form a spectrum of phenotypes that resemble virtually all of the currently recognized stages in normal lymphocyte differentiation (Fig. 11.1). The immunobiology of these tumors is currently providing a fascinating view of this important group of human neoplasms. Human lymphomas often retain immunologic functions (Jaffe and Green, 1977) and also display intriguing immunoregulatory disturbances that occur either primarily or secondarily to the "immuno-oncologic" events. Understanding the biology of these lymphomas offers the potential of providing the basis for future therapeutic strategies that utilize modalities such as immunotherapy and biological response modification (BRM) (Hersh, 1981). Selected aspects of current interest in the immunobiology of human lymphoid neoplasia will be considered in the following sections. A more comprehensive review of this subject was recently published elsewhere (Twomey and Good, 1978).

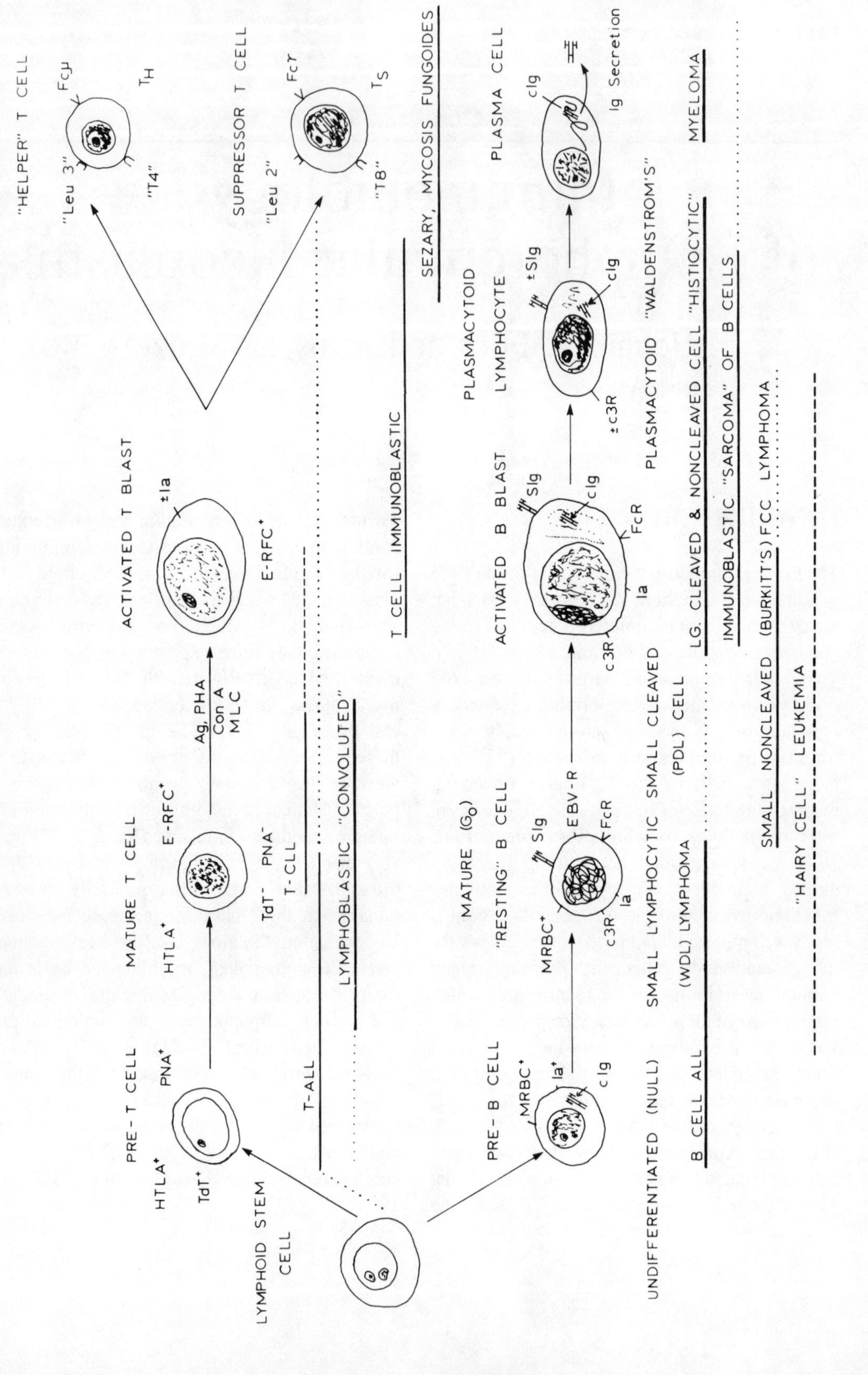
LYMPHOID STEM CELL
PRE - T CELL
HTLA⁺
TdT⁺
PNA⁺
MATURE T CELL
HTLA⁺
E-RFC⁺
TdT⁻ PNA⁻
T-CLL
Ag, PHA
Con A
MLC
ACTIVATED T BLAST
±Ia
E-RFC⁺
"HELPER" T CELL
"Leu 3"
Fcμ
"T4"
T_H
SUPPRESSOR T CELL
"Leu 2"
FcY
"T8"
T_S
T-ALL
LYMPHOBLASTIC "CONVOLUTED"
T CELL IMMUNOBLASTIC
SEZARY, MYCOSIS FUNGOIDES
PRE - B CELL
MRBC⁺
Ia⁺
c Ig
MATURE (G_o)
"RESTING" B CELL
MRBC⁺
SIg
EBV-R
FcR
c3R
Ia
ACTIVATED B BLAST
SIg
cIg
FcR
Ia
c3R
PLASMACYTOID LYMPHOCYTE
±SIg
cIg
±c3R
PLASMA CELL
cIg
Ig Secretion
UNDIFFERENTIATED (NULL)
SMALL LYMPHOCYTIC SMALL CLEAVED
(WDL) LYMPHOMA
(PDL) CELL
B CELL ALL
PLASMACYTOID "WALDENSTROM'S"
MYELOMA
LG. CLEAVED & NONCLEAVED CELL "HISTIOCYTIC"
IMMUNOBLASTIC "SARCOMA" OF B CELLS
SMALL NONCLEAVED (BURKITT'S) FCC LYMPHOMA
"HAIRY CELL" LEUKEMIA

Etiologic Considerations and Factors Predisposing to Neoplasia in the Human Immune System

The etiology of human lymphoma remains one of the fascinating riddles of medical science. Aside from the basic conundrum posed by neoplasia and its causes, lymphoma as a neoplasm of the immune system represents an undermining, in a sense, of the body's primary defenses. Like the "horror autotoxicus" of Ehrlich's concept of autoimmune disease, the lymphomatous process reverses the defensive role of the immune system. This reversal gives rise to a dual threat to the body; it poses both the lack of its front-line defense against the environment and the loss of whatever type of surveillance mechanism that the immune system provides. Virtually all immune surveillance theories are predicated on the notion that the immune system is the sentinel against neoplastic transformation (Chapter 12). But it is clear from the incidence of lymphomatous diseases in the human population that the defender is also one of the most frequent targets. In fact, if one considers the natural killer (NK) cell system as the currently popular candidate for the putative surveillance effector system (Chapter 12), it would appear from the NK target cell repertoire that one of its major functions may be the elimination of neoplastic lymphoid (e.g., lymphoma) cells. It remains unclear, however, whether this reflects an actual function of the NK system to control the high risk of lymphomagenesis or simply is due to an increased susceptibility of lymphoma target cell lines to NK-mediated lysis in vitro. Although little is known as to why the immune system has a propensity to give rise to neoplastic transformations, it is interesting to speculate as to the possible causes. Recent studies involving the NK system and the mediator interferon (IF) have provided a new perspective from which to view regulatory and apparent surveillance aspects of the immune system (Taylor-Papadimitriou, 1980). These factors, together with the much studied T cell suppressor networks are beginning to unravel the intricate pathways that mediate immunologic damping mechanisms. If our current concepts regarding these mechanisms are correct, one might expect that the combination of NK cell stimulation through the mediation of type I IF and the secretion of type II (immune) IF by various kinds of lymphoid cells would be a major inhibitory component in the immunologic armamentarium against nascent malignantly transformed lymphoid cells. While such notions are superficially attractive and considerable indirect evidence can be mustered to support such contentions, virtually no direct proof is available to implicate these systems in human lymphomagenesis. One of the problems involved is, of course, identifying the individuals at risk to develop lymphoma at the appropriate time to evaluate their immunologic capabilities. Such studies may provide some insight into the immunologic mileau in which lymphoid neoplasia arises, because a number of immunoregulatory disturbances have been described in lymphomatous conditions (Louie et al., 1980). It is still not clear, however, what the relationship of these disturbances to the neoplasms is with respect to cause or effect. Recently, Klein has proposed a general hypothesis for the development of human lymphomas, using the Epstein-Barr (EB) virus–Burkit's lymphoma model system (Klein, 1979). This model system is based on the extensive studies on EB virus and its associated pathologic manifestations that have been reported by Klein and his coworkers over the last decade (Klein, 1980). Basically, Klein envisions a concatenation of events similar in many respects to the older tumor progression model of Foulds (1958) more than 20 years ago. These events involve three basic steps, the first of which is a chronic infection with EB virus that gives rise to "immortalized" B lymphocytes. This step is

Fig. 11.1 Schematic diagram of normal human T and B lymphocyte differentiation as currently envisioned. Various types of lymphomas and lymphocytic leukemias, according to their cell surface marker phenotype, are shown as "frozen" stages of differentiation corresponding to their normal lymphocyte counterparts. Abbrev: E-RFC$^+$—sheep red cell rosette forming cell; PNA—Peanut agglutinin Leu 3, T4 etc.,—monoclonal antibody-defined antigens, Tdt—terminal transferase.

analogous to the ''initiation'' step of chemical carcinogenesis. The second step is again analogous to the carcinogenesis model and involves an environmental stimulus provided by malaria infestation leading to chronic antigenic stimulation of the immortalized B cells. This step would correspond to the ''promoter'' step in the carcinogenesis model. The final step involves the omnipresent reciprocal 8:14 chromosomal translocation associated with Burkitt's lymphoma (Zech et al., 1976), by some unspecified mechanism. This model clearly has much circumstantial support from the epidemiology and virology of Burkitt's lymphoma and incorporates a number of associations previously noted in other models of animal as well as human lymphoma, such as chronic antigenic stimulation (Metcalf, 1961) and viral association (Rowe, 1973). Unfortunately, the vast majority of patients observed to develop lymphoma exhibit no history of exotic infections that can be correlated with such a progressive pathogenesis. The only real pathogenetic clue may be in the last step of Klein's hypothesis, the nonrandom chromosomal translocation involving chromosome 14. There is no strong evidence that the Epstein-Barr virus, or any other virus, for that matter, is causally associated with human lymphoma, except, paradoxically, for a ''malignant'' form of infectious mononucleosis that gives rise to a polyclonal lymphoproliferative process that can closely resemble lymphoma pathologically. This condition is usually X-linked and familial and probably results from the inability of suppressor or cytotoxic T cells to control a usually self-limited infection of B lymphocytes by the EB virus, as is the usual case in infectious mononucleosis (Purtilo et al., 1979).

Recently, however, there has been considerable interest generated by another group of viruses; these are the RNA tumor viruses or retroviruses. These viruses are related to oncogenic viruses which cause leukemias and lymphomas in many animal species and contain the so-called ''ONC'' genes which are responsible for neoplastic transformation both in vitro and in vivo (Duesberg, 1980). Recently Gallo's laboratory at the National Institutes of Health has described a human ''ONC'' gene homologous to the transforming gene of the simian sarcoma virus (SSV) (Dalla Favera et al., 1981). This finding may indicate that such cellular genes could be involved in neoplastic transformation if promoter sequences from the genomes of certain ''oncogenic'' viruses are inserted in the host genome near such genes. The model system for this speculation is the avian leukosis virus which is associated with lymphoma development in infected birds. Recent studies have shown that lymphomagenesis occurs when a promoter sequence for RNA polymerase II (found in all known retroviruses flanking the viral genes) is inserted adjacent to one of the ''ONC'' genes which are related to the ''transforming'' genes of certain retroviruses (Neel et al., 1981). This promoter-insertion model could explain the difficulty that viral oncologists have had over the years in establishing a viral association with human lymphomas and leukemias. Recently, cell lines from human cutaneous T cell lymphomas established with IL-2 (TCGF) by Gallo and coworkers have yielded type C retroviruses (Poiesz et al., 1980). Other human lymphoma cell lines established in Kaplan's laboratory from patients with diffuse ''histiocytic'' lymphoma have also been reported to contain retroviruses (Kaplan et al., 1977).

If one considers the 14q+ translocations as the one apparently reproducible finding in the common B cell non-Hodgkin's lymphomas (although the 14 chromosome is also involved in some T cell lymphomas), what does this clue tell us about the etiology of human lymphoma? Unfortunately it does not tell nearly enough to provide even a modicum of understanding of the pathogenesis involved. At this stage, about all that can be deduced is that the B cell is the apparent target in most of the human non-Hodgkin's lymphomas and that the neoplastic B cells in most (if not all) of such cases have chromosomal translocations involving the 14 chromosome (Rowley and Fukuhara, 1980). The cause or effect question here is immediately apparent in regard to these translocations. One of the hopeful prospects is that there is some evidence that chromosome 14 contains the genes for the heavy chain of human immunoglobulins (Croce et al., 1979) and that many of the genes that control B cell proliferation and differentiation may be located at or near the site of the translocated chromosomal segments. If this is true, then perhaps we are at least in the right area of the haystack to look for the proverbial needle. It is interesting to note that we may not be as far away from being able to analyze these possibilities as it may seem, due to the rapidly progressing studies involving gene expression which have focused significantly on the B lymphocyte and the genes encoding immunoglobulin synthesis (Early et al., 1980). It is quite possible that the technology and molecular probes that have been devised for delineating normal gene structure and function can be extended to the neoplastic counterparts of these cells, which in turn may provide significant information relating to the etiology of these neoplasms.

Morphologic and Microenvironmental Aspects of Lymphoid Neoplasia within the Immune System

Lymphoma in its simplest definition is a monoclonal expansion of neoplastic lymphoid cells, generally within the confines of the lymphoid system. Generations of pathologists, including the authors, have spent years microscopically studying the morphologic characteristics of the various types of lymphoma cells and trying to sort them into meaningful morphologic classifications. As most clinicians involved with the treatment of lymphoma patients will surely agree, this area of pathology has become chaotic. In recent years, many pathologists have felt obliged to replace the older but clinically well established Rappaport classification (Rappaport, 1966) with a new, more scientifically accurate immunologic classification. These attempts have been rather unsuccessful, due primarily to the intrinsic limitations of morphology in delineating the lineage and functional or biologic characteristics of lymphoid cells. Of course, cellular atypia is present in many neoplastic lymphoid cells; this allows the experienced pathologist to confidently diagnose such cells as lymphoma. Such distinctions, in fact, formed the basis of the Rappaport and other older lymphoma classifications. In this discussion, however, we will be concerned with some of the newer methodologies for studying human lymphoma cells that may augment our current diagnostic modalities in the future.

If we consider classical morphology, there is no question that studies by Lukes, Lennert and a number of others (Lukes et al., 1978; Lennert et al., 1975) have widely expanded our abilities to recognize neoplastic lymphoid cells and the patterns of lymphomatous involvement that occur within the human lymphoid system. The concepts and hypotheses put forth by these pathologists have attempted to place the morphologic description of lymphomatous lesions into immunologic perspective by pointing out the relationship of these lesions to T and B cell-dependent areas in the lymphoid system. This in itself has been a major accomplishment, as it has stimulated a reconsideration of these diseases as tumors of the immune system, rather than as their former designation as one of the types of neoplastic disease of the hematopoietic system. Unfortunately, however, normal and neoplastic lymphoid cells appear to be morphologically similar, with a rather narrow range of variation generally observed. As with normal lymphocytes, this leads to problems with lymphoma cells, in that they can be divided into a relatively small number of morphologic categories that are generally recognizable. Another problem is that not all neoplastic lymphoid cells are distinguishable from their normal counterparts and those that are recognizable as lymphoma cells do not always behave in a clinically similar manner within a histopathologically defined subgroup. In practice, the lesions that are most readily diagnosed as malignant are those that show maximal effacement of the lymphoid organ structure by a monomorphic replacement or infiltration, with neoplastic lymphoid cells displaying at least some cellular atypia. The type of lesion that generally presents the most difficulty is often the "early" lesion, showing only minimal structural effacement of the lymph node or other lymphoid organ, or the lesion that either develops from or contains a prominent reactive or hyperplastic component. These lesions are often polymorphic overall but contain varying numbers of atypical cells, often in monomorphic clusters. Such lesions are often virtually impossible to diagnose accurately by morphology alone and force the pathologist to equivocate with terms like "atypical hyperplasia," although these lesions often ultimately turn out to represent either incipient or frank neoplasia. These situations underscore the need for better methods of diagnosing human lymphoid neoplasias utilizing newer, more sophisticated diagnostic methodologies.

In the last decade, lymphocyte cell membrane immunologic markers have been described that allow for the determination of T cell or B cell lineage of normal lymphocytes (Chess and Schlossman, 1977). This major advance in lymphocyte identification was later applied to neoplastic human lymphoid cells and found to identify a large percentage of such neoplasms as to their putative cellular origins (Thierfelder et al., 1977). Membrane markers such as the sheep red blood cell (E_N) receptor for T lymphocyte and the surface immunoglobulin receptor (SIg) for B lymphocyte lineage have proved to be reliable cell markers and have formed the basis for most studies involving human lymphoid neoplasias (Table 11.1). Other markers such as the complement receptor(s) (CRL) and Fc receptors have proven to be less reliable primarily due to the lack of cell-specific distribution of these receptors (Winchester et al., 1975).

One of the principle features of neoplastic lymphoid cells is their monoclonal nature (Fialkow et al., 1973). Studies on both B and T cell lymphomas and lymphocytic leukemias, using glucose-6-phosphatase dehydrogenase (G6PD) isozymes and cell surface or cytoplasmic Ig for the neoplastic B cells, have shown that virtually all of these neoplasms consist of monoclonal neoplastic cellular proliferations. Most of the studies on these tumors have been performed on cell suspensions derived from lymph nodes or other tissues involved with the neoplasm. Levy and his colleagues (Levy et al., 1977) have described an immunofluorescent technique for light-chain typing lymphomatous lesions on frozen sections. This technique is particularly useful as it allows for not only the confirmation of the clonality of B cell lymphomas, thereby distinguishing monoclonal neoplastic lesions from polyclonal hyperplastic proliferations, but also

Table 11.1 Immunologic Markers in Non-Hodgkin's Lymphomas, M. D. Anderson Hospital Cases, 1978–1980.

		B Cell[b]						
Lymphona Type[a]	Cases (N)	μ	γ	C′	T Cell[c]	Tdt[d]	Null Cell[g]	MØ
Well differentiated lymphocytic	27[e]	19	3	20	1	ND	4	0
Nodular poorly differentiated lymphocytic	28	25	3	16	0	ND	0	0
Nodular large cell	6	4	2	1	0	ND	0	0
Diffuse large cell ("histiocytic")	23	18	2	5	0	ND	2	1
Nodular mixed cell	4	2	0	1	0	ND	0	0
Burkitt's	4	4	0	ND	0	ND	0	0
Undifferentiated, non-Burkitt's	5	3	0	0	0	ND	1	0
Lymphoblastic ("convoluted")	6	0	0	0	4	3	2	0
Hairy cell	8	3	0	1	0	ND	4	1
Mycosis fungoides	3	0	0	0	3	0	0	0
Diffuse poorly differentiated lymphocytic	6	3	0	2	2	1	1	0

[a]Modified Rappaport Classifrcation.
[b]Defined as >50% SIg+ cells with monoclonal light chain predominance ±C′ receptor.
[c]Defined as <15% SIg+ cells, >50% E_N+ ± αTdt and αTdt.
[d]Defined as >60% FITC −α Tdt.
[e]Values refer to actual number of cases of the particular type of lymphoma indicated which displayed the categorized marker.
[f]Not done.
[g]Defined as <20% SIg+, E_N+, and C′+ cells.

for determining the pattern and extent of involvement in these tumors. Monoclonality of B cell lymphomas and leukemias when correlated with characteristic cytogenetic abnormalities and the appropriate histopathologic morphological criteria form the current basic diagnostic criteria for identifying these neoplasms.

Although these markers have provided a means for determining the probable cellular origin of most human lymphomas and thus have greatly expanded our understanding of these neoplasms vis-a-vis the normal immune system, they have not provided the much-needed and greatly sought after method for dissecting the immune system into functional subsets or into prognostically significant subgroups. This is perhaps not surprising in that this often serendipitously discovered group of receptors probably represents only a first generation of cell membrane markers: as such, they should not be expected to provide great precision in separating lymphocytes of various types. These cell membrane markers, in addition to a number of histochemical techniques for identifying the monocyte/macrophage lineage of cells, as well as lymphocytes (Knowles, 1980) include alpha naphtyl acetate (nonspecific) esterase and acid phosphatase. Combinations of these markers have provided the basic armamentarium for establishing the immunologic identity of human lymphoid neoplasms until very recently.

In the 1980's there is already an indication that we may expect a quantum jump in the diagnosis and understanding of human lymphomatous disease. This optimistic view is based on several observations and suppositions that seem reasonable at this time. These include the development of new methods for better normal lymphocyte identification and functional characterization that appear to be applicable to neoplastic lymphoid cells. These methods principally involve the use of monoclonal antibody technology and the application of in vitro methods similar to those used in cellular immunology for assessing the functional capabilities of lymphoma cells. Such new methodology should allow for the first time the correlation of cell surface phenotype with functional capabilities of human lymphoma cells. In addition, a number of other techniques, such as flow cytofluorimetry (Silvestrini et al., 1977) and DNA molecular hybridization analysis (Hieter et al., 1981), have been developed to the stage where they can now be used to provide meaningful data on lymphoma cells and their similarities or differences when compared to their normal lymphocyte counterparts.

The advent of hybridoma technology and the use of monoclonal antibodies (MCA) are having a profound impact on human lymphoma studies even though the use of these techniques is still barely in its infancy. It is generally predicted that monoclonal antibody reagents should provide for, not only better discrimination between neoplastic lymphoid cell types, but also identification of clinically significant subgroups within histopathologically defined morphological types of lymphoma cells. The realization of such a prediction would clearly revolutionize this field of study, biologically as well as clinically. The first fruits of these endeavors have already been reported, as a number of B cell-specific MCA have been shown to react with various types of human lymphomas that had been identified as B cell type by conventional cell membrane marker analysis (Nadler et al., 1980, Abramson et al., 1980). Of considerable interest is the unexpected finding that a number of MCA that are apparently specific for normal T cells and unreactive with normal B cells react with some types of B cell lymphomas (Aisenberg and Wilkes, 1980). This finding could be interpreted a number of ways, of course, but it may indicate that such neoplastic cells are derived from quite primitive lymphoid precursors, such as lymphoid stem cells before they theoretically bifurcate into the T and B cell differentiation pathways. Alternatively, one can offer other explanations, such as the aberrant expression of normally repressed genes by neoplastic cells or possibly the presence of an oncofetal antigen that crossreacts with normal T cell specificities. Trivial explanations aside, MCA promise to greatly expand our capability to probe the cell surface of lymphoma cells and to identify tumor-associated, if not tumor-specific, antigens present on these cells. At the very least, this should greatly reduce the number of operationally defined but poorly characterized "null cell" type lymphomas that are an important group of these tumors, comprising a significant percentage of the cases in some series. At present, it is unclear what the ultimate level of cellular discrimination will be with MCA, as many of the studies so far have identified either uncharacterized or poorly characterized antigenic specificities that may or may not ultimately prove to be significant. In this regard, another type of hybridoma holds promise. This is the human lymphoma-myeloma cell hybridoma which has been described in murine-human lymphoma hybrids by Levy and his colleagues (Levy and Dilley, 1978). Since a lymphoma-specific antigen has not as yet been described in humans, the most specific and distinctive type of antigenic specificity presently identifiable is the idiotype of the cell surface immunoglobulin (SIg) receptor. The variable region of this receptor contains specificites (idiotopes) virtually unique to the neoplastic clone (Hough et al., 1976). Hybrids between a B cell type lymphoma cell and an appropriately selected myeloma cell line will yield hybridomas secreting immunoglobulins identical to the cell surface receptor of the lymphoma cell. Large amounts of this SIg receptor type immunoglobulin can be obtained and purified without difficulty. With this neoplastic clonal product, one can make anti-idiotype antibodies in rabbits or goats that upon proper absorption will react only with the idiotypic specificity found on the lymphoma in question. In this sense, such an idiotype-specific antibody is virtually tumor-specific and is therefore unique for a particular lymphoma. Such antibodies can then be used as diagnostic reagents for that particular lymphoma, which will identify even cryptic lymphoma cells in bone marrow or in other areas where small numbers of such cells are often concealed among normal or reactive lymphoid cells. Anti-idiotype reagents also have possible usefulness as antitumor agents, either alone or when a cytotoxic substance such as ricin toxin is attached to them (Blythman et al., 1981), as well as other applications in tumor imaging, etc. These newer methods for obtaining more precise immunodiagnostic reagents to identify human lymphoma cells, when combined with our present diagnostic modalities, should greatly improve lymphoma diagnosis in the near future.

Another poorly understood but important area of lymphoma research that appears to be coming into our experimental purview is an understanding of the homing and microenvironmental characteristics of lymphoma cells. The peregrinating behavior of normal T and B lymphocytes is now well known and lymphocyte homing studies in experimental animals have demonstrated T and B cell compartmentalization of the lymphoid system (Weissman et al., 1978). Similar cell trafficking, compartmentalization and homing proclivities have also been described for neoplastic human lymphoid cells (Warnke and Levy, 1978). This retention of homing behavior by neoplastic lymphocytes may be viewed simply as evidence that the neoplastic cells have not lost the cell surface structures (antigens, receptors, etc.) responsible for the homing behavior of their normal counterparts and thus migrate (or infiltrate) selectively according to their cell surface phenotype. It is unclear whether the dissemination of lymphoid malignancies involves obligatory homing into microenvironmentally suitable areas, where specific cell interaction or the production of necessary growth factors potentiate the cell's proliferative capacity; this is a distinct possibility. Perhaps the most obvious example of lymphoma cell homing is with the cutaneous T cell lymphomas (CTCL) such as the Sezary syndrome and Mycosis fungoides. The reason for this dermal tropism is unclear in these diseases, but recent studies using in vivo homing methodology with Indium-labeled Sezary cells indicates that the neoplastic cells enter the skin from the circulation (Miller et al., 1980). These and other studies suggest that the neoplastic cells do not arise in the skin but migrate from other sites, perhaps from lymph nodes that may contain a subset of T cells that normally migrates to the dermis in response to immunologic stimuli. Unfortunately, very little is known about the dynamics of lymphoma cell interactions in vivo or in vitro. One of the recent findings that is intriguing in this respect is the identification of clonal "excess" in the peripheral blood of patients with nodal but apparently nonleukemic lymphoma (Ault et al., 1980), implying that the neoplastic clone may be more widely disseminated than is morphologically identifiable in most cases. If this is the case and the neoplastic lymphoid cells are not limited to the lymphoid tissue per se but are instead constantly recirculating even when they are not obvious in the peripheral blood smear, we may have to change our concepts regarding the basic nature of lymphomatous disease as a primarily localized disease of lymphoid tissues. Suffice it to say that this subject needs much study; this should be aided by the recent introduction of in vitro Indium-oxine labeling of normal human lymphocytes, which can be reinjected subsequently into the donor and identified in vivo with the use of a gamma camera (Wagstaff et al., 1981a). This technology can also be extended to neoplastic lymphoid cells which will allow us to follow a patient's own lymphoma cells in vivo and to determine their migratory pathways and homing propensities (Wagstaff et al., 1981b). This is an exciting prospect, as it may provide some explanation for the variation in migratory behavior and tissue distribution often seen with morphologically similar types of neoplastic lymphoid cells. But perhaps of equal importance, it should allow us to better appreciate the dynamic nature of the lymphomatous disease processes, which in the past have often been viewed as isolated proliferations of lymphoid cells in a single or small group of lymph nodes, rather than as systemic processes, as most recent studies seem to indicate. New findings in the area of experimental lymphocyte homing, involving the differential gating capacity of the high endothelial (post capillary) venules in lymph nodes and the presence of specific cell membrane receptors on migrating lymphoid cells, apparently for recognition and entrance into the lymph node, could have interesting and significant correlations in the cellular dynamics of neoplastic state (Butcher et al., 1979).

Human Lymphomas as Representing Stages in T and B Lymphocyte Differentiation

As has been discussed in Chapters 1 and 2, both T and B lymphocytes undergo a differentiative process as they develop from primitive precursors into mature effector cells (Fig. 11.1). The concatenation of events involved in these processes are complex and, at best, incompletely defined. Differentiation in both the T and B cell lineage is dependent, at least in part, on accessory cells of various types that provide regulatory molecules (lymphokines, monokines, etc.) which control at least some aspects of the differentiation process (Broder and Waldmann, 1978). With the advent of immunologic membrane markers, it has become possible to relate the various morphologic types of lymphoma cells to their cell surface phenotype to establish a putative stage in normal B cell differentiation to which the lymphoma cell corresponds (Salmon and Seligmann, 1974). Since these neoplastic lymphoid cells do not under most circumstances have the capability to differentiate further than the observed cell surface phenotype, it has been suggested that such cells are "frozen" at a particular stage in differentiation by the neoplastic process and thus proliferate continuously without concomitant differentiation. This view has attained some credence in the last few years; most neoplastic lymphoid cells do resemble normal stages in T and B cell maturation by cell membrane marker analysis and such tumor cells have not been shown to demonstrate generalized gene derepression for cell surface marker molecules. These considerations militate against the trivial explanation that correlations between normal and neoplastic cell surface phenotypes occur by the chance expression of aberrant cell surface phenotypes by the malignant clones. An interesting question arises, however, in regard to lymphoma cell differentiation potential, as to whether the expressed cell surface phenotype represents the stage at which the malignant transformation event occurred or, alternatively, simply identifies the stage beyond which further differentiation is blocked for the particular malignant clone. It is possible in this latter regard that many (if not all) lymphoid tumors are derived from an oncogenic event occurring quite early in lymphocyte ontogeny, when the rapidly proliferating lymphoid precursor pool may be more susceptible to neoplastic transformation. Such malignantly transformed lymphocytes could then proliferate and differentiate to a finite extent that is either genetically preprogrammed or is dependent on the availability of accessory cell help needed for subsequent progressive steps in the differentiation process. Unfortunately, the late stages of human B cell maturation are poorly defined and the number of actual steps involved between the activated B cell blast and the mature plasma cell is still undefined, as are the factor(s) that drive this process. Such a hypothetical scheme might explain the paradoxical in vitro behavior of most human neoplastic lymphocytes that respond poorly, if at all, to mitogens or other stimulatory agents without the presence of appropriate accessory cells (Robert et al., 1980). It may be that the proliferating (stem cell) pool in these neoplasms is small but gives rise to progeny with a finite differention potential, which then mature to the stage represented by the lymphoma cell surface phenotype, thus yielding a population of tumor cells apparently blocked at that stage of differentiation. Alternatively, as suggested by the work of Fu and his collaborators (Fu et al., 1979), the problem may lie with the accessory cell requirements for differentiation in some lymphoid neoplasms. These studies showed that one particular type of chronic lymphocytic leukemia (CLL), of the B cell type, lacked adequate T cell help for terminal differentiation, which could be reversed when normal allogeneic T helper cells were provided. This implies that a regulatory cell anomaly may be responsible for at least some apparent maturation arrests seen in these neoplasms and that such cells can differentiate if provided with the appropriate immunoregulatory signal. If this turns out to be the case, it may be a harbinger of the use of immunotherapeutic or biologic response modifier (BRM) therapy for such neoplasms. This type of tumor cell modification by BRM might, for instance, be able to alter tumor cells with an unfavorable cell surface phenotype into a less aggressive form of the disease or one more amenable to conventional therapy. Finally, we should not overlook the potential of human T and B cell lymphomas as models for putative stages in normal lymphocyte differentiation. As previously stated, we currently recognize relatively few defined stages in the differentiation processes of these cells. It is possible that B cell lymphomas, such as Waldenstrom's macroglobulinemia and hairy cell leukemia, for example (Fig. 11.1), correspond to normal stages in B cell differentiation that have been heretofore unrecognized. Lymphoma cells could also provide homogeneous populations of cells characteristic of various stages of both T and B cell maturation. These cells could then be analyzed for cell surface structures either biochemically or with monoclonal antibodies or for gene expression by molecular biologic techniques (C-DNA probes, chromosomal protein analysis, etc.).

Functional Capabilities of Neoplastic Human Lymphoid Cells

As described in the previous section, human lymphoma and lymphocytic leukemia cells usually retain cell surface phenotypic and in some cases morphologic similarity to their normal T and B cell counterparts (Fig. 11.1). If this mimicry actually reflects true cellular homology between normal and neoplastic lymphoid cells, one might predict that functional characteristics associated with normal lymphocytes at the corresponding differentiation stage would also be retained. This is in fact the case, particularly in the T cell lymphomas, which have been shown to possess a variety of effector functions characteristic of subsets of normal T lymphocytes (Broder and Bunn, 1980). These functions are of interest not only for the immunobiologic characterization of the tumor cells, but also for the possible clinical manifestations that such tumor cells may elicit by interactions with normal immune cells within the host's lymphoid system or even possibly in nonlymphoid organs beyond the confines of the immune system.

The best studied example of immunologically functional human lymphoid neoplasm is the Sezary syndrome, which comprises a form of the cutaneous T cell lymphomas (CTCL), composed of skin-seeking neoplastic T lymphocytes displaying peculiar cerebriform nuclei that are also found in the peripheral blood of these patients. These patients often also show very high serum levels of IgA, which is believed to be an immunoglobulin isotype that is highly thymic-dependent, requiring considerable T cell help for B cells to become IgA-secreting plasma cells. Interestingly, Broder and his colleagues (Broder et al., 1976) have shown that leukemic T cells from Sezary patients have the capacity to function as polyclonally active T helper cells for immunoglobulin (Ig) synthesis in vitro by purified normal B cells. Subsequent recent studies have confirmed the T helper cell phenotype of these cells utilizing monoclonal antibodies specific for these normal T cell subsets (Haynes et al., 1981). These findings imply that the functional tumor cells may account for the IgA serum elevations by subserving an immunoregulatory role that is abnormal in the sense that the helper cells are not members of the usual normal T helper subset regulating antibody synthesis. Perhaps of more importance, however, is the implication that such abnormal regulatory cells are not sensitive to the feedback suppression by normal immunoregulatory networks, which under normal circumstances provide the essential damping signals when excessive immune responses occur. It is by no means clear at this time that such neoplastic regulatory cells are in fact intrinsically refractory to suppressor cell signals, factors or other inhibitory influences, which may simply be absent or present in very low concentrations when the immune system is commandeered by neoplastic clones. In addition to the Sezary syndrome, mycosis fungoides, an aleukemic form of CTCL, has also been shown, at least in some cases, to be composed of neoplastic T helper cells (Berger et al., 1979) with similar functional properties.

Helper functions, however, are apparently not the only regulatory activity characteristic of the CTCL, as there have been a number of recent reports of Sezary cases where suppression rather than help was found when the lymphoma cells were assayed in a pokeweed mitogen (PWM)-driven in vitro Ig synthesis assay system, similar to that used for the T helper cases (e.g., Hopper and Haren, 1980). The T suppressor Sezary cases appear to be clinically and pathologically similar to the T helper cases, although the suppressor cases have been single case reports and thus may reflect rare or unusual occurrences. Also, the T suppressor Sezary cases have not been assayed for T cell surface markers such as Fc receptor for Ig isotype ($T\mu$ or T_γ) or monoclonal antibodies specific for the T suppressor subset that could verify that the suppressor activity observed actually corresponded to a T suppressor phenotype of the neoplastic Sezary cells. If this latter situation could be unequivocally demonstrated, it would signify an interesting functional heterogeneity within the CTCL that could indicate that there is more functional diversity present in such neoplastic T cell clones than has previously been evident. In addition to these apparent suppressor cell variants of the Sezary syndrome, a number of other neoplasms of probable suppressor T cell origin have been described. These include the subacute T cell leukemia found chiefly in southern Japan (Uchiyama et al., 1977) which occurs in adults and consists of atypical appearing T lymphoid cells that form spontaneous sheep cell (E_N) rosettes and show some predilection for skin involvement. In a significant percentage of these cases, the leukemia cells behave as suppressor cells when cocultured with normal cells in polyclonally activated in vitro Ig synthesis assays. In addition, supernatants from short term culture of the leukemic cells also suppressed Ig synthesis by normal lymphocytes in vitro. These cases appear to represent neoplastic T lymphoid cells expressing a mature suppressor phenotype that is also functionally active. Such cases are in marked contrast to a number of childhood T cell acute lymphocytic leukemia (ALL) cases studied by Broder (Broder et al., 1978), in which the author contends that the leukemic cell was not a mature suppressor cell. In this case, the leukemic cells belong to an apparently precommitted T cell precursor, termed a pro-suppressor T cell, that requires interaction with a normal inducer (helper) T cell to express the suppressor effector function. Here again we have evidence that the neoplastic lymphoid cell is not necessarily an autonomous and unregulated malignant cell, but actually requires an accessory cell to achieve functional maturation. This type of leukemia may actually be mimicking a component of the normal T cell suppressor system which represents an aspect of immunoregulatory networks that is just beginning to be appreciated in the human immune system. Functional activity in the B cell lymphomas and lymphocytic leukemias is limited essentially to the production of immunoglobulin by the neoplastic cells, since this is by far the most characteristic product of the B cell series. As in the case of normal B cells, neoplastic B lymphoid cells appear to form a morphologic spectrum with regard to ability to synthesize and secrete immunoglobulin. If one studies a population of antigen or mitogen-stimulated normal B cells in vitro a week or more after establishing the culture, using fluorescent antibody techniques that allow for morphologic correlation (Wu et al., 1976), a spectrum of cell types are found to contain and usually secrete immunoglobulin. This spectrum usually includes large SIg-positive blast cells with varying degrees of plasmacytoid features (eccentric nuclei, rough endoplasmic reticulum development, etc.) at the least differentiated extreme and the smaller characteristic plasma cell at the fully differentiated extreme. Some neoplastic B cells morphologically appear to roughly parallel the normal condition, with lymphomas such as immunoblastic sarcoma, plasmacytoid lymphocytic (Waldenstrom's lymphoma) and myeloma representing the terminal stages in B cell differentiation with Ig-synthesizing capabilities (Lukes et al., 1978).

However, this correlation between cell morphology and Ig expression is not rigorous, as a number of lymphomas and lymphocytic leukemias without morphologic evidence of plasmacytoid differentiation have been found to contain and secrete Ig (Kim et al., 1973). This group of B cell lymphoid tumors usually involves the so-called well differentiated (small lymphocytic) lymphocyte lymphomas and a subset of CLL that often presents with a monoclonal gammopathy.

Growth Factors and Their Effects on Human Neoplastic Lymphoid Cells

One of the major impediments to studying the biology of both normal and neoplastic human lymphoid cells has been the inability to routinely grow these cells in vitro. Until recently, the normal human lymphocyte was thought to be capable of only progressing through several rounds of in vitro replication by means of exposure to antigens (and/or mitogens), given the appropriate accessory cell interactions. Long-term in vitro culture of normal lymphoid populations was believed to be restricted to either those conditions of EB virus infection (B cell) or repeated allogeneic stimulation (T cell). The situation with neoplastic cells is surprisingly even more restrictive in that these neoplastic cell populations frequently were shown to be refractory to mitogen exposure. The establishment of proliferating cell populations is essentially limited to EB virus-transformed B lymphoblastoid cells and the apparent ability of a few neoplastic T cell populations derived from patients with acute lymphoblastic leukemia (ALL) to spontaneously adapt to in vitro growth. The ability to maintain normal lymphoid cells in culture has, however, significantly changed since the recent discovery of growth factors for the lymphoid cells (Morgan et al., 1976). Among the multiple factors reported, the most pertinent for the present discussion are the monokine, lymphocyte activity factor (LAF), and the lymphokine, T cell growth factor (TCGF). These growth factors are now frequently referred to as Interleukin 1 (IL-1) and Interleukin 2 (IL-2), respectively [for review, see Ruscetti and Gallo (1981)]. Examination of the necessary and sufficient conditions for stimulation of optimal normal T cell mitogenesis has revealed that these two growth factors operate in a bimodal amplification type network (Smith et al., 1980). Following antigenic (and/or mitogenic stimulation), a subset of normal T lymphocytes is thought to respond to IL-1 exposure with the subsequent production of IL-2. IL-2 is believed to represent the actual mitogenic stimulus that initiates responding (activated) T cells to progress through the replicative cycle (Maizel et al., 1981). Utilization of IL-2 in various stages of purity has allowed for the cloning and continual culture of normal human T cells for extended periods of time. This has not only greatly aided the study and characterization of normal T cell subpopulations, but has provided new insight into the mechanism of lymphocyte activation and factors controlling proliferation.

The role of the low molecular weight soluble growth factors in human malignant T lymphocyte cell proliferation remains to be fully elucidated. To assess the current data, one must consider the information derived from cells grown both in primary tissue culture and those malignant T cells grown in long term in vitro culture. The majority of available human long term malignant T cell lines have been grown and maintained as log phase cultures without the influence of either antigenic or monocytic (IL-1) intervention. These cells may be maintained, in a serum-dependent environment, with a population doubling time of 18 to 24 hours. Many of the established human T cell lines fail to constitutively produce IL-2-like activity and have been shown to be refractory to lectin exposure in regard to the production of IL-2 (Gillis and Watson, 1980). Yet, screening of multiple human T cell lines has revealed a population of cells (Jurkat cell line) which, upon lectin stimulation, retains the ability to produce IL-2 (Gillis and Watson, 1980). The role of IL-2 in this malignant T cell proliferation is still somewhat obscure in light of the fact that the induction of IL-2 production is associated with significant cell death (Gillis and Watson, 1980). Furthermore, several clones derived from the Jurkat line continue to grow as log-phase cultures, yet have lost the ability to produce detectable quantities of IL-2 (Maizel and Ford, unpublished observations). Whether the cells that no longer actively release IL-2 may produce small quantities of this moiety to which they are sensitive or whether these cells actually produce intracellular IL-2-like compounds that mediate proliferation remains to be determined. Similar data have been accumulated in those studies examining long-term murine lymphoma and leukemia cell lines (Gillis et al., 1980). Several lines have been found which demonstrate the ability to produce IL-2 activity upon lectin or phorbol ester stimulation and/or demonstrate augmentation or appearance of that activity after lectin plus IL-1 stimulation (Gillis and Mizel, 1981; Smith et al., 1980). Yet, interpretation of the proliferative role of IL-2 in these systems is complicated by the fact that many murine T cell lines fail to constitutively produce IL-2 activity and fail to produce activity upon exogenous lectin stimulation (Poiesz et al., 1980; DeVries et al., 1981). In addition, subclones may be derived from the IL-2 producing lines that continue to grow as log phase cultures yet no longer produce significant IL-2-like activity (Smith et al., 1980).

Work on human malignant T cells in primary in vitro culture represents a somewhat different picture. Although, as with long term cultures, these T cells do not require exogenous antigen or IL-1 exposure, the primary cell cultures of unfractionated putative malignant T cells from Sezary syndrome, Mycosis fungoides, T cell acute lymphoblastic leukemia (ALL) and T cell chronic lymphocytic leukemia (CLL) have demonstrated some mitogenic responsiveness to IL-2 stimulation alone (Poiesz et al., 1980; DeVries et al., 1981. What role normal tumor-activated T cells play in this IL-2 responsiveness remains to be fully determined. Furthermore, a small percentage of these cell populations become independent of the need for IL-2 supplementation and this independence has been used as documentation for the purported malignant nature of the cells grown (Poiesz et al., 1980). Another series of experiments has revealed that lectin stimulation of terminal deoxynucleotidyl transferase-positive leukemic blasts resulted in IL-2 production (Gillis and Watson, 1980). Additions of exogenous purified human IL-2 to these leukemic cells resulted in a significant diminution of leukemic cell proliferation (Gillis and Watson, 1980). Therefore, the ultimate role, in malignant T cell proliferation, of those soluble factors that are

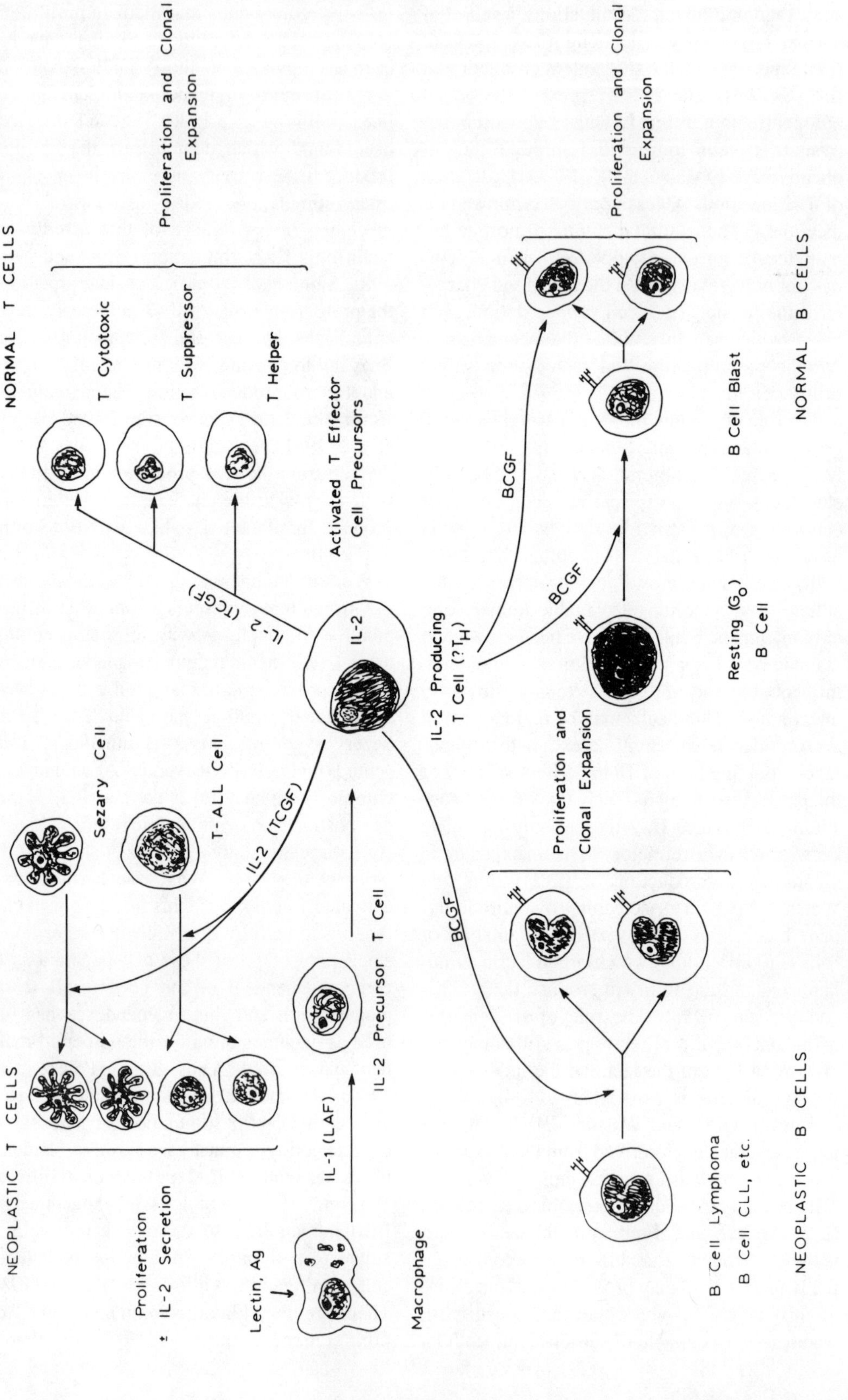
NORMAL T CELLS
T Cytotoxic
T Suppressor
T Helper
Proliferation and Clonal Expansion
Activated T Effector Cell Precursors
IL-2 (TCGF)
IL-2
IL-2 Producing T Cell (?T_H)
NEOPLASTIC T CELLS
Proliferation
± IL-2 Secretion
Sezary Cell
T-ALL Cell
IL-2 (TCGF)
Lectin, Ag
Macrophage
IL-1 (LAF)
IL-2 Precursor T Cell
BCGF
BCGF
BCGF
Resting (G_o) B Cell
B Cell Blast
NORMAL B CELLS
Proliferation and Clonal Expansion
Proliferation and Clonal Expansion
B Cell Lymphoma
B Cell CLL, etc.
NEOPLASTIC B CELLS

necessary for normal T cell proliferation requires significant clarification. It will be interesting to ascertain in the future the exact relationship of the interleukins to neoplastic T cell growth. At this juncture, the data are somewhat contradictory, yet future experimentation in this area may reveal that malignant T cells retain aspects of normal growth control involving the interleukins in part of its biologic history (Fig. 11.2).

The effect of growth factors on normal human B cells is a subject that is just beginning to be explored, although considerable information exists in the murine system (Anderson and Melchers, 1981; Swain et al., 1981). Human B cells require "helper" signals from T cells and macrophages for proliferation and probably differentiation (see Chapter 2 and Ballieux et al., 1979). In vitro, normal human B cells, like the other lymphocytes, do not grow well under normal culture conditions and usually die within a week. Human B cells do, however, possess a membrane receptor for EBV (one of the most specific markers for this lymphocyte lineage). Cultured B cells, as stated above, are often transformed by this ubiquitous virus, giving rise to immortalized B lymphoblastoid cell lines (Nilsson, 1979). A similar situation is seen with neoplastic human B cells and usually only those containing the EBV genome (usually Burkitt's lymphoma cells) can be established in continuous culture. With the exception of viral transformation, the lack of in vitro growth appears to be a result of the auxotrophic nature of normal and possibly neoplastic human B cells, in that they require specific "helper" factors produced by accessory cells. Recent studies in our laboratory (Ford et al., 1981) indicate that lectin-stimulated peripheral blood lymphocyte-conditioned media fractionated by ammonium sulfate precipitation, DEAE sepharose and ultragel chromatography contains a factor that apparently copurifies with TCGF (IL-2), which stimulates proliferation in human B cells. This factor appears to be different from TCGF in that absorption studies have shown that T cells do not apparently absorb the B cell-stimulatory activity and B cells do not absorb the T cell-stimulatory activity (Maizel, Mehta and Ford, in press). These results imply that a B cell growth factor (BCGF) analogous to TCGF is needed to activate human B lymphocytes. This factor(s) (BCGF) is probably derived from T helper cells (T_H) and represents at least one of the T_H cell products obtained when unseparated populations of lymphocytes are stimulated with mitogens or antigen. Interestingly, we have found that this factor(s) occasionally stimulates proliferation of neoplastic human B cells in vitro (Fig. 11.3). In this regard, we have demonstrated that some human B cell lymphomas and leukemias retain the capability of responding to putative normal immunoregulatory signals. We have been able to culture neoplastic B cells for extended periods in B cell growth factor-containing culture media and have obtained colonies of apparently neoplastic B cells from lymphomatous lymph nodes using soft agar cloning techniques augmented with growth factors. These preliminary results indicate that the soluble factors in lectin-stimulated conditioned media have the potential for greatly expanding our understanding of both normal and neoplastic B cells in much the same manner as they have recently contributed to a better understanding of T cell biology (Fig. 11.2). The prospect of neoplastic B cell culture and cloning is particularly exciting both clinically and biologically, as this may open completely new vistas for studying these neoplasms.

Fig. 11.2 The human interleukin system, showing our current concepts of the various growth factors and their target cells. Both normal and neoplastic lymphoid cells appear to be sensitive to these factors, which in some cases appear to be obligatory for cell proliferation. Abbrev: Il-I—Interleukin I;IL-2—Interleukin 2 (T cell growth factor (TCGF); BCGF—B cell growth factor; LAF—Lymphocyte activating factor (IL 1).

Summary

In this brief review, we have considered some of the newer aspects of human lymphoid neoplasia that are providing interesting insights into these diseases. It is becoming increasingly clear that these neoplasms are composed of cells that are

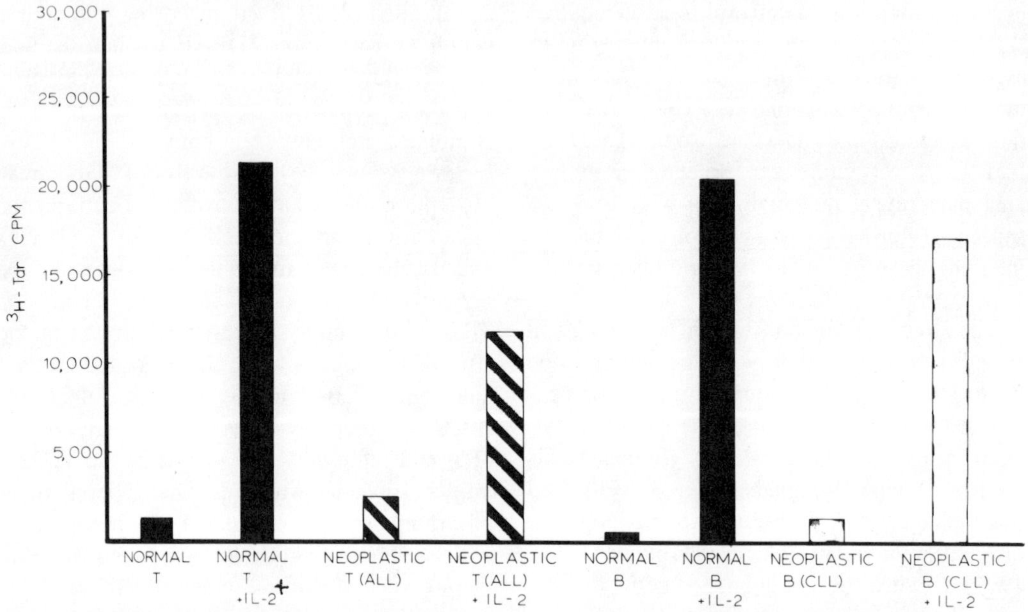

Fig. 11.3 Reactivity of Human Interleukin 2 on Normal and Neoplastic Human Lymphocytes. Purified populations of lymphoid cells, were cultured for 72 hrs. *in vitro* with ultrogel purified IL-2 and labelled with O.Sμ of ^{3}H-Tdr twenty four (24) hours prior to harvest.

often not as biologically aberrant as was previously believed. Instead, in many cases, these neoplasms retain phenotypic characteristics and sensitivity to normal immunoregulatory cells similar to their normal lymphocytic counterparts. These findings suggest that new techniques currently being developed in cellular immunology and the development of therapeutic modalities involving biologic response modifier therapy will find fertile ground in this interesting group of human tumors.

Acknowledgments

The authors would like to thank Shashi Mehta for his help in the experimental work referred to in this chapter. We also thank Ms. Robin Agee for typing the manuscript and Ms. Julie Collins for the illustrations. This work was supported in part by National Institutes of Health grants CA 25411 and CA 21927, and a grant from the King Faisal Foundation.

References

Abramson, C., Kersey, J., and LeBien, T., 1981. A monoclonal antibody reactive with cells of human B lymphocyte lineage. J Immunol 126:88–88.

Aisenberg, A.C., and Wilkes, B. 1980. Unusual human lymphoma phenotype by a defined monoclonal antibody. J Exp Med 152:1125–1131.

Anderrson, J., and Melchers, F. 1981. T cell dependent activation of resting B cells: Requirement for both non-specific unrestricted and antigen-specific Ia-restricted soluble factors. Proc Natl Acad Sci USA 78:2497–2501.

Ault, K.A. 1979. Detection of small numbers of monoclonal B lymphocytes in blood of patients with lymphoma. N Engl J Med 300:1401–1405.

Ballieux, R.E., Hiejnen, C.J., Uytdehaag, F., and Zegers, W. 1979. Regulation of B cell activity in man: Role of T cells. Immunol Rev. 45:3–40.

Berger, C.L., Warburton, D., Raafat, J., LoGerfo, P. and Edelson, R. 1979. Cutaneous T cell lymphoma: Neoplasm of T cells with helper activity. Blood 53:642–651.

Blythman, H., Casellas, P., Gros, O., Gros, P. Jansen, F., Paducci, F., Pau, B., and Vidal, H. 1981. Immunotoxins: Hybrid molecules of monoclonal antibodies and a toxin subunit specifically kill tumor cells. Nature 290:145–146.

Broder, S., and Bunn, P.A. 1980. Cutaneous T-cell lymphomas. Semin Oncol 7:310–331.

Broder, S., Poplack, D., Whang-Peng, et al. 1978. Characterization of a suppressor-cell leukemia. N Engl J Med 298:66–72.

Broder, S., and Waldemann, T.A. 1978. The suppressor-cell network in man. N Engl J Med 299:1281–1284.

Butcher, E.C., Scollay, R.G., and Weissman, I.L. 1979. Lymphocyte adherence to high endothelial venules: Characterization of a modified *in vitro* assay and examination of the binding of syngeneic and allogeneic lymphocyte populations. J Immunol 123:1996–2003.

Chess, L., and Schlossman, S.F. 1977. Human lymphocyte subpopulations. Adv Immunol 25:213–240.

Croce, C.M., Shander, M., Martinis, J., Cicurel, L., D'Ancona G., Dolby, T., and Koprowski, H. 1979. Chromosomal location of the genes for human immunoglobulin. Proc Natl Acad Sci USA 76:3416–3419.

DallaFavera, R., Gelmann, E.P., Gallo, R.C., and Wong-Staal, F. 1981. A human "onc" gene homologous to the transforming gene (v-sis) of Simian sarcoma virus. Nature 292:31–35.

DeVries, J.E., Vyth, F.A., and Mendelsohn, J. 1981. T cell growth factor-mediated proliferation of lymphocytes from a T-chronic lymphocytic leukemia patients lacking mitogen and alloantigen responsiveness. Clin Exp Immunol 43:302–310.

Duesberg, P.H. 1980. Cold Spring Harbor Symposium Quantitative Biology 44:13–28.

Early, P. Huang, H., Davis, M., Calame, K., and Hood, L. 1980. An immunoglobulin heavy chain variable region gene is generated from three segments of DNA: V_H, D, J_H. Cell 19:981–992.

Failkow, P.J., Klein, E., Klein, G., Clifford, P., and Singh, S. 1973. Immunoglobulin and G-6-PD as markers of cellular origin in Burkitt lymphoma. J Exp Med 138:89–99.

Ford, R.J., Mehta, S., Franzini, Montagna, R., Lachman, L. and Maizel, A. 1981 Nature 294:261–263.

Ford, W.L. 1971. Lymphocyte migration and immune responses. Prog Allergy 1–79.

Foulds, L. 1958. The natural history of cancer. J Chronic Dis 8:2–37.

Fu, S.M., Chiorazzi, H., Kunkel, H., Halper, J.P., and Harris, S.R. 1978. Induction of *in vitro* differentiation and immunoglobulin synthesis of human leukemic B lymphocytes. J Exp Med 148:1570–1578.

Gillis, S., and Mizel, S. 1981. T cell lymphoma model for the analysis of interleukin 1-mediated T cell activation. Proc Natl Acad Sci USA 78:1133–1137.

Gillis, S., Scheid, M., and Watson, J. 1980. Biochemical and biologic characterization of lymphocyte regulatory molecules. III. J Immunol 125:2570–2578.

Gillis, S., and Watson, J. 1980. Biochemical and biological characterization of lymphocyte regulatory molecules. V. Identification of an IL-2-producing human T cell line. J Exp Med 152:1709–1719.

Haynes, B.F., Metzger, R.S., Minna, J.D., and Bunn, P.A. 1981. Phenotypic characterization of cutaneous T cell lymphoma. N Engl J Med 304:1319–1324.

Hersh, E.M. 1981. Perspectives for immunological and biological therapeutic intervention in human cancer. In: Immunological Aspects of Cancer Therapy, ed. E. Mehich. In press.

Hieter, P.A. Korsmeyer, S.J., Waldmann, T.A., and Leder, P. 1981. Human immunoglobulin K light-chain genes are deleted or rearranged in λ-producing B cells. Nature 290:368–372.

Hopper, J.E., and Haren, J.M. 1980. Studies on a Sezary lymphocyte population with T-suppressor activity. Clin Immunol Immuno Path 17:43–54.

Hough, D.W., Eady, R.P., Hamblin, F.D., Stevenson, F.K. and Stevenson, G.T. 1976. Anti-idiotype sera raised against surface immunoglobulin of human neoplastic lymphocytes. J Exp Med 144:960–966.

Katz, D.H. 1977. Lymphocyte differentiation, recognition, and regulation. Academic Press; New York.

Kim, H., Heller, P., and Rappaport, H. 1973. Monoclonal gammopathies associated with lymphoproliferative disorders: A morphologic study. Am J Clin Pathol 59:282–294.

Klein, G. 1979. Lymphoma development in mice and humans: Diversity of initiation is followed by convergent cytogenetic evolution. Proc Natl Acad Sci USA 2442–2446.

Klein, G. 1980. Immune and non-immune control of neoplastic development. Cancer 45:2486–2499.

Knowles, D.M. 1980. Non-Hodgkin's lymphomas. Immunologic and enzymatic markers useful in their evaluation. In: Progress in Surgical Pathology, vol. II, pp. 71–105, ed. C.M. Fenoglio and M. Wolff.

Lennert, K., Stein, H., and Kaiserling, E. 1975. Cytological and functional criteria for the classification of malignant lymphomath. Br J Can (Suppl.) 31:29–43.

Levy, R., and Dilley, J. 1978. Rescue of immunoglobulin secretion from human neoplastic lymphoid cells by somatic cell hybridization. Proc Natl Acad Sci USA 75:2411–2415.

Levy, R., Warnke, R., Dorfman, R.F., and Haimovich, J. 1977. The monoclonality of human B-cell lymphomas. J Exp Med 145:1014–1028.

Louie, S., Daoust, P.R., and Schwartz, R.S. 1980. Immunodeficiency and the pathogenesis of non-Hodgkins lymphoma. Semin Oncol 7:267–284.

Lukes, R.J., Parker, J.W., Taylor, C.R., et al. 1978. Immunologic approach to non-Hodgkin's lymphomas and related leukemias. Semin Hematol

15:322.

Maizel, A.L. Mehta, S.R., Hauft, S., Franzini, D., Lachman, L.B., and Ford, R.J. 1981. Human T lymphocyte/monocyte interaction in response to lectin: Kenetics of entry into the S-phase. J Immunol 127:1058–1064.

Maizel, A.L., Sahasrabudde, C. Mehta, S., and Ford, R., 1982.Isolation of a human B cell mitogenic factor. Proc Nat Acad Sci (USA) In press.

Meir, J.W., and Gallo, R.C. 1980. Purification and some characteristics of human T-cell growth factor from phytohemagglutinin-stimulated lymphocyte conditioned media. Proc Natl Acad Sci USA 77:6134–6138.

Metcalf, D. 1961. Reticular tumors in mice subjected to prolonged antigenic stimulation. Br J Cancer 15:769–779.

Miller, R.A., Coleman, C.N., Fawcett, H.D., Hoppe, R.T., McDougall, I.R. 1980. Sezary syndrome: a model for migration of T lymphocytes to skin. N Engl J Med 303:89–92.

Minowada, J. 1978. Markers of human leukemia-lymphoma cell lines reflect haemtopoietic cell differentiation. In: Human Lymphocyte Differentiation: Its Application to Cancer, ed. B Serrou and C. Rosenfeld. Elsevier/North Holland; New York.

Morgan, D.A., Ruscetti, F., and Gallo, R.C. 1976. Selective *in vitro* growth of T lymphocytes from normal human bone marrows. Science 193:1007–1008.

Nadler, L., Stashenko, P., Hardy, R., and Schlossman, S.F. 1980. A monoclonal antibody defining a lymphoma associated antigen in man. J Immunol 125:570–577.

Neel, B.G., Hayward, W.S., Robinson, H.L., et al. 1981. Avian leukosis virus-induced tumors have common proviral integration sites and synthesize discrete new RNAs; Oncogenesis by promoter insertion. Cell 23:323–334.

Nilsson, K. 1979. The nature of lymphoid cell lines and their relationship to the virus. In: The Epstein-Barr Virus, pp. 225⅓266, ed. M.A. Epstein and B.G. Achong. Springer-Verlag; New York.

Poiesz, B.J., Ruscetti, F.W., Gazdar, A.F., Bunn, P.A., Minna, J.D., and Gallo, R.C. 1980. Detection and isolation of type C retrovirus particles from fresh and cultured lymphocytes of a patient with T-cell lymphoma. Proc Natl Acad Sci USA 77:7415–7419.

Poiesz, B.J., Ruscetti, F.W., Mier, J.W., Woods, A.M., and Gallo, R.C. 1980. T cell lines established from human T-lymphocytic neoplasias by direct response to T-cell growth factor. Proc Natl Acad Sci USA 77:6815–6819.

Purtilo, D.T., Paquin, L., DeFlorio, D., Virzi, F., and Sakhuja, R. 1979. Immunodiagnosis and immunopathogenesis of the X-linked recessive lymphoproliferative syndrome. Semin Hematol 16:309–343.

Quesenberg, P., and Levitt, L. 1979. Hematopoietic stem cells. N Engl J Med 301:755–763.

Rappaport, H. 1966. Tumors of the hematopoietic system. In: Atlas of Tumor Pathology. AFIP article 8, Washington D.C.

Robert, K.H., and Nilsson, K. 1979. Covariances of mitogenic responses in leukemic blood lymphocytes: A functional marker system for the human B lymphocyte differentiation. Scand J Immunol 10:127–133.

Rowe, W.P. 1973. Genetic factors in the natural history of murine leukemia virus infection. Cancer Res 33:3061–3068.

Rowley, J.D., and Fukuhara, S. 1980. Chromosome studies in non-Hodgkin's lymphomas. Semin Oncol 7:255–266.

Ruscetti, F.S., and Gallo, R.C. 1981. Human T-lymphocyte growth factors; Regulation of growth and function of T lymphocytes. Blood 57:379–394.

Salmon, S., and Seligmann, M. 1974. B-cell neoplasia in man. Lancet 2:1229–1233.

Silvertrini, R., Piazza, R., Riccardi, A., and Rilke, F. 1977. Correlation of cell kinetic findings with morphology of non-Hodgkin's lymphomas. J Natl Cancer Inst 58:499–510.

Smith, K.A., Gilbride, K.J., and Favata, M.F. 1980. Lymphocyte actuating factor promotes T-cell growth factor production of cloned murine lymphoma cells. Nature 287:853–855.

Smith, K.A., Kachman, L.B., Oppenheim, J.J., and Favara, M.F. 1980 The functional relationship of the interleukins. J Exp Med 151:1551–1556.

Sprent, J., Miller, J.F.A.P., and Mitchell, G.F. 1971. Antigen induced selective recruitment of circulating lymphocytes. Cell Immunol 2:171–180.

Swain, S.L., Dennert, G., Warner, J.F., and Dutton, R.W. 1981. Culture supernatants of a stimulated T-cell line have helper activity that acts synergistically with interleukin 2 in the response of B cells to antigen. Proc Natl Acad Sci USA 78:2517–2521.

Taylor-Papadimitriou, J. 1980. Effects of interferons on cell growth and function. In: Interferon 2, pp. 13–46. Academic Press; New York.

Thierfelder, S., Rodt, H., and Thiel, E., eds. 1977. Immunological Diagnosis of Leukemias and Lymphomas. Springer-Verlag; New York.

Twomey, J.J., and Good, R.A., eds. 1978. The Immunobiology of Lymphoid Neoplasms. Plenum Press; New York.

Uchiyama, T., Yodoi, J., Sagawa, K., Takatsuki, K., and Uchino, H. 1977. Adult T cell leukemia: Clinical and hematologic features in 16 cases. Blood 50:481–492.

Wagstaff, J., Gibson, C., Thatcher, N., Ford, W.L., Sharma, H., Benson, W., and Crowther, D. 1981a. A method for following human lymphocyte traffic using indium-111 oxine labelling. Clin Exp Immunol 43:435–442.

Wagstaff, J., Gison, C., Thatcher, N., Ford, W.L., Sharma, H., Benson, W., and Crowther, D. 1981b. Human lymphcyte traffic assessed by indium-III oxine labelling: clinical observations. Clin Exp Immunol 43:443–449.

Zech, L., Hoglund, U., Nilsson, K., Klein, G. 1976. Characteristic chromosomal abnormalities in biopsies and lymphoid cell lines from patients with Burkitt's and non-Burkitt's lymphomas. Int J Cancer 17:47–60.

Chapter 12

Immunologic Defenses against Cancer

Ronald B. Herberman

Introduction

The role of the immune system in resistance to tumor growth has been a subject of intense interest in the last 10 years. To a large extent, attention has been focused on this issue by the convincing documentation that some tumors in mice have tumor-associated antigens that can be recognized by the host and can thereby induce specific resistance to progressive tumor growth (Gross, 1943; Foley, 1953; Prehn and Main, 1957; Klein et al., 1960). In addition to such tumor-associated transplantation antigens, early workers in tumor immunology looked for and described tumor-specific antigens, i.e., antigens on tumor cells which appeared to be qualitatively different from those on normal cells. Such antigens were reported to be present on a variety of human tumors [for review, see Herberman and McIntire (1979) and Herberman (1979)] as well as on tumors of experimental animals. A further impetus to the field was provided by the development of in vitro assays for detecting humoral and cell-mediated immune responses to tumor-associated cell surface antigens. Considerable reactivity was detected in tumor-bearing or tumor-immune individuals, which was often assumed to be directed against the tumor-associated transplantation antigens [reviewed by Herberman (1974, 1979)]. These findings led to extensive efforts in immunotherapy and immunodiagnosis of cancer, based on the expectation that these immunologic approaches would lead to major advances in the clinical management of patients with cancer.

Actual progress in this direction generally has been disappointing; this has led to considerable skepticism regarding the relevance of the immune system to cancer. However, to realistically appraise the situation and the problems, it is important to realize that several different and rather separate issues are involved. Among the issues of major clinical relevance are the possible importance of immune surveillance in prevention of detectable tumor development and growth; the possible efficacy of immunotherapy; the possible value of immunologic tests and tumor markers for the detection, diagnosis and management of cancer patients; and the possible immunosuppressive effects of tumor growth, which could compromise immunologic reactivity against a wide range of microbial and other antigens. In this review, I will focus primarily on immune surveillance and immunotherapy and discuss how immune parameters may serve as useful clinical correlates and aids in assessing prognosis.

A further consideration in regard to possible interactions between the immune system and cancer is the complexity of the immune system. Until recently, almost all attention was directed toward T and B cells. There is now a need to consider a heterogeneous array of potential effector mechanisms, each of which, alone or in concert with other parts of the immune system, could play an important role in host defenses against tumors.

Effector Mechanisms that may be Involved in Resistance against Tumor Growth

There is abundant evidence that T cells and B cells can react against tumor-associated antigens on a variety of experimental and human tumors. There is also a family of other natural effector mechanisms that may play an important part in host defenses. The major components in the natural immune system are natural killer (NK) cells, natural antibodies, macrophages and granulocytes. Below I will briefly discuss and compare some of the salient features of these effector mechanisms.

Tumor-associated Antigens and their Recognition by T and B Cells

Central to a possible involvement of T or B cells in resistance to tumor growth is the expression of immunogenic tumor-associated antigens on neoplastic cells. A tumor-associated antigen is an antigen that is found on a tumor cell and is undetectable on the cells of an adult normal individual. Most studies here focused on tumor-associated antigens on the cell surface, i.e., tumor-associated surface antigens (TASA).

One of the main functions of T cells is to be able to directly interact with and cause the lysis of target cells bearing antigens to which the T cells have been previously sensitized. One of the principal in vitro assays for the study of T cell immunity to TASA has been the ^{51}Cr release cytotoxicity assay. T cells have virtually no detectable spontaneous cytotoxic or other form of reactivity against tumor cells; rather they must be activated, usually by being exposed to the specific antigens, often presented on accessory cells like macrophages. Thus, there is a considerable latent period, of 7 to 10 days or more, in which to develop initial or primary reactivity. Reactivity then most often subsides to low or undetectable levels. Upon re-exposure to the antigen, a characteristic feature of T cells is to show an accelerated memory response, with development of high levels of activity within 2 to 5 days (Holden et al., 1975; Plata et al., 1975; Glaser and Herberman, 1976; Ting and Bonnard, 1976).

It appears, at least in some systems, that proliferation of lymphocytes is needed for generation of cytotoxic T cells against TASA (e.g., Bernstein et al., 1977). Direct evidence for lymphoproliferative responses to TASA has been obtained in a variety of tumor systems, particularly human tumors (Vànķy and Stjernswärd, 1979; Dean, 1979). Immune T cells may also respond to TASA by production and release of a variety of lymphokines, such as migration-inhibitory factors (McCoy, 1979), macrophage activating factors (Holden et al., 1979) and interferon. These lymphokines can activate or otherwise change the function of a variety of cell types; this may be an important mechanism for interaction between immune T cells and other effector cells for a more effective antitumor response.

The main manifestation of B cell response to TASA is production of specific antibodies. Immunization with tumor antigens usually leads to the formation of antibodies, as well as to cell-mediated immune responses. In addition to their direct effects on tumor cells, antibodies to TASA may act in cooperation with certain lymphocytes, macrophages or granulocytes which bear receptors for the Fc portion of immunoglobulin, especially IgG, to produce antibody-dependent cell-mediated cytotoxicity (ADCC). The extensive literature on antibodies to tumors has been reviewed in detail (Ting and Herberman, 1976; Hirshaut, 1977). Only a few selected points will be discussed here, particularly because there is relatively little evidence for a major role of antibodies in defense against tumors.

Macrophages and Polymorphonuclear Leukocytes (PMN)

Macrophages, monocytes and PMN are the other main categories of well known effector cells. These cells share many characteristics, but in most regards they are quite divergent from T cells. Macrophages and monocytes represent different stages of differentiation of the same cell type, and they and PMN are derived from common myelomonocytic bone marrow stem cells. In contrast to T cells, both macrophages and PMN have natural, spontaneous cytotoxic (cytolytic and/or cytostatic) reactivity against tumor cell lines (Keller, 1978; Mantovani et al., 1979; Tagliabue et al., 1979; Korec, 1980). In addition, they are rapidly activatable, within hours to 1 day, to considerably higher levels of cytotoxic activity (Sbarra and Strauss, 1980). Most of the activating factors are nonspecific and include lymphokines [e.g., macrophage-activating factor and interferon for macrophages (David and Remold, 1979)], phorbol esters for both cell types (De Chatelet et al., 1976; Nathan et al., 1979) and microbial products, particularly bacterial endotoxin for mouse macrophages (Doe and Henson, 1979). Stimulation of macrophages and PMN, in addition to leading to augmented cytotoxicity, causes a variety of biochemical and other changes. Activated macrophages have been shown to act as nonspecific suppressors of immune functions (Oehler et al., 1978; Jerrells et al., 1978) and to produce a series of immunomodulating products. These include lymphocyte-activating factor, which has activating effects on T cells (Oppenheim et al., 1980); interferon (Rabinovitch et al., 1977); prostaglandins, particularly of the E series (PGE) (Allison, 1978); and colony-stimulating factor (CSF). The production of interferon, PGE and CSF is of particular interest, since each of these molecules can appreciably affect the growth or functions of macrophages themselves as well as of other cell types.

In contrast to T cells, the interaction of macrophages and PMN with target cells does not depend on well defined antigenic specificities. They can kill a wide range of syngeneic, allogeneic and xenogeneic target cells, but some selectivity for certain targets, which are mainly malignant cells, has been demonstrated (Korec, 1980; Keller, 1980). There is no evidence for a clonal distribution of cells reacting with particular target cells or for a need to recognize products of the major histocompatibility complex on the targets.

Natural Killer (NK) Cells

NK cells share a number of features with T cells, being nonadherent and nonphagocytic and having some T cell-associated markers. However, NK cells are not thymic-dependent, with high levels of activity being detectable in athymic nude or neonatally thymectomized mice and rats (Herberman and Holden, 1978; Herberman, 1980). NK cells also share some properties with macrophages and PMN and they therefore represent a cell population that is quite difficult to categorize. NK cells have been found in most normal individuals of a wide range of mammalian and avian species (Herberman et al., 1978; Herberman, 1980). They express surface receptors for the Fc portion of IgG and they thereby appear to also function as K cells, mediating ADCC against tumor target cells (Ojo and Wigzell, 1978; Landazuri et al., 1979). Although NK cells clearly are not typical T cells, they have been found to share a variety of T cell-associated markers. About half of human NK cells express receptors for sheep erythrocytes (West et al., 1977) and the majority react (Ortaldo et al., 1981) with some monoclonal antibodies (9.6 and 3A1) to T cell-associated antigens. Similarly, at least one-half of mouse NK cells were shown to express Thy 1 (Mattes et al., 1979) and about 20% reacted with a monoclonal antibody to LyT1 (Koo and Hatzfeld, 1980). Also the monoclonal antibody, OX8, directed against a subpopulation of rat T cells with suppressor activity has been shown to react with a large proportion of rat NK cells (Reynolds et al., 1981a). NK cells have also been shown to grow in response to TCGF (Dennert, 1980; Ortaldo and Timonen, 1981) and they may also produce TCGF (Domzig et al., 1981). Furthermore, a highly enriched population of human NK cells has been shown to proliferate in response to T cell mitogens, phytohemagglutinin and concanavalin A (Timonen et al., 1981a). In contrast to such evidence for the relationship of NK cells to T cells, NK cells have also been shown to share some cell surface markers with macrophages and PMN. In the human, each of these cell types reacts with OKM1 and antibodies to asialo GM1 and Mac 1 (Zarling and Kung, 1980; Kay and Horwitz, 1980; Breard et al., 1981; Ault and Springer, 1981; Ortaldo et al., 1982) and in the mouse, one group has detected a macrophage-associated antigen, Mph 1, on a considerable portion of NK cells (Lohmann-Matthes and Domzig, 1980).

Particularly because of the conflicting evidence as to the relationship of NK cells to well known categories of lymphoid cells, much effort has been directed toward the identification of markers restricted to, or, at least, highly selective for, NK cells. The best such marker to date has been a morphologic one. Recent evidence has indicated that virtually all human and rat NK activity is mediated by large granular lymphocytes (LGL) (Timonen et al., 1981b; Reynolds et al., 1981b), which comprise only about 5% of the peripheral blood or splenic leukocytes in man and other species. LGL can be readily identified on cytocentrifuge preparations of lymphoid cells and they can be highly enriched by centrifugation on density gradients of Percoll (Timonen and Saksela, 1980; Timonen et al., 1981; Reynolds et al., 1981b). It now appears that LGL account for a high proportion of human T_G cells (Ferrarini et al., 1980), the relationship of which to typical T cells also has recently been questioned (Reinherz et al., 1980b). A monoclonal antibody, OKT10, has been found to react with most human LGL, but not with other peripheral blood leukocytes (Ortaldo et al., 1981). However, this antigen is not entirely specific for LGL, since it is also expressed on most thymocytes and a subpopulation of bone marrow cells (Reinherz et al., 1980a). Several surface antigens have also been found to be expressed, with some selectivity, on most or all mouse NK cells (Glimcher et al., 1977; Cantor et al., 1979; Kasai et al., 1980; Young et al., 1980; Tai and Warner, 1980). However, none of these markers have been shown to be restricted only to NK cells. Further, in contrast to LGL, which account for virtually all of the natural cytotoxic reactivity against a wide range of target cells (Landazuri et al., 1981), most of the alloantigenic markers on mouse NK cells have not been found on the related natural cytotoxic (NC) effector cells that react with some solid tumor target cells (Stutman et al., 1980; Burton, 1980).

In regard to their functional characteristics, NK cells share a number of features with macrophages and PMN. As with these other effector cells, NK cells have spontaneous activity in normal individuals and their activity can be rapidly augmented, particularly by interferon (Herberman et al., 1980; Saksela et al., 1980), but also by other stimuli (Goldfarb and Herberman, 1981b; Herberman et al., 1981c). However, like T cells and in contrast to macrophages and PMN, NK cells can proliferate in response to TCGF. As with all of the other types of effector cells, the activity of NK cells appears to be well regulated, subject to a variety of inhibitory cells and factors (Herberman et al., 1981c). The nature of the target cell recognition by NK cells seems to be intermediate between the exquisite specificity of T cells and the ill-defined or absent specificity of macrophages or PMN (Ortaldo and Herberman, 1981). NK cells can react against a wide variety of syngeneic, allogeneic and xenogeneic cells. Susceptibility to cytotoxic activity is not restricted to malignant cells, with fetal cells, virus-infected cells and some subpopulations of thymus cells, bone marrow cells and macrophages also being sensitive to lysis. It appears that NK cells can recognize at least several widely distributed antigenic specificities and that such recognition is clonally distributed (Ortaldo and Herberman, 1981). Despite this analogy with antigen recognition by T cells, recognition by NK cells does not seem to require expression of products of the major histocompatibility complex on target cells and there is no evidence for a memory response by NK cells. However, some similarity to a memory response has been seen with NK cells, since in vivo or in vitro exposure to NK-susceptible cell lines can rapidly activate NK cells via induction of interferon (Djeu et al., 1981). The nature of this recognition for interferon production and for cytotoxic interactions of NK cells with target cells is not clear. Some investigators have suggested that NK cells have T cell-like receptors (Kaplan and Callewaert, 1980), whereas others have postulated lectin-like receptors (Stutman et al., 1980a).

Similar to each of the other effector cell types, NK cells have been found not only to have direct cytotoxic effects against target cells, but also to produce and release soluble factors. Best documented is the ability of NK cells to produce interferon (Trinchieri and Santoli, 1978; Saksela et al., 1980; Djeu et al., 1981). In recent studies with highly enriched populations of human LGL, various tumor cell lines, viruses, mitogens and bacterial and other adjuvants were shown to induce considerable production of interferon after culture overnight (Djeu et al., 1981). Of particular note was that during these short-term incubations, only the LGL and not T cells or monocytes produced interferon in response to most of the stimuli. Human LGL, upon incubation with concanavalin A plus phorbol ester, also were found to produce substantial levels of TCGF (Domzig et al., 1981). These observations are of considerable interest for at least three reasons. First, they indicate that NK cells may be able to serve as important immunoregulatory cells, providing accessory function for a variety of immune responses that are affected by interferon or TCGF. Secondly, it appears that NK cells may be able to react with foreign materials in a multifaceted way, by producing soluble factors that can induce antiviral resistance and cytostasis of tumor cells, as well as by direct cytotoxic effects. Further, the ability of NK cells to rapidly produce interferon and TCGF provides a mechanism for positive self regulation.

Is the Immune Surveillance Hypothesis Valid?

The general role of the immune system in preventing or limiting tumor growth has been emphasized by many investigators, perhaps beginning with Ehrlich (1909). Burnet (1957) stated, "It is by no means inconceivable that small accumulations of tumor cells may develop and because of the possession of new antigenic potentialities provoke an effective immunological reaction with regression of the tumor and no clinical hint of its existence." Thomas (1959) extended the concept further, postulating that the mechanisms for homograft rejection were evolved primarily as a natural defense against neoplasia. This theory of immune surveillance has generated many experimental studies and much discussion and controversy. One of the reasons for the controversy is that the concept is rather complex and leads to a series of predictions. Some of the major predictions are as follows. a) Tumor cells have antigens, i.e., structures that could be recognized by the immune system and could result in reactivity of the host against the tumor, leading to its eventual elimination. b) The part of the immune system that is involved in resistance against tumor growth is the same as that involved in rejection of transplants of normal tissues. c) Immune depression is a necessary antecedent event to the development of detectable tumors. Along this line, d) immunosuppression would be expected to cause increased susceptibility to tumor development and e) one requisite action of carcinogens and/or tumor promoters might be to suppress host defenses.

The main support for the immune surveillance hypothesis has come from evidence related to prediction d, since naturally occurring or induced immunodepression has been associated with a higher incidence of some types of tumors. In experimental animals, this has been most clearly demonstrated with tumors induced by oncogenic viruses. Polyoma virus is widespread in nature, yet wild mice do not develop polyoma tumors (Huebner, 1963). However, administration of the virus to newborn mice of some inbred strains, when their immune system is not fully developed, results in neoplastic growth. Suppression of immunity, particularly by procedures which affect thymus-dependent immune responses, has been shown to greatly increase the incidence of polyoma tumors (Law, 1965, 1966; Law and Ting, 1965; Allison and Law, 1968; Allison, 1970). Similarly, neonatal thymectomy of chickens results in an increased frequency of tumors in strains which are genetically resistant to the malignant effects of Marek's disease virus (Payne, 1972). Treatment with antilymphocyte serum potentiated murine leukemia virus-induced tumors and shortened the latent period of spontaneous leukemia in AKR mice (Allison and Law, 1968). There is also considerable clinical evidence that immunodepression is associated with an increased incidence of tumors. Several studies have pointed out the association of immune deficiency diseases and lymphomas and leukemia (Fraumeni, 1969; Doll and Kinlen, 1970). Gatti and Good (1971) estimated that the incidence of tumors in these patients was about 10,000 times that seen in the general age-matched population. Allograft recipients receiving immunosuppressive agents, mainly prednisone and azathioprine, have also been found to have an increased incidence (approximately 100 times that of the general age-matched population) of tumors (Penn and Starzl, 1972; Greene et al., 1981). Again lymphomas have been prominent, but the majority of the tumors have been of epithelial origin.

Similarly, patients with Hodgkin's disease or other types of cancer, or patients with arthritis or other benign diseases who received chemotherapeutic (mainly alkylating) agents, have been found to subsequently develop primary malignancies, mainly leukemias and lymphomas, with relatively high frequency (Hyman, 1969; Canellos et al., 1974; Roberts and Bell, 1976; Tchernia et al., 1976; Puri and Campbell, 1977; Reimer et al., 1977).

The effects of immunosuppression on tumor induction in experimental animals by chemical carcinogens have been even less clear-cut (Stutman, 1975). In some studies, an increased incidence of tumors was seen (e.g., Grant, 1966; Balner and Dersjant, 1969). Lappé (1971), in a study involving isografts of methylcholanthrene-treated skin, found fewer tumors in immunocompetent mice and also found evidence for microscopic regressions of tumors. However, Haran-Ghera and Lurie (1971) did not find an increased incidence of tumors due to dimethylbenzanthracene in mice treated with antilymphocyte serum. Similarly, there has been a general failure to observe more rapid tumor growth or even higher incidences of carcinogen-induced tumors in nude mice (Stutman, 1979). One possible explanation for such negative findings has been that the carcinogenic agents themselves are immunosuppressive and additional suppression may not have an incremental effect. However, the data on this point (prediction e) in regard to possible effects on mature T cells and humoral immunity have been conflicting (summarized by Stutman, 1975).

A likely explanation for many of the discrepant results concerning the possible association of immune depression and tumor development is that various effector mechanisms may be involved in host resistance; results may vary with the type of effector mechanism that plays a predominant role with each form of cancer and with the nature and extent of the immune deficiency.

Such a likelihood of diversity of effector mechanisms that might be involved in immune surveillance may be offered as a response to most of the criticisms that have been raised against the hypothesis. When information about thymus-dependent immunity became known, and particularly when T cells were found to play a central role in allograft rejection, the immune surveillance hypothesis was modified to stress the key role of this effector mechanism in antitumor resistance (Burnet, 1970). Related to this has been the emphasis placed on expression in tumors of tumor-associated transplantation antigens, since such structures would have to be recognized by T cells in order to get effective T cell-mediated resistance to tumor growth. However, it has only been possible to obtain strong evidence for a major in vivo role of T cells in immunity to virus-induced tumors (e.g., Collavo et al., 1974; Gorczynski and Norbury, 1974; Berenson et al., 1975; Glaser et al., 1976) and little comparable evidence exists for spontaneous tumors or even for transplantable chemical carcinogen-induced tumors. Much attention has been given to the decreased incidence of mouse mammary tumors in neonatally thymectomized mice (Yunis et al., 1969; Stutman, 1975). There has also been a failure to detect tumor-associated transplantation antigens on many spontaneous tumors (Hewitt et al., 1976). These observations have led to the suggestion (Klein and Klein, 1977) that immune surveillance may only be operative against tumors induced by oncogenic viruses, which have strong transplantation antigens and for which immune T cells have been shown to be important in resistance. Other investigators have reacted to such information in a more pessimistic way; Nossal (1980), for instance, suggested that immune surveillance and tumor immunology in general were moribund if not terminally ill. The major exceptions to the central role of immune T cells in resistance to tumor growth have led to a counter-theory of immunostimulation (Prehn and Lappé, 1971), which suggests that the immune system may have mainly enhancing effects on tumor induction and growth. However, when T cell-mediated immunity is viewed as only one of a series of possible host defense mechanisms, the evidence summarized above need not be viewed in such a negative light. Target cell structures other than tumor-associated transplantation antigens might be involved in recognition by other types of effector cells; in T cell-deficient individuals, the other effector mechanisms might still be functional and capable of resisting tumor growth.

What then are the likely alternatives to T cell-mediated immunity in antitumor resistance and immune surveillance? A variety of possibilities need to be seriously considered, such as macrophages, NK cells and other related natural effector cells and ADCC. The evidence in support of a role for each is summarized below.

Possible Role of Macrophages in Immune Surveillance

Observations that activated macrophages could have substantial cytotoxicity against a variety of tumor cell lines and the evidence that transformed cells were selectively susceptible to such attack led rapidly to suggestions that macrophages might play an important role in antitumor defenses and might be primarily responsible for immune surveillance against tumors (Hibbs et al., 1972a and b, 1978; Hibbs, 1974a; Baldwin, 1976; Currie, 1976; Fidler et al., 1978; Adams and Snyderman, 1979). It has been pointed out by several authors that an immune surveillance role of macrophages would overcome most of the arguments that have been raised against the immune surveillance hypothesis (e.g., Adams and Snyderman, 1979) and that the characteristics of cytotoxicity by macrophages fit most of the requirements for an ideal model antitumor effector cell (Hibbs et al., 1978).

To continue to seriously consider a possible role for the macrophage in antitumor defense, it is important to go beyond the theoretical considerations and generate experimental data in support of various testable predictions regarding macrophages. Among such predictions are that macrophages should be able to enter the site of tumor growth, that selective depression of macrophage function should be associated with an increased incidence of tumors, that selective augmentation of macrophage function or selective adoptive transfer of macrophages should be associated with a decreased incidence of tumors, and that one of the requisite effects of carcinogen-inducing tumors controlled by macrophages should be to depress macrophage function. It is particularly important to obtain experimental data concerning these predictions in regard to the development of spontaneous or carcinogen-induced primary tumors. However, most of the available information has been from studies with transplantable tumor lines; often it is based on a therapy protocol rather than a protocol for prevention of tumor development. Nevertheless, it is worthwhile to consider the available data and their limitations and discuss the further experiments that are needed.

There is abundant evidence that macrophages can accumulate in considerable numbers in a variety of transplantable tumors (Evans, 1972; Eccles and Alexander, 1974) and in many primary tumors (Gauci and Alexander, 1975; Alexander, 1976; Levy and Wheelock, 1974). The possibility of a functional antitumor role for such cells was supported by observations that the degree of in situ infiltration of primary tumors by macrophages was inversely correlated with a tendency toward metastic spread of the tumors (Alexander, 1976). However, more extensive examination of this issue has resulted in a considerable amount of contradictory evidence, indicating no correlation between the number of macrophages within a tumor and its metastic potential [summarized by Evans and Haskill

(1981).] This had led to the opposite suggestion, that the presence of macrophages within some tumors may promote their growth and metastasis (Evans, 1978, 1979).

A frequent experimental approach has been to examine the effects of macrophage-depressive treatments on the growth of tumors. Growth of some transplantable tumors, and particularly their tendency to metastasize, was found to be increased when the recipients were treated with silica, carrageenin, trypan blue or gold salts (Ghose, 1957; Faraci et al., 1975; McBride et al., 1975; Keller, 1976; Sones and Castro, 1977), which are agents which have been shown to deplete macrophages or interfere with their functions (Allison et al., 1966; Hibbs, 1974b and 1975; Ghaffar et al., 1976). Similarly, Wood and Gillespie (1973) showed that in vitro damage to macrophages in a tumor inoculum resulted in an increased incidence of metastases. Such treatments have also been shown to augment the development of some primary tumors. Silica treatment of mice during the period of exposure to ultraviolet light was shown to increase the incidence of resultant skin tumors (Norbury and Kripke, 1979) and treatment with silica, carrageenin or antimacrophage serum enhanced Friend virus-induced leukemogenesis (Marcelletti and Furmanski, 1978). Similarly, repeated inoculations of silica into AKR mice resulted in earlier development of spontaneous leukemia (Chow et al., 1979). It should be noted that there are some major limitations to such evidence. Silica and carrageenin, and possibly the other depressive treatments as well, may not be entirely selective in their effects. They may in fact cause increases in some functions, particularly suppressor activity, by macrophages or other cells (Cudkowicz and Hochman, 1979). These agents can directly or indirectly depress the functions of other cell types, e.g., NK cells (Oehler and Herberman, 1978; Djeu et al., 1979). The effects of such treatments on tumor growth are not always in the same direction, even with the same tumor. For example, Mantovani et al. (1980) found that treatment of mice with silica or carrageenin increased the incidence of pulmonary metastases but inhibited the growth of the primary tumors. Evans (1979) observed a parallel retardation of growth of the tumors by using another treatment, sublethal irradiation with 400 R, which resulted in a decrease for several weeks in the macrophage content in fibrosarcomas.

The converse line of evidence, indicating a decrease in tumor growth after treatment with agents that can stimulate the function of macrophages, has often been taken as a further demonstration of the important role of macrophages in antitumor defenses (e.g., Levy and Wheelock, 1974). For example, administration of pyran copolymer (Norbury and Kripke, 1979) has been shown to inhibit the development of ultraviolet light-induced skin tumors. However, a major limitation to such an approach is that almost all of the agents used for stimulation of macrophages also can have substantial effects on the activity of other potential effector mechanisms. In particular, such treatments usually cause interferon production and a consequent augmentation of NK activity (Herberman et al., 1979, 1981b).

A more direct approach has involved the adoptive transfer of activated macrophages. Fidler (1974) showed that transfer of macrophages that had been activated in vitro could interfere with the metastatic spread of tumor cells. Similarly, transfer of in vivo activated macrophages had protective effects (Sones and Castro, 1977; Liotta et al., 1977). However, even such data do not conclusively demonstrate a direct effector role for macrophages, since activated macrophages are known to produce interferon and other products that might act to stimulate other effector cells, particularly NK cells (e.g., Djeu et al., 1979a).

There are some other suggestive pieces of evidence to be considered in regard to the possible role of macrophages in antitumor defense. Although there are some exceptions, there is generally higher reticuloendothelial activity in strains of mice with low tumor incidence than in those strains with high tumor incidence [summarized by Stern (1981)]. It is also of note that a variety of agents that are taken up by the reticuloendothelial system and that have been shown to be macrophage-toxic can induce tumors. Administration of trypan blue to mice has been shown to cause hepatic sarcomas of the Kupffer cells (Papacharalampous, 1960) and reticulum cell sarcomas (Gillman et al., 1973). Similarly, carrageenin, polyvinylpyrrolidone, dextran and CM cellulose have been shown to induce sarcomas, reticulum cell sarcomas or lymphosarcomas (Hueper, 1959, 1961; Walpole, 1962). However, these results may not bear on the issue of the involvement of macrophages in immune surveillance; at least some of the tumors appear to involve macrophages themselves and, therefore, seem to be a reflection of transformation following direct damage to this cell population. Of greater interest is whether other types of carcinogens which cause tumors of other cell types cause depression of macrophage function during the latent period, prior to the detectable appearance of tumors. Most studies measured reticuloendothelial clearance or phagocytosis by macrophages in vitro rather than macrophage-mediated cytotoxicity or other functions and the results have been mixed. Some carcinogens (methylcholanthrene and acetylaminofluorene) have been shown to decrease reticuloendothelial functions (Argus et al., 1962; Faraci et al., 1975; Thor et al., 1977; Tewari et al., 1979; Stern, 1981), whereas others (dimethylbenzanthracene, urethane and methylnitrosourea) have had no detectable effect (Franceschi et al., 1972; Zwilling et al., 1978).

Overall, the available evidence regarding the role of macrophages in immune surveillance is fragmentary and incomplete. Adams and Snyderman (1979) have summarized the current status well. "The extant data support but do not controvert the hypothesis that macrophages exert surveillance. However, the experiments to test this proposition vigorously have not been performed." What then are the needed experiments? Perhaps the most compelling series of experiments would be to produce a selective depression in macrophage function or to utilize animals with a selective genetic defect in macrophage function to determine whether such animals have an increased incidence of spontaneous tumors or of carcinogen-induced tumors. To overcome the likelihood that in most cases the abnormalities would not be limited to macrophages, it would be important to show that selective reconstitution of the animals with macrophages could decrease or eliminate any increased incidence of tumors. Another approach would be to obtain extensive evidence as to whether carcinogens cause a decrease in macrophage function, especially cytotoxic activity, during the latent period and, if so, whether a selective restoration of macrophage function would interfere with carcinogenesis. Yet another direction would be to identify treatments which could selectively increase macrophage functions without altering other effector functions (e.g., non-interferon-inducing agents) and to then determine whether this is associated with a decrease in the incidence of spontaneous or carcinogen-induced tumors.

Possible Role of NK Cells or Other Related Natural Effector Cells to Immune Surveillance

There is substantial evidence for an important role of NK cells in in vivo resistance against established cell lines of tumors, particularly those that show susceptibility to in vitro cytolysis by NK cells.

A major approach has been to look for correlations between in vivo resistance to the growth of the tumor cell lines and the levels of NK activity in the recipients. In several different situations, a good correlation was observed. Some NK-sensitive tumor lines have produced a lower incidence of tumors and have grown more slowly in nude or thymectomized mice than in euthymic mice with the same genetic background (Kiessling et al., 1976; Herberman and Holden, 1978; Riesenfeld et al., 1980). Fewer transplantable tumors have also been induced in 5- to 10-week-old mice at the peak of NK activity than in older mice with low NK activity (Sendo et al., 1975; Herberman and Holden, 1978). Some recent studies have examined the effects of age on growth of several transplantable tumors in nude mice. A much higher incidence of metastases after either intravenous or subcutaneous transplantation was seen in 3-week-old nude mice which had low NK activity than in 6-week-old mice which had high NK activity. A high rate of pulmonary metastases in young nude mouse recipients was seen with xenogeneic as well as allogeneic tumor cell lines (Hanna, 1980;

Hanna and Fidler, 1981). Augmentation of NK activity in the 3-week-old nude mice by treatment with poly I:C or *C. parvum* inhibited the development of metastases. The apparent major role of NK cells in resistance against growth of transplantable tumors in nude mice and the ability to circumvent this by using nude mice with low NK activity has practical implications in the utilization of nude mice for growth of human tumors. Many investigators have noted the difficulty with which some tumors grow in nude mice and the rarity of metastases, even when metastatic deposits of human tumors are transplanted (Rygaard and Poulsen, 1969; Castro, 1972; Ozzello et al., 1974; Schmidt and Good, 1976; Maguire et al., 1976; Sharkey and Fogh, 1979). The findings that some human tumor cells are susceptible to mouse NK activity (Haller et al., 1977; Nunn and Herberman, 1979) are consistent with a role for NK cells in this resistance.

Kiessling and his associates (Kiessling et al., 1975b; Petrányi et al., 1976) performed an extensive series of experiments which demonstrated a correlation between the levels of NK activity in different strains of mice and the resistance of F_1 hybrids between each strain and A mice to the A strain lymphoma, YAC, the cultured line of which is highly sensitive to NK activity. Mice which were thymectomized, irradiated, and reconstituted with fetal liver also showed this resistance (Kiessling et al., 1976). Haller et al. (1977) extended this approach by transferring bone marrow cells from high or low NK strains to lethally irradiated low NK recipients. Recipients of cells from high NK donors developed high NK activity and had increased resistance to growth of YAC.

The various types of correlation described above have only been observed with tumor lines with some susceptibility to lysis by NK cells. The growth of completely NK-resistant cell lines has not been affected by the levels of NK activity in the recipients (e.g., Riesenfeld et al., 1980). It is of interest in this regard that in a study of two sublines of a mouse lung tumor the metastatic subline was resistant to NK activity, whereas the nonmetastatic subline showed some susceptibility (Gorelik et al, 1979).

Beige mice with low NK activity associated with their recessive point mutation (Roder and Duwe, 1979) have also provided a convenient model for examining the role of NK cells in resistance to growth of transplantable tumor lines. Talmadge et al. (1980) found that an NK-susceptible syngeneic melanoma cell line grew more rapidly and produced more metastases in beige compared to normal mice. This difference was not seen with an NK-resistant subline of the same tumor. Using a similar approach, Kärre et al. (1980) found that two NK-susceptible syngeneic lymphomas produced a higher incidence of tumors and grew more rapidly in beige than in normal heterozygous littermates.

Another approach to the in vivo role of NK cells in the growth of transplantable tumors has been the attempt to transfer increased resistance by NK cell-enriched populations. Kasai et al. (1979) enriched for Ly 5+ spleen cells and depleted Thy 1+ and B cells and showed that this small subpopulation of cells had high NK activity. Mixture of these Ly 5+ with an NK-sensitive lymphoma cell line resulted in reduced tumor incidence after transplantation. Similarly, local adoptive transfer of NK-1+ cells suppressed growth of the YAC lymphoma (Tam et al., 1980). Systemic adoptive transfer of cells with the characteristics of NK cells from normal or nude mice was also found to increase protection against a transplantable leukemia in an immunochemotherapy model system (Cheever et al., 1980).

In an alternative approach that utilized information about selective markers on mouse NK cells, Habu et al. (1981) administered anti-asialo GM1 to nude mice. The treated mice had almost no detectable NK activity and showed increased susceptibility to transplantation of syngeneic, allogeneic and human tumors.

Although the above studies point to a significant role of NK cells in resistance against tumor growth, they do not conclusively show that NK cells are the actual in vivo effector cells. Since these studies relied on measurement of tumor incidence or growth rate at a considerable time after tumor challenge, one cannot rule out the possibility that NK cells helped to induce or recruit other effector mechanisms, such as T cells or activated macrophages. To obtain more direct information about the role of NK cells in the direct and rapid in vivo elimination of tumor cells, ^{125}I-iododeoxyuridine- (^{125}IUdR) labeled tumor cells were inoculated intravenously and clearance from the lungs and other organs was measured (Riccardi et al., 1979, 1980a and b). In young mice of strains with high NK activity, there was a greater clearance of radioactivity when measured at 2 to 4 hours after inoculation than was seen in strains with low reactivity. In parallel with the decline of NK activity in mice after 10 to 12 weeks of age, in vivo clearance of intravenously inoculated tumor cells was also found to decrease. Furthermore, treatment of mice with a variety of agents that produced augmented or decreased in vitro reactivity also resulted in similar shifts in in vivo reactivity. Such correlations were observed with several NK-susceptible tumor lines but not with some completely NK-resistant lines (Riccardi et al. 1980b).

As further confirmation of the role of NK cells in resistance to growth of NK-susceptible transplantable tumors, transfer of NK cell-containing populations into mice with cyclophosphamide-induced depression of NK activity was shown to significantly restore both in vivo clearance and NK reactivity (Riccardi et al., 1981a and b). The effectiveness of the transfer correlated with the levels of NK activity of donor cells in a variety of situations: NK-reactive spleen cells were able to transfer reactivity, whereas NK-unreactive thymus cells were ineffective; spleen cells from young mice of high NK activity strains were considerably more effective than cells from older mice or from strains with low NK activity; the cells responsible for transfer had the characteristics of NK cells, being nonadherent and nonphagocytic, expressing asialo GM1 and lacking easily detectable Thy 1 antigen; and cells from donors with drug-induced depression of NK activity were unable to transfer reactivity. These results extend the recent findings of Hanna and Fidler (1980), who showed that the transfer of NK-reactive spleen cells to cyclophosphamide-treated mice could decrease the number of metastases developing in the lungs after challenge with NK-susceptible solid tumor cells.

A similar pattern of results was obtained when radio-labeled cells were inoculated subcutaneously into the footpads of mice (Gorelik and Herberman, 1981a). Clearance correlated in several ways with the levels of NK activity in the recipients; cells with the characteristics of NK cells were effective in local adoptive transfer. However, in contrast to NK activity and the results with intravenously inoculated tumor cells, no decrease in clearance was observed in older or beige mice. Those results suggest that other effector cells may also be involved in reactivity in subcutaneous tissues ([e.g., the natural cytotoxic cells described by Stutman et al. (Paige et al., 1978; Stutman et al., 1980b and c)] or that in some situations local factors may augment the NK cell activity.

Although the results in some studies, particularly those with intravenously inoculated radio-labeled tumor cells, suggested that NK cells may be particularly involved in resistance against hematogenous metastatic spread of tumors (Hanna and Fidler, 1980), the results with the footpad assay (Gorelik and Herberman, 1981) and the various demonstrations of NK-related differences in outgrowth of subcutaneous tumors indicate that natural effector cells can also enter and be active at sites of local tumor growth. This is supported by the direct demonstration of NK cells in cell suspensions prepared from small tumors growing at subcutaneous or intramuscular locations (Gerson, 1980). Thus, NK cells have the potential to be involved in the primary line of defense against both the local outgrowth as well as the metastatic spread of transplanted tumors. However, it appears that the effectiveness of this natural resistance mechanism is rather limited. Even with tumor cells that are highly susceptible to NK activity, development of progressively growing tumors can occur in animals with high NK activity.

From the available evidence as summarized above, it seems likely that NK cells play an important role in resistance to growth and metastatic spread of some tumor cell lines. Although such results are encouraging, they do not indicate whether NK cells also can have a similar role in defense against growth and metastasis of primary tumors. To obtain evidence in support of such a function, it would be desirable to document the following predictions. Primary tumor cells should have some demonstrable susceptibility to recognition by NK cells. The NK cells of tumor-bearing individuals should be able, under some circumstances, to interact with the autologous tumor. Selective alterations in NK activity in tumor-bearing individuals should affect the growth or degree of metastatic spread of the tumors.

Unfortunately, information relevant to any of these points is quite scanty and, to my knowledge, no clear data exist for the last prediction. Before reviewing the available evidence regarding NK reactivity against primary tumor cells, I would like to point out the difficulties that would be anticipated were NK cells to play a significant role in growth of primary tumors. For such studies, one would have to obtain tumors of sufficient size to prepare adequate numbers of tumor cells. By definition, such tumors must have been at least relatively successful in evading host defense mechanisms. Therefore, if NK cells play an important role in resistance, one would predict that tumor outgrowth would only occur in the face of relative resistance to lysis by NK cells and/or depression of NK activity. Thus, the results most consistent with these qualifications of the stated predictions would be detectable but low levels of interaction between NK cells and tumor cells.

Some evidence has accumulated. The majority of spontaneous mammary tumors of C3H mice (Serrate and Herberman, 1981) and of spontaneous lymphomas in AKR mice (Nunn et al., 1977) have been found to have detectable, albeit low, susceptibility to lysis by NK cells. Similarly, some human leukemias (Rosenberg et al., 1972; Axberg et al., 1980; Zarling et al., 1979), a myeloma (Axberg et al., 1980) and some carcinomas, sarcomas and melanomas (Vánky et al., 1980; Mantovani et al., 1981) have been significantly lysed by NK cells. Such lysis has been appreciably augmented, and thereby evident with a higher proportion of tumors, when the effector cells were pretreated with interferon (Zarling et al., 1979; Axberg et al., 1980; Vánky et al., 1980; Mantovani et al., 1981). As further support for the ability of NK cells to recognize primary tumor cells, Ortaldo et al. (1977) showed that a variety of human tumor cells could cold target inhibit the lysis of radiolabeled K562 cells. Most of these positive results were obtained with NK cells from normal allogeneic donors. In fact, Vánky et al. (1980) detected NK reactivity only against allogeneic human tumor cells and concluded that the NK cells of the tumor-bearing individual lacked the ability to recognize the autologous tumor cells. They postulated that recognition of foreign histocompatibility antigens was involved in lysis by NK cells, particularly those stimulated by interferon. If correct, their hypothesis would virtually preclude a role for NK cells in resistance against primary tumor growth. However, such restriction of NK reactivity to allogeneic tumors does not fit the many examples of tumor cell lines susceptible to syngeneic NK cells (e.g., Herberman et al., 1975; Kiessling et al., 1975a). Similarly, normal C3H mice have been found to be reactive against some syngeneic mammary tumors (Serrate and Herberman, 1981) and some cancer patients also have had detectable, interferon-augmentable NK activity against their autologous tumor cells (Mantovani et al., 1981). The reason for the discrepancies among the human studies is not clear. The positive results were obtained with ovarian carcinoma cells, mainly in 20-hour cytotoxicity assays (Mantovani et al., 1981), whereas the allo-restricted results involved other types of tumors tested only in 4-hour assays. The greater sensitivity of the prolonged assay seems sufficient to account for the differences. In addition, it is possible that the subpopulation of NK cells that are required to interact to certain types of tumors may be selectively inhibited in the autologous tumor-bearing host.

Another line of evidence in support of the possibility for NK cells to interact in vivo with autologous primary tumor cells is the demonstration that NK cells can enter and accumulate at the site of tumor growth. NK cells have been detected in small spontaneous mouse mammary carcinomas (Gerson, 1980) and in small primary mouse tumors induced by murine sarcoma virus (Gerson, 1980; Becker, 1980). In contrast, NK activity has usually been undectable in large tumors in mice (Gerson, 1980) or in clinical tumor specimens. This may be due, at least in part, to the presence of suppressor cells, which have been demonstrated in some cell suspensions from some tumors (Vose and Moore,

1979; Gerson, 1980; Eremin, 1980; Gerson et al., 1981; Allavena et al., 1981).

To further support the possible role of NK cells in resistance against the growth of primary tumors, it would be very helpful to examine the effects of selective alterations of NK activity in tumor-bearers. However, very few experiments specificially designed to examine this issue have been reported. Suggestive evidence has come from the administration of indomethacin to mice bearing primary murine sarcoma virus-induced tumors (Brunda et al., 1980). With a treatment schedule that augmented the depressed NK reactivity, tumor incidence and size were reduced and a higher proportion of tumors completely regressed. Similarly, one could invoke the therapeutic efficacy of interferon for some primary tumors, a treatment known to augment NK reactivity. The limitations of such data are that such agents have pleiotropic effects and it is not possible to determine whether the alterations in other functions had the more important influence on tumor growth. Studies with more selective alterations in NK activity will be needed to settle this issue. Such experiments probably should be performed in individuals with only a small amount of tumor present, to allow the detection of effects on tumor growth that might be more likely during a phase when the host is not already overwhelmed by extensive tumor burden.

Of paramount interest is whether NK cells may be involved in immune surveillance against the initial development of spontaneous or carcinogen-induced tumors. Thus far, very few well-designed experiments have been performed to address this issue directly.

However, first it is of interest to summarize several pieces of circumstantial evidence consistent with or suggestive of a role for NK cells. NK activity has been shown to be substantially augmented by retinoic acid (Goldfarb and Herberman, 1981a), which has been reported to retard the development of some primary tumors (Lotan, 1980). In support of this possibility, cells with the characteristics of NK cells have been found to inhibit the in vitro proliferation of autologous EBV-infected B cells (Shope and Kaplan, 1979). Patients with the genetically determined Chediak-Higashi syndrome have a high risk of development of lymphoproliferative diseases (Dent et al., 1966). In recent detailed studies on several patients with this disease (Roder et al., 1980, 1981), all were found to have profound deficits in NK and K cell activities, whereas a variety of other immune functions, including cytotoxicity against tumor cells by T cells, monocytes and granulocytes, was essentially normal. Similarly, beige mice, which have an analogous genetic defect, also have a substantial (Roder et al., 1979; Roder and Duwe, 1979) but incomplete (Brunda et al., 1980b; Cudkowicz, 1981) selective deficiency in NK activity. A small colony of aged beige mice has recently been reported to have a high incidence of lymphoma (Loutit et al., 1980). Another human genetic abnormality, X-linked lymphoproliferative disease (Purtilo et al., 1977), has been associated with a defect in the ability to control proliferation of B cells infected with Epstein Barr virus (EBV). Recently, low NK activity has been found in such individuals; this deficit has been suggested to be involved in the pathogenesis of the disease (Sullivan et al., 1980). Patients on immunosuppressive therapy after kidney allotransplants have a high risk of developing both reticuloendothelial tumors and a variety of carcinomas (Penn and Starzl, 1972). Patients on such treatment regimens have recently been found to have very low NK activity and this has been suggested as a contributing factor in the subsequent development of tumors (Lipinski et al., 1980; Tursz et al., 1981). Each of these lines of evidence fits one of the major predictions of the immune surveillance theory, which is that tumor development would be associated with, and in fact preceded by, depressed immunity.

In regard to the prediction of the immune surveillance theory that carcinogenic agents cause depressed immune function, the initial fragmentary data on NK cells are promising. Urethane, which produces lung tumors only in some strains of mice, caused transient and marked depression of NK activity in a susceptible strain (Gorelik and Herberman, 1981b) but not in resistant strains (Gorelik and Herberman, 1981c). Administration of normal bone marrow cells, which can reconstitute NK activity, to urethane-treated mice reduced the subsequent development of lung tumors (Kraskovsky et al., 1973; Gorelik and Herberman, unpublished observations). Also, infection during the latent period with various viruses, each known to induce interferon and thereby augment NK activity, also reduced the incidence of lung tumors induced by urethane. Carcinogenic doses of dimethylbenzanthracene also were found to produce depression of NK activity during the latent period (Ehrlich et al., 1980). Sublethal irradiation of mice has been found to cause considerable depression of NK activity (Hochman et al., 1978). Of particular interest, the schedule of multiple low doses of irradiation of C57BL mice, which has been highly effective in inducing leukemia in this strain, was found to produce a substantial deficit in NK activity (Parkinson et al., 1981; Gorelik and Herberman, unpublished observations). The depressed NK activity could be restored by transfer of normal bone marrow cells (Gorelik and Herberman, unpublished observations), a procedure which has been reported to interfere with radiation-induced leukogenesis (Kaplan et al., 1953). In contrast, transfer of bone marrow from beige mice did not restore NK activity. NK activity also has been strongly inhibited by two different classes of potent tumor promoters, phorbol esters (Keller, 1979; Goldfarb and Herberman, 1981a) and teleocidin (Goldfarb, Sugimura and Herberman, unpublished observations). All of these observations support the possibility that one of the requisites for tumor induction by carcinogenic agents may be interference with host defenses, including those mediated by NK cells.

Further studies are needed to more directly demonstrate a role for NK cells in immune surveillance. Ideally, one would like to show increased tumorigenesis when NK activity is selectively depressed and reduced tumor formation when such deficiencies are selectively reconstituted or normal levels of reactivity are selectively augmented. However, there are several practical problems which limit vigorous pursuit of such experimental protocols. In addition to the long periods of time needed for such studies and difficulties in identifying the most relevant experimental carcinogenesis models, completely selective and sustained alterations of NK activity are not easily found or produced. For example, as discussed above, much attention is currently being given to the beige mouse model as a test system for oncogenesis in NK-deficient animals. However, beige mice have some residual NK activity, which can be augmented by interferon (Brunda et al., 1980b) and can approach normal levels upon prolonged incubation with target cells (Cudkowicz, 1981). Furthermore, they appear to have normal levels of natural cytotoxic activity in vitro against some monolayer tumor target cells (Burton, 1980) and in vivo against subcutaneous inoculations of both lymphoma anc carcinoma cell lines (Gorelik and Herberman, 1981a). In addition, the rate of cytotoxicity by macrophages is also somewhat retarded (Mahoney et al., 1980), so that an increased tumor incidence in beige mice could not be definitely attributed to the deficit in NK activity. Conversely, induction of interferon or other procedures to augment NK activity generally also alter other immune functions. Yet another, and perhaps the most central, limitation to the use of beige mice or other NK-deficient mice to evaluate the role of NK cells in prevention of carcinogenesis is that many of the carcinogens themselves can strongly inhibit NK activity. Thus, after treatment with a carcinogen, the normal recipients may have NK activity as low as the beige mice; therefore differences in tumor development might not be seen. The most convincing protocol might be to reconstitute animals with depressed NK activity by adoptive transfer of purified NK cells and determine the effects on carcinogenesis.

In addition to the above evidence for an NK cell role in antitumor defense, there are also some recent indications of a possible role for the related NC cells in mice that have been found to react primarily with solid tumor cell lines (Paige et al., 1978; Stutman et al., 1980a; Burton, 1980). A good correlation has been seen between in vitro susceptibility to lysis by NC cells of recently derived transplantable chemically induced fibrosarcomas and the cell dose required to produce local tumors in vivo (Stutman et al., 1980b). These investigators also tested the prediction that if NC cells were involved in immune surveillance, tumors induced in vivo by chemical carcinogens would be more resistant to lysis by NC cells than would in vitro transformed cells not exposed to such selective pressure by in vivo NC cells. Indeed, several in vitro transformed lines were quite susceptible to lysis by NC cells. A further tested prediction was that NC cells should be able to enter the site of locally growing tumors; indeed, they were detected within two transplantable sarcomas (Stutman et al., 1980c). Such evidence is clearly quite scanty and does not bear directly on the possible involvement in immune surveillance, but does support the possible involvement of NC cells in in vivo antitumor resistance.

Possible Role of ADCC in Immune Surveillance

In addition to any direct cytotoxic effects on tumor cells, macrophages (Haskill and Fett, 1976; Key and Haskill, 1981), PMN (Gale et al., 1974; Hafeman and Lucas, 1979; Levy et al., 1979) and NK (K cells) (Ojo and Wigzell, 1978; Landazuri et al., 1979; Timonen et al., 1981) may also act in cooperation with antibodies to produce ADCC. ADCC has been detected against a variety of experimental (Pollack et al., 1972; Landazuri et al., 1974; Harada et al., 1975; Lamon et al., 1975; Haskill and Fett, 1976; Blair et al., 1976) and human tumors (Hakala et al., 1974; Jondal and Gunven, 1977). Also, phagocytosis of tumor cells by macrophages or PMN may occur and be dependent on the presence of antitumor antibodies (Key and Haskill, 1980). However, there is still little evidence of a significant role for ADCC or antibody-dependent phagocytosis in in vivo antitumor resistance. This is probably due in large part to difficulties in distinguishing between ADCC and the direct antitumor effects of antibodies or various effector cells. In vivo administration of antibodies has, in a variety of experimental tumor systems (reviewed by Ting and Herberman, 1976; Herlyn et al., 1980), resulted in some protection against progressive tumor growth. It has often been suggested that ADCC is a major mechanism for the observed effects. However, in only a few studies has evidence been provided to support this possibility. Furthermore, most of the supportive data are indirect and not conclusive. For example, tumor cells isolated from antibody-producing mice have been shown to be coated with antibodies and thereby susceptible to cytotoxicity by macrophages (Haskill and Fett, 1976). Also, mice inoculated with tumor-protective hyperimmune serum along with an ascites tumor cell line have been shown to have considerable numbers of rosettes of macrophages with tumor cells (Langlois et al., 1981); this correlated with in vivo evidence for macrophage-mediated ADCC. Phagocytosed tumor cells within macrophages have also been noted at the site of tumor growth (Key and Haskill, 1981). Shin and his associates (Shin et al., 1975, 1976, 1978) used a somewhat more direct approach to support an in vivo role for ADCC by alloantibodies. IgG antibodies were shown to have limited effects on mice with larger tumor burdens. This appeared to be related to a shortage of macrophages at the tumor site, since efficacy could be restored by local addition of macrophages. Although it has been quite difficult to obtain convincing evidence of an in vivo antitumor role for ADCC, the following approach might be expected to provide substantially better insight into the possible importance of this mechanism. In a tumor system in which in vivo administration of antibodies can be shown to have protective effects, normal recipients of antibodies and tumor cells could be compared with animals selectively depleted of one or another type of potential effector cell. Loss of efficacy of antibodies, for example, in animals with selective deficits in NK cells or macrophages would point toward an important collaboration between these components of the immune system. Further evidence for mediation of antitumor effects by ADCC would be provided by restoration of antibody activity by adoptive transfer of a purified effector cell population into the deficient recipients.

Clearly, since there is such a paucity of evidence for an in vivo role of ADCC with tumor cell lines, the question of a possible involvement of this mechanism in immune surveillance becomes highly speculative. However, this effector mechanism should at least be kept in mind and appropriate studies should be done to investigate. This is particularly relevant for the natural effector cells, since treatments which alter their direct cytotoxic activity have also tended to cause a parallel alteration in their capacity for ADCC. Furthermore, in addition to the possible role of antibodies specifically induced by tumor-associated antigens, natural antitumor antibodies have been demonstrated (Martin and Martin, 1975; Menard et al., 1977; Chow et al., 1979, 1981; Houghton et al., 1980), which might interact with effector cells and mediate ADCC. It should be noted that virtually all of the evidence discussed above for a possible role of macrophages or NK cells in immune surveillance would also be compatible with the mediation of their effects by collaboration with such natural antibodies.

Mechanisms by Which Tumors may Escape Immune Attack

Despite the multiplicity of potential antitumor effector mechanisms, it is important to note that once tumors become detectable, they usually grow progressively and result in the death of the host. Therefore, much attention needs to be given to the mechanisms for the frequent failure of the immune system to adequately control tumor growth. A variety of mechanisms has been observed or suggested to account for insufficient host defenses; these will be briefly discussed below.

Immunoresistance of Tumor Cells

One major factor may be resistance of tumor cells to attack by immune mechanisms, rather than an actual lack of the necessary structures and factors for possible recognition and interaction. It has been found in a number of studies that for tumor cells to be able to react with antibodies or immune cells they need to have sufficient quantities or densities of the relevant tumor-associated cell surface antigens (e.g., Klein et al., 1966; Ting et al., 1972). Tumor cells with subthreshold amounts of these antigens are immunoresistant. The loss or rapid shedding of cell surface antigens from tumor cells has been suggested as a possible explanation for the failure of such antigens to function as tumor-associated transplantation antigens (Baldwin and Price, 1976). One well-studied mechanism in this area is antigenic modulation (Old et al., 1968). This mechanism was originally described with TL antigen. This tumor-associated surface antigen is quite immunogenic in some strains of mice but does not function as a transplantation antigen, since exposure of tumor cells to anti-TL antibody causes a reversible loss of antigen. Some oncofetal antigens have been shown to undergo antigenic modulation (Ortaldo et al., 1974) and this may explain why they usually fail to be involved in resistance against tumor growth. Similarly, surface antigens associated with Gross leukemia virus have been found to be lost, or at least described in expression, during in vivo growth of tumors, but returned upon in vitro cultivation (Aoki and Johnson, 1973; Ioachim et al., 1974).

This issue of immunoresistance has also been shown to be relevant for the interaction of NK cells with tumors. Even highly NK-susceptible tumor lines have been shown to become relatively NK-resistant after growth in vivo (Becker et al., 1978; Durdik et al., 1980). The nature of this resistance is not well defined, but there have been some indications for reversibility (Becker et al., 1978), thereby making such examples apparently analogous to antigenic modulation. In other instances, growth in vivo may select for a stable resistant tumor cell variant (Durdik et al., 1980). Treatment of some NK-resistant cell lines with inhibitors of RNA or protein synthesis has been found to make them sensitive to lysis by NK cells (Collins et al., 1981; Kunkel and Welsh, 1981). Interferon has been found to be one of the mediators of induction of NK resistance of target cells, since pretreatment of some NK-sensitive target cells with interferon can render them resistant (Trinchieri and Santoli, 1978; Welsh and Kiessling, 1980).

Resistance of tumor cells to lysis by NC cells (Stutman et al., 1980c) or by macrophages (Rhodes, 1980) has also been found to occur. This may also be associated with more efficient tumor growth.

Inhibition of Effector Functions

Another major category of possible mechanisms for lack of effective host resistance is deficiency or inhibition of effector functions. As discussed above, the tumor-bearing state or even the latent period prior to overt tumor growth is often associated with some immunodepression. Although in some instances there may be a decrease in a particular effector cell population or an intrinsic defect in its function, more often the depressed reactivity has been found to be attributable to inhibition or suppression of function, either by host-derived suppressor cells or factors or by tumor-produced suppressor factors.

Suppressor Cells

Almost all effector mechanisms have been found to be well regulated, with cells or factors inhibiting their activity as well as other cells or factors acting in an accessory or augmenting capacity.

Suppression of T Cell-mediated Immunity to Tumor Antigens. There is substantial evidence for suppressor cells that can either specifically or nonspecifically inhibit immune response to tumor-associated antigens. The specific suppressor cells mainly have been found to be within a particular subpopulation of T cells; such suppressor T cells have been found to be involved in several experimental tumor systems (Fujimoto et al., 1976a and b; Takei et al., 1976; Daynes and Spellman, 1977; Fisher and Kripke, 1978; Berendt and North, 1980). A particularly good and well-studied tumor system in which suppressor T cells appear to play a central role in tumor development is that of ultraviolet light-induced tumors in mice (Daynes and Spellman, 1977; Fisher and Kripke, 1978). Such tumors have been shown to be highly antigenic and are usually rejected upon transplantation into normal syngeneic recipients (Kripke, 1974). However, these tumors grow progressively in mice treated with ultraviolet light (Kripke and Fisher, 1976). Spleen and lymph node cells from ultraviolet light-treated mice were shown to contain suppressor T cells that could adoptively transfer inhibition of tumor rejection by normal recipients (Daynes and Spellman, 1977; Fisher and Kripke, 1978). The T suppressor cells in this and some other tumor systems appear to bear antigens of the I-J region of the major histocompatibility complex, with in vivo administration of anti-J sera interfering with the suppressor cell activity and leading to some retardation of tumor growth (Greene et al., 1977; Perry et al., 1980).

Macrophages represent the other category of suppressor cells for antitumor immune responses. Macrophage suppressor cells have been shown nonspecifically to inhibit lymphoproliferative responses to tumor-associated antigens (reviewed by Oehler et al., 1978; Herberman et al., 1980; Herberman, 1981), the primary or secondary generation of antitumor cytotoxic T cells (Oehler and Herberman, 1979) and the production of lymphokines (Varesio et al., 1979, 1980). However, in contrast to the above discussed evidence for an in vivo role of T suppressor cells, there is as yet little comparable evidence of an important role for suppressor macrophages in interfering in vivo with antitumor T cell immunity.

There is considerable evidence in cancer patients for the presence of suppressor macrophages which can inhibit antitumor lymphoproliferative responses, as well as responses to mitogens or alloantigens (reviewed by Herberman, 1981). In contrast, there is little documentation in cancer patients of suppressor T cells which can specifically inhibit antitumor responses. However, Vose (1980) recently reported that suppressor lymphocytes, particularly T cells, which could suppress mixed lymphocyte-tumor cell interactions were present at the site of growth of some human tumors and in regional lymph nodes.

Suppression of NK Activity. Much of the inhibition in NK activity that is seen after in vivo treatment with a variety of agents appears to be due to the presence of suppressor cells. Suppressor cells have been detected in mice after treatment with carrageenin, corticosteroids, x-irradiation, adriamycin, *C. parvum*, pyran copolymer and other immune adjuvants (Cudkowicz and Hochman, 1979; Lotzova and Gutterman, 1979; Santoni et al., 1980a and b). The nature of the suppressor cells in these various situations has not been adequately defined, but adherent cells have usually been found to be responsible. The suppressor cells induced by pyran copolymer appear to be phagocytic as well as adherent and therefore are presumed to be macrophages (Santoni et al., 1981a). The mechanism(s) by which these suppressor cells inhibit NK activity has not been defined, but with pyran-induced suppressor cells, soluble factors appear to be involved (Santoni et al., 1981a).

In considering the effects of some agents on NK activity, it is important to note that either augmentation or inhibition can be produced, depending on a variety of circumstances (Santoni et al., 1980b). Such opposite effects by the same agent have been seen with *C. parvum*, BCG, pyran copolymer, adriamycin and glucan. The route of inoculation appears to be an important variable with some agents [e.g., *C. parvum*, glucan (Lotzová and Gutterman, 1979; Lotzová, 1980)], with depression of NK activity particularly associated with intravenous inoculation and boosting of reactivity mainly seen after intraperitoneal inoculation. It is possible that, depending on the route, different cells come in contact with the agent; consequently, different effects may be seen. This is not the entire explanation for opposite results, however, since treatment by the same route and with the same dose of an agent can result in both augmentation and depression of NK activity. This may in part be due to differences in the kinetics of augmenting and depressing effects. Augmentation tends to occur early, within 1 to 4 days after treatment, whereas induction of depression tends to occur later. With the macrophage-activating agents, this may be related to the more rapid induction of IFN production than the activation of suppressor activity. Also, as seen with pyran copolymer and adriamycin (Santoni et al., 1980b), the status of the recipients may in some way determine the direction of the effect of the same treatment on NK activity. There are some indications that this may be related to the baseline levels of activity of NK cells and suppressor cells. At various sites and times, NK cells may vary in their responsiveness to augmentation by IFN or to depression. Similarly, macrophages and other suppressor cells may vary in their ability to be activated. Much more information seems to be required in this area before one can predict with confidence the magnitude, or even the direction, of a response to a particular in vivo treatment. Understanding of such variables is likely to provide much insight into the basic factors involved in regulation of NK activity.

In studies of the maintenance of mouse NK activity upon overnight incubation at 37°C, a role for suppressor cells from normal mice has been detected (Brunda et al., 1981a). Peritoneal macrophages from normal mice, either resident cells obtained without any stimuli or elicited by various materials, markedly suppressed NK activity of effector cells incubated alone or with IFN. This suppressor activity appeared restricted to peritoneal macrophages, since splenic adherent cells were inactive. The peritoneal macrophages of several strains had suppressor activity, including those from high NK strains and from nude mice. This type of suppressor activity appeared quite distinct from that seen with activated macrophages. The normal peritoneal cells did not suppress the effector phase of NK activity, and peritoneal macrophages from *C. parvum*-treated mice, which were cytotoxic and able to suppress lymphoproliferative responses, had diminished ability to suppress the in vitro maintenance of NK activity (Brunda et al., 1981b).

Immunosuppressor Products of Tumor Cells

Another factor to be considered in the depressed immunity and ineffective host defense to some tumors is immunosuppression by the tumor cells or products of the tumors. In some transplantable tumors in experimental animals, the inhibitory properties of the tumor cells could be attributed to contamination by passenger viruses (e.g., Campbell et al., 1977; Bonnard et al., 1976). In addition, tumor cells appear to be able to produce a variety of immunosuppressive factors (e.g., DeLustro and Argyris, 1976; Pike and Snyderman, 1977; Rhodes et al., 1978; Mizel et al., 1980), which might play an important role in evading host defenses. Some tumor cells may also make considerable amounts of prostaglandins (Easty and Easty, 1976; Bennett et al., 1977; Grinwich and Plescia, 1977) which, as discussed below, can be immunosuppressive. However, there is very little evidence that such tumor-produced factors contribute to progressive tumor growth in vivo.

In addition to induction of suppressor cells by various treatments, suppressor cells for NK activity have also been detected in some natural situations. The low NK activity in newborn mice (Cudkowicz and Hochman, 1979; Santoni, Riccardi and Herberman, unpublished observations) may be attributable, at least in part, to the presence of suppressor cells. Furthermore, some strains of mice with genetically determined low NK activity have been found to have suppressors for NK activity. In careful kinetic studies of NK activity in A and SJL mice of various ages, it has been noted that 4- to 6-week-old mice have levels of NK activity comparable to those of other strains, but that by 8 weeks of age their reactivity is substantially depressed (Riccardi et al., 1981b). Adherent spleen cells of normal SJL mice have been found to inhibit the NK activity of spleen cells of high NK strains (Riccardi et al., 1981b). In in vivo studies of adoptive transfer of NK activity, SJL recipients also have been found to inhibit full expression of the reactivity of donor NK cells (Riccardi et al., 1981b; G. Cudkowicz, personal communication). It is of interest that other investigators have independently noted that the macrophages of SJL mice are functionally hyperactive (Gallily and Haran-Ghera, 1979).

Suppressor cells for NK activity have also been found in some tumor-bearing individuals with low NK activity. For example, mice bearing progressively growing primary tumors induced by murine sarcoma virus and low or undetectable NK activity in situ, but removal of adherent or phagocytic cells led to a marked increase in activity (Gerson et al., 1981). A role for suppressor macrophages within the tumor was supported by mixing experiments, in which cells from the tumor inhibited the activity of normal spleen cells. Similar evidence for suppressor cells has been obtained with some human tumors (Gerson, 1980; Vose, 1980; Eremin, 1980).

Other Inhibitory Factors

Inhibition by Serum Factors. Serum from tumor-bearing individuals has frequently been found to inhibit various antitumor effector mechanisms. In regard to specific cell-mediated cytotoxicity against tumor-associated antigens, serum factors have been shown to specifically or nonspecifically interfere with reactivity (Sjögren, 1974; Baldwin et al., 1976; Glaser et al., 1976;Bansal et al., 1976; Hellström and Hellström, 1976). Although most serum blocking factors, particularly those which appeared to act specifically, were initially thought to be antibodies, increasing evidence for a role of circulating antigens and antigen-antibody complexes has also been obtained (Thomson, 1975; Prather and Lausch, 1976; Nepom et al., 1976).

Serum blocking factors have also been described in other assays of specific cell-mediated immunity to tumor antigens, with sera of tumor-bearing individuals able to inhibit lymphoproliferative responses (Stjernswärd and Vánky, 1972; Gutterman et al., 1973; Mavligit, 1973) and production of lymphokines (Halliday, 1972).

Serum factors have also been found to be able to inhibit NK activity. Nair et al. (1980) recently reported that preincubation of normal mouse spleen cells in serum could interfere with their cytotoxic activity and that sera from tumor-bearing individuals were more inhibitory than those from normal donors. Studies of Sulica et al. (submitted for publication) with human NK cells have indicated an inhibitory role of monomeric cytophilic IgG. Incubation of cells with serum or IgG inhibited reactivity, whereas incubation in medium lacking IgG led to an increase in NK activity.

There have been some indications that antibodies or other serum factors can interfere with host resistance in vivo. Administration of serum from tumor-bearers has often been shown to cause enhancement of growth of syngeneic tumors (reviewed by Ting and Herberman, 1977).

Although in most instances the mechanisms for enhancement have not been elucidated, there have been suggestions of a correlation between enhancing activity and serum factors blocking specific cell-mediated cytoxicity (e.g., Bansal et al., 1972). Furthermore, "unblocking" sera from tumor-free individuals, with the ability to counteract the serum-blocking factors in cytoxicity assays, were found to have some protective effects upon in vivo transfer to tumor-bearers (Bansal and Sjögren, 1972). Such observations have led to clinical approaches for treatment of cancer patients. A trial with patients with malignant melanoma was initiated to examine the effects of repeated infusion of sera found to contain unblocking factors (Wright et al., 1976), but no clinical benefits have been reported. Another approach has been to pass the plasma of cancer patients over columns containing *Staph. aureus* protein A to remove some circulating IgG. Such a protocol has been shown to have some antitumor effects in dogs with spontaneous tumors (Terman, 1981) and clinical trials are now under way in several institutions. It should be noted, however, that the nature of the alteration in the plasma that may lead to reduction in tumor size has not been defined and the mechanism involved might be quite different from removal of blocking antibodies or immune complexes.

Prostaglandins. Prostaglandins, particularly of the E series (PGE), may be produced by stimulated macrophages or by tumor cells and have been shown to have various immunosuppressive effects. Indomethacin, an inhibitor of prostaglandin synthesis, has been shown to reverse some of the suppression by monocytes or macrophages of lymphoproliferative responses of tumor-bearing mice or cancer patients (Goodwin et al., 1977; Herberman et al., 1980). PGE may also inhibit cytostatic activity of macrophages (Schultz et al., 1979) or may interfere with the maintenance of their cytolytic activity (Russell, 1981). Similarly, PGE and some other prostaglandins have been shown to be inhibitors of both spontaneous and interferon-boosted human and mouse NK activity (Droller et al., 1978; Brunda et al., 1980).

Production of prostaglandins in vivo may have a significant effect on tumor growth. Administration of inhibitors of prostaglandin synthesis (either indomethacin or aspirin) to mice bearing murine sarcoma virus-induced tumors led to partial restoration of their NK activity (Brunda et al., 1980) and also to reduced tumor growth (Strausser and Humes, 1975; Brunda et al., 1980). Such treatment has also been shown to reduce the growth of several other experimental tumors and to augment the antitumor effects of some immunostimulants (Plescia et al., 1975; Lynch et al., 1978; Lynch and Salomon, 1979). Conversely, administration of prostaglandins has been found to facilitate carcinogenesis in mice by methylcholanthrene (Lupulescu, 1978).

Neuroendocrine Factors. Neuroendocrine factors have been found to have inhibitory effects on various immune functions. For example, with NK cells, corticosteroids (Oehler and Herberman, 1978; Djeu et al., 1979b), transportation stress (Herberman and Holden, 1978) and left cerebral decortication (Bardos et al., 1981) have been shown to inhibit cytotoxic reactivity. Similarly, Riley (1981) has found that stress-induced elevation in circulating corticosteroids was associated with suppression of T cell numbers and functions. The most impressive indication that this may have important implications for in vivo host resistance to tumor growth has come from a study of spontaneous mammary carcinogeneis in mice maintained under low or high stress conditions (Riley, 1975). Mice exposed to chronic stress had an incidence of mammary tumors at 400 days at age of 92%, whereas only 7% of mice housed in a low stress protective environment developed tumors by that time. The latter group did, however, develop tumors with high frequency with a median latent period of 566 days.

Prognostic Significance of Tumor-Host Interactions

In addition to the possible importance of the immune system in resistance to tumor growth, various assays of immune function and of reactivity to tumor-associated antigens might be expected to have clinical value for the detection or diagnosis of cancer, for assessing prognosis and for monitoring the clinical course of disease (reviewed by Herberman, 1979). For example, if most tumors of a particular type contained common immunogenic tumor-associated antigens, one might expect a high incidence of specific reactivity in cancer patients and little or no reactivity among non-tumor-bearing individuals. However, most results to date have not fit these predictions. The major problems have been related to the findings of NK activity and other forms of natural immunity to tumors and also to reactivity against a variety of different tissue antigens, only some of which are tumor-associated. In addition to difficulties in discriminating between specific antitumor cytotoxicity and NK activity, other assays have revealed similar problems. For example, studies with leukocyte migration inhibition assays have usually shown substantially higher reactivity among cancer patients than controls against organ site-associated antigens (reviewed by McCoy, 1979). However, there has also been some reactivity against antigens on nonmalignant tissues, some reactivity of cancer patients against antigens on nonmalignant tissues and reactivity of some normal individuals and patients with benign diseases against tumor extracts (McCoy, 1979). Assays of lymphoproliferative responses to tumor cells or tumor extracts appear to detect tumor-associated antigens, but clear interpretation of results has been limited to autologous tests (Vánky and Stjernswärd, 1979, Dean, 1979) and therefore the potential for diagnosis is quite limited.

In view of these limitations, most of the emphasis has been focused on the possible value of these assays in assessing prognosis and monitoring cancer patients, particularly during the course of immunotherapy trials.

Overall, the correlations between circulating antibodies and clinical parameters have not been impressive. There have been virtually no large scale prospective studies of the actual prognostic value of these assays. Several studies have detected elevated levels of immune complexes in the sera of an appreciable number of patients with cancer of various types (Jose and Seshadri, 1974; Carpentier et al., 1977, 1978; Teshima et al., 1977; Höffken et al., 1978; Brandeis et al., 1978; Baldwin et al., 1979; Theofilopoulos and Dixon, 1979; Eiras et al., 1980). Although it is usually assumed that such complexes are of tumor-associated antigens and antibodies, little documentation of this possibility has yet been obtained. Despite this, some studies have indicated a correlation between levels of circulating complexes and clinical course (Jose and Seshadri, 1974; Carpentier et al., 1977, 1978; Rossen et al., 1977; Höffken et al., 1978; Brandeis et al., 1978; Baldwin et al., 1979; Eiras et al., 1980). For example, in the studies of Carpentier et al., circulating complexes were associated with extensive disease and, in patients with acute leukemia, were correlated with poorer response to chemotherapy and short survival. Such results appear promising, but there have as yet been no reports of a large prospective trial based on levels of circulating complexes. These would probably be difficult to perform adequately, since there are indications of lack of agreement among different assays for immune complexes and of loss of discrimination when sera are collected under conditions other than those routinely used in the small pilot studies (Herberman et al., 1981a).

Clinical Correlations of Immunologic Assays in Cancer Patients

Humoral Assays

There have been relatively few attempts to correlate the presence of circulating antibodies to tumor-associated antigens with the extent of tumor burden or with the clinical course of disease. The reports that considered these issues had rather heterogeneous and sometimes divergent results. In malignant melanoma, some workers found a loss of detectable antibodies in advanced disease (Lewis et al., 1971), whereas others did not see a correlation with disease status (Morton et al., 1968; Nairn et al., 1972). In patients with sarcomas, the measurement of serum antibodies appeared to have some clinical value. Patients who had definitive surgery and remained tumor-free had high levels of antibody, as measured by complement-fixation assays (Morton et al., 1970; Sethi and Hirshaut, 1976). In one of these studies (Morton et al., 1970), but not in the other (Sethi and Hirshaut, 1976), declining antibody titers were associated with recurrence of disease or metastatic spread. In patients with Burkitt's lymphoma, antibodies to the membrane antigen associated with Epstein-Barr virus were found to have some clinical correlates (Klein, 1978). Several patients in long term remission were found to have a fall in antibody titers some time before recurrence of tumor; however, the correlation between relapse and change in antibody titers was not complete.

Assays of Cellular Immunity to Tumor-associated Antigens

Several studies of skin tests for delayed hypersensitivity reactions to tumor extracts have indicated some clinical correlations. Reactivity to leukemia-associated antigens correlated with clinical state (Char et al., 1973). There have also been some indications for application to initial diagnosis. Skin tests with soluble and partially purified extracts of malignant melanoma were evaluated for use in the differential diagnosis of ocular melanoma. Although the initial tests appeared very promising (Char et al., 1974), subsequent tests on a larger series of patients indicated that, although the tests could significantly discriminate between patients with melanoma and those with simulating ocular lesions, the incidence of false positives and negatives was too high for clinical use (Char et al., 1977). A major limitation to large scale evaluation of the delayed hypersensitivity skin tests and other procedures dependent on tumor extracts is the need for large amounts of tumor. This is a concern because antigenicity and specificity have been found to vary substantially among different extracts (Weese et al., 1978). A possible solution to this problem is the use of established cell lines derived from tumors which contain skin-reactive antigens (Roth et al., 1976; Weese et al., 1978). However, further serious drawbacks to this approach are the logistical and technical difficulties in performing the skin tests and in accurately quantitating the degree of reactivity.

Some assays of lymphoproliferative responses to autologous tumor cells or tumor extracts have indicated a correlation with local disease or good prognosis. For example, such findings were obtained in patients with acute leukemia (Gutterman et al., 1973) and with some carcinomas (Mavligit et al., 1973). More recently, analysis of followup information from patients with breast cancer who were tested shortly after resection of the primary tumor indicated a significant correlation, even among patients with stage I disease, between high reactivity and a prolonged disease-free interval (Cannon et al., 1981). The association between recurrence and low or undetectable reactivity was not attributable to a generalized depression in lymphocyte reactivity, since mixed leukocyte responses were normal in most of these poor prognosis patients.

Several groups have examined the correlation between reactivity in leukocyte migration inhibition assays with tumor extracts and clinical parameters, but the results have been divergent. Cochran et al. (1972, 1974) found decreased reactivity in patients with advanced disease and in most patients in the immediate postoperative period. McCoy et al., (1974, 1977) also observed the effect of surgery, but did not find a good correlation with stage of disease. In contrast, Black et al. (1974) observed that reactivity of breast cancer patients was associated with early disease and good prognosis. Similarly, Kjaer (1974) found reactivity in renal cancer patients with localized disease but not in those with metaststic disease.

Using the leukocyte adherence inhibition assay, some investigators have also noted a correlation between reactivity and good prognosis. In studies with the tube modification of the assay, Thomson et al. (1979) noted a decreased frequency of reactivity in patients with advanced disease; after resection of primary tumors, persistent or recurrent reactivity was associated with residual or metastatic disease. In contrast, reactivity as measured by the original hemocytometer method was observed in patients at all stages of disease and it often persisted for long periods after tumor removal (Maluish, 1979). However, specific serum blocking factors appeared to be indicative of residual or recurrent tumor.

Despite the various reports of useful results with migration inhibition and adherence inhibition assays, it should be noted that most of the assays are technically difficult and not entirely reliable for assessment of the reactivity of an individual. There has been considerable variability among tumor extracts used for testing (e.g., Kjaer and Christensen, 1977; Cannon et al., 1978). It has therefore been quite difficult to standardize the assays for large scale testing. In addition, most of the data cited above are from population-based studies and thus far these tests have only been useful in this context. Their use for longitudinal monitoring of individual patients for correlation with clinical parameters is still quite limited.

Depressed K cell-mediated ADCC activity has also been observed in cancer patients. Ting and Terasaki (1974) found significantly less killing by cells from cancer patients than by those from normal donors or patients with benign diseases. However, there was no apparent correlation between reactivity of the cancer patients and stage of disease. Recently, a more extensive study was performed to examine this issue (McCredie and MacDonald, 1980). K cell activity was found to be decreased in a considerable proportion of patients with advanced cancer, whereas patients with early stages of cancer were indistinguishable from the nonmalignant controls. One suggestion for a prognostic correlation in this study was a persistence of radiation-induced depression in reactivity among patients with persistent tumor or metastases, in contrast to recovery of reactivity among patients with complete tumor regression.

There have only been a few reports of clinical correlation with assays of cytotoxicity by monocytes or PMN. Jerrells et al. (1979) observed decreased monocyte-mediated cytostasis in cancer patients. Similarly, Korec (1980) found decreased cytostasis by PMN from cancer patients with tumor present, but no depression in patients without evidence of disease.

Assays of NK Cells and Other Natural Effector Cells

Depressed NK activity has been observed in mice (Herberman et al., 1975; Becker and Klein, 1977) and patients (McCoy et al., 1973; Takasugi et al., 1977; Hersey et al., 1979, 1980; Forbes et al., 1980; Pross and Baines, 1980; Tursz et al., 1981) bearing various types of tumors; this has been particularly associated with large tumor burdens. Possibly determination of NK activity in cancer patients might have prognostic value; however, there have been no reports of studies designed directly to address this question.

Use of Assays for Monitoring of Immunotherapy Trials

One of the major objectives of immunotherapy for cancer is to restore deficient immunologic function or to augment reactivity above the existing levels. However, most of the trials of immunotherapy have been essentially empirical, with various agents given either at maximal tolerable or available doses or at arbitrary doses and schedules. In fact, it should be noted that there is little reason to expect that more of a particular agent will be better. The relevant principles for immunomodulation are likely to be quite different from those that have been developed for treatment with chemotherapeutic agents, where the highest possible dose is given. Although it is very difficult to choose among the various possible effector mechanisms, some hypotheses must be developed in order to formulate rational strategies for biological response modification. Prior to conducting large-scale clinical trials, it would seem essential to determine the dose and schedule for a particular agent that optimally augments for a sustained period one or more of the effector mechanisms considered important. This is of particular concern since a variety of agents may not only augment the activity of a particular immunologic function, but under some conditions also cause depression via induction or activation of suppressor cells (e.g., Santoni et al., 1980b). One possible approach would be to determine the optimal immunomodulating dose for each of several effector functions and then set up and compare the therapeutic results of protocols based on such information. For example, one might compare the optimal schedule for augmenting macrophage cytolytic activity with that for augmenting NK or ADCC activity. The primary concern then in a phase I trial with a putative biological response-modifying agent would be to carefully monitor for the effects of the agent at various doses and schedules of administration. This would appear to be an obvious and straightforward approach. However, this has not been the case with agents that have been brought to the clinical level so far.

A major technical issue to be raised in regard to the monitoring of the effects of various agents on effector activity is the problem of substantial spontaneous fluctuation in reactivity in the assays over a period of time. Some of this may be attributed to technical variation from day to day in the assay itself, e.g., with varying susceptibility of a target cell to lysis. In addition, there may be considerable biological fluctuation in reactivity. The experience in my laboratory has been that such variation is more marked in cancer patients than in normal donors; this can only in part be ascribed to treatment-induced alterations. Thus, there is a real need to carefully control the monitoring.

In regard to controlling the technical variations in the assays, several steps have been quite helpful. First is testing within each experiment of specimens from three or more normal donors. This allows a comparison between the results of the cancer patients and those of the normal controls and the relative degree of reactivity for each test specimen can thereby be calculated. For example, with lymphoproliferative assays, a relative proliferation index (RPI) has been calculated (Dean et al., 1978). Expression of the patient data as RPI has reduced the range of values and has allowed better discrimination of abnormal results. Similar adjustments can be made for any of the other immunologic assays. The principal limitation of this approach is the possibility for considerable variation in the levels of reactivity among the small numbers of different randomly selected donors used as controls. This can be solved by using the same donors repeatedly or, as a much more convenient and practical procedure, obtaining large numbers of lymphoid cells by leukapheresis and cryopreserving them in multiple aliquots. For each experiment, aliquots of cryopreserved cells from the same set of normal donors can be thawed and tested as the standard controls. This approach has proven very useful for all of the cell-mediated immunity assays currently being performed in my laboratory. It has been more difficult to adequately cryopreserve NK activity than lymphoproliferative responsiveness or monocyte-mediated cytotoxic activity, but by screening multiple batches of frozen cells it has been possible to select ones with well preserved NK activity. Secondly, temporal variations in the susceptibility of target cells to cell-mediated cytotoxicity can be avoided by the use of cryopreserved target cells (Holden et al., 1976) in each assay. Finally, as an alternative to the immediate testing of serial specimens from patients, all of the test specimens can be cryopreserved and then all of the serial samples from a given patient can be tested in the same experiment. This allows comparison among samples without any problem with day-to-day variation in the assays. It should be noted, however, that there are two main concerns regarding this approach. First, there is the possibility of technical failure in an experiment with a consequent loss of all test results for a given patient. This can be avoided by having additional cryopreserved aliquots of the same specimens, to permit repetition of the entire experiment if necessary. In addition, successful utilization of this approach depends on the reliable and consistent ability to cryopreserve and recover immunologic reactivity, with the relative differences among serial samples being as noticeable with the frozen specimens as with fresh ones. As mentioned, in tests in my laboratory, this has been a problem with NK activity. Therefore, this function is evaluated on fresh samples from patients, whereas all other assays are now performed with cryopreserved specimens.

Certain steps can also be taken to control for problems with spontaneous, immunotherapy-unrelated variations in the immunologic reactivity of patients. Multiple baseline pretreatment values can be obtained to get an accurate estimate of the degree of spontaneous fluctuation in immunologic reactivity of each patient. Ideally, these baseline specimens should be obtained at the same intervals and over the same time period as the specimens to be obtained after administration of the immunotherapeutic agent. From this repeated pretherapy testing, it is possible to determine whether an agent would induce a change in reactivity that is beyond the confidence intervals of the spontaneous reactivity of the patient. In addition, it would be very helpful to test in parallel a group of patients not receiving immunotherapy who are comparable to the treated patients in terms of type and stage of disease and any prior therapy. By including such controls in an evaluation of the effects of BCG or *Corynebacterium parvum* on NK activity of cancer patients (Herberman et al., 1981b), we have observed that considerable and usually unexplainable shifts in reactivity occur in some control patients during a period of 2 to 3 weeks. Patients with initially low reactivity tended to show an increase, whereas patients with initially very high reactivity tended to show a decrease. Such variations could, at least in part, be a reflection of the statistical principle of reversion to the mean. If for some reason a patient has a transient period of depressed or augmented reactivity (e.g., due to intercurrent infection or residual effects of previous therapy or even to stress), it would not be surprising to have a later shift to values in the normal range. In any event, these possible sources of biologic variation in immunologic reactivity of cancer patients need to be kept in mind and controlled for in order to avoid attributing them to the effects of immunotherapy.

Summary

The above discussion has pointed out the heterogeneity of immunologic effector mechanisms potentially important for host resistance against tumor growth. It probably is not realistic to try to decide which among these mechanisms is most important; rather it seems best to consider the possibility that several or even all may be involved. For some tumors, one effector mechanism may predominate and for others a different mechanism may be more important. Also, it seems likely that several different effector mechanisms may act in concert in the defense against some types of tumors. This may provide a backup system in the event of escape from the predominant or first line effector mechanism. Thus, immunologic defenses against tumors may be quite complicated and multifocal, requiring detailed and prolonged investigation to adequately understand host-tumor interactions. However, this complexity may add considerable flexibility to the system and, in terms of attempts to augment host resistance against tumors, it may be possible to favorably alter the balance by affecting any one of the several effector mechanisms that are involved.

References

Adams, D.O., and Snyderman, R. 1979. Do macrophages destroy nascent tumors? J Natl Cancer Inst 62:1341–45.

Alexander, P. 1976. The functions of the macrophage in malignant disease. Annual Rev Med 27:207–24.

Allavena, P., Introna, M., Mangioni, C., and Mantovani, A. 1981. Inhibition of natural killer activity by tumor-associated lymphoid cells from ascitic ovarian carcinomas. J Natl Cancer Inst. In press.

Allison, A.C. 1970. Potentiation of viral carcinogenesis by immunosuppression. Brit Med J 4:419–20.

Allison, A.C. 1978. Mechanisms by which activated macrophages inhibit lymphocyte responses. Immunol Rev 40:3–27.

Allison, A.C., Hammington, J.S., and Birbeck, M. 1966. An examination of the cytotoxic effects of silica on macrophages. J Exp Med 124:141–53.

Allison, A.C., and Law, L.W. 1968. Effects of antilymphocyte serum on virus oncogenesis. Proc Soc Exp Biol Med 127:207–11.

Aoki, T., and Johnson, P.A. 1973. Suppression of G (Gross) leukemia cell surface antigens: A kind of antigenic modulation. J Natl Cancer Inst 49:183–89.

Argus, M.F., Hudson, M.T., Seepe, T.L., Kane, J.F., and Ray, F.E. 1962. Effect of rapid tissue growth on the uptake of fluorene-2,7-di(sulfonamide-2-naphthalene)-S^{35} by the liver and spleen of rats and hampsters. Brit J Cancer 16:494–99.

Ault, K.A., and Springer, T.A. 1981. Cross-reaction of a rat-anti-mouse phagocyte-specific monoclonal antibody (anti-Mac-1) with human monocytes and natural killer cells. J Immunol 126:359–64.

Axberg, I., Gidlund, M., Orn, A., Pattengale, P., Riesenfeld, I., Stern, P., and Wigzell, H. 1980. In: Thymus, Thymic Hormones and T Lymphocytes, ed. F. Aiuti, pp. 154–64. Academic Press; New York.

Baldwin, R.W. 1976. Role of immunosurveillance against chemically induced rat tumors. Transplant Rev 28:62.

Baldwin, R.W., Byers, V.S., and Robins, R.A. 1979. Circulating immune complexes in cancer: Characterization and potential as tumor markers. Behring Inst Mitt 64:63–77.

Baldwin, R.W., and Price, M.R. 1976. Immunobiology of rat neoplasia. Ann NY Acad Sci 276:3–10.

Balner, H., and Dersjant, H. 1969. Increased oncogenic effect of methylcholanthrene after treatment with anti-lymphocyte serum. Nature 224:376–78.

Bansal, S.C., Bansal, B.R., and Boland, J.P. 1976. Blocking and unblocking factors in neoplasia. Current Topics Microbiol Immunol 75:45–63.

Bansal, S.C., Hargreaves, R., and Sjögren, H. 1972. Facilitation of polyoma tumor growth in rats by blocking sera and tumor eluate. Int J Cancer 9:97–106.

Bansal, S.C., and Sjögren, H. 1972. Counteraction of the blocking of cell-mediated tumor immunity by inoculation of unblocking sera and splenectomy. Immunotherapeutic effects on primary polyoma tumor in rats. Int J Cancer 9:490–99.

Bardos, P., Biziere, K., Degenne, D., and Renoux, G. Regulation of NK activity by the cerebral neocortex. In: NK Cells: Fundamental Aspects and Role in Cancer/Human Cancer Immunology, vol. 6, eds. B. Serrou and R.B. Herberman. Elsevier North-Holland; Amsterdam. In press.

Becker, S. 1980. Intratumor NK reactivity. In: Natural Cell-Mediated Immunity against Tumors, ed. R.B. Herberman, pp. 985–96. Academic Press; New York.

Becker, S., Kiessling, R., Lee, M., and Klein, G. 1978. Modulation of sensitivity to natural killer cell lysis after *in vitro* explantation of a mouse lymphoma. J Natl Cancer Inst 61:1495–98.

Becker, S., and Klein, E. 1977. Decreased "natural killer"—NK—effect in tumor bearing mice and its relation to the immunity against oncorna virus determined cell surface antigens. Eur J Immunol 6:892–98.

Bennett, A., Deltacia, M., Stamford, I.F., and Zebro, T. 1977. Prostaglandins from tumors of human large bowel. Brit J Cancer 35:881–84.

Berendt, M.J., and North, R.J. 1980. T cell-mediated suppression of anti-tumor immunity. An explanation for progressive growth of an immunogenic tumor. J Exp Med 151:69–80.

Berenson, J.R., Einstein, A.B., Jr., and Fefer, A. 1975. Syngeneic adoptive immunotherapy and chemotherapy of Friend luekemia: Requirement for T cells. J Immunol 115:234–38.

Bernstein, I.D., Cohen, E.F., and Wright, P.W. 1977. Relationship of cellular proliferation and the generation of cytotoxic cells in an *in vitro* secondary immune response to syngeneic rat lymphoma cells. J Immunol 118:1090–95.

Black, M.M., Leis, H.P., Shore, B., and Zachrau, R.E. 1974. Cellular hypersensitivity to breast cancer: Assessment by a leukocyte migration procedure. Cancer 33:952–58.

Blair, P.B., Lane, M.A., and Mar, P., 1976. Antibody in the sera of tumor-bearing mice that mediates spleen cell cytotoxicity toward the autologous tumor. J Immunol 116:606–609.

Bonnard, G.D., Manders, E.K., Campbell, D.A., Jr., Herberman, R.B., and Collins, M.J., Jr. 1976. Immunosuppressive activity of a subline of the mouse EL-4 lymphoma. Evidence for minute virus of mice causing the inhibition. J Exp Med 143:187–205.

Brandeis, W.E., Helson, L., Wang, Y., Good, R.A., and Day, N.K. 1978. Circulating immune complexes in sera of children with neuroblastoma. Correlation with stage of disease. J Clin Invest 62:1201–9.

Breard, J., Reinherz, E.L., O'Brien, C., and Schlossman, S.F. 1981. Delineation of an effector population responsible for natural killing and antibody-dependent cellular cytotoxicity in man. Clin Immunol Immunopathol 18:145–50.

Brunda, M.J., Herberman, R.B., and Holden, H.T. 1980a. Inhibition of murine natural killer cell activity by prostaglandins. J Immunol 124:2682–87.

Brunda, M.J., Holden, H.T., and Herberman, R.B. 1980b. Augmentation of natural killer cell activity of beige mice by interferon and interferon inducers. In: Natural Cell-Mediated Immunity against Tumors, ed. R.B. Herberman, pp. 411–15. Academic Press; New York.

Brunda, M.J., Taramelli, D., Holden, H.T., and Varesio, L. 1981a. Peritoneal macrophages from normal mice suppress natural killer cell activity. Fed Proc. 40:1094.

Brunda, M.J., Taramelli, D., Holden, H.T., and Varesio, L. 1981b. Effects of resting and activated macrophages on natural killer cell activity and lymphoproliferation. Proc Amer Assoc Cancer Res. 22:310

Burnet, F.M. 1957. Cancer—a biological approach. Brit Med J 1:779–86; 841–47.

Burnet, F.M. 1970. The concept of immunological surveillance. Progr Exp Tumor Res 13:1–27.

Burton, R.C. 1980. Alloantisera selectively reactive with NK cells: Characterization and use in defining NK cell classes. In: Natural Cell-Mediated Immunity against Tumors, ed. R.B. Herberman, p. 19–35. Academic Press; New York.

Campbell, D.A., Jr., Manders, E.K., Oehler, J.R., Bonnard, G.D., Oldham, R.K., and Herberman, R.B. 1977. Inhibition of *in vitro* lymphoproliferative responses by *in vivo* passaged rat 13762 mammary adenocarcinoma cells. I. Characteristics of inhibition and evidence for an infectious agent. Cell Immunol 33:364–77.

Canellos, G.P., DeVita, V.T., and Arsenau, J.C. 1974. Carcinogenesis by cancer chemotherapeutic agents: Second malignancies complicating Hodgkin's disease in remission. Recent Results Cancer Res 49:108–14.

Cannon, G.B., Dean, J.H., Herberman, R.B., Keels, M., and Alford, C. 1981. Lymphoproliferative responses to autologous tumor extracts as prognostic indicators in patients with resected breast cancer. Int J Cancer 27:131–38.

Cannon, G.B., McCoy, J.L., Connor, R.J., Jerome, L., Keys, L., Dean, J.H., and Herberman, R.B. 1978. Use of the leukocyte migration inhibition assay to evaluate antigenic differences on human breast cancers and melanomas. J Natl Cancer Inst 60:969–78.

Cantor, H., Kasai, M., Shen, H.W., LeClerc, J.C., and Glimcher, L. 1979. Immunogenetic analysis of natural killer activity in the mouse. Immunol Rev 44:1–32.

Carpentier, N., Lambert, P.H., and Miescher, P.A. 1978. Circulating immune complexes in patients with malignancies. In: Current Trends in Tumor Immunology, eds. R. Reisfeld, S. Ferrone, and R.B. Herberman. STPM Garland Press; New York.

Carpentier, N.A., Lange, G.T., Fiere, D.M., Fournie, G.J., Lambert, P.H., and Miescher, P.A. 1977. Clinical evidence of circulating immune complexes in human leukemia. J Clin Invest 60:874–84.

Castro, J.E. 1972. Human tumours grown in mice. Nature New Biol 239:83–84.

Char, D.H., Hollinshead, A., Cogan, D.G., Ballantine, E., Hogan, M.J., and Herberman, R.B. 1974. Cutaneous delayed hypersensitivity reactions to soluble melanoma antigen in patients with ocular melanoma. New Eng J Med 291:274–77.

Char, D.H., Hollinshead, A., and Herberman, R.B. 1977. Skin tests with soluble melanoma antigens in patients with choroidal tumors. Cancer 40:1650–54.

Char, D.H., LePourhiet, A., Leventhal, B.G., and Herberman, R.B. 1973. Cutaneous delayed hypersensitivity responses to tumor associated and other antigens in acute leukemia. Int J Cancer 12:409–19.

Cheever, M.A., Greenberg, P.D., and Fefer, A. 1980. Therapy of leukemia by nonimmune syngeneic spleen cells. J Immunol 124:2137–42.

Chow, D.A., Greene, M.I., and Greenberg, A.H. 1979. Macrophage-dependent, NK cell-independent natural surveillance of tumors in syngeneic mice. Int J Cancer 23:788–97.

Chow, D.A., Wolosin, L.B., and Greenberg, A.H. 1981. Immune natural anti-tumor antibodies. II. The contribution of natural antibodies to tumor surveillance. Int J Cancer 27:459–69.

Cochran, A.J., Grant, R.M., Spilg, W.G., Mackie, R.M., Ross, C.E., Hoyle, D.E., and Russell, J.M. 1974. Sensitization of tumor-associated antigens in human breast carcinoma. Int J Cancer 14:19–25.

Cochran, A.J., Spilg, W.G., Mackie, R.N., and Thomas, C.E. 1972. Post-operative depression of tumor directed cell-mediated immunity in patients with malignant disease. Brit Med J 2:67–70.

Collavo, D., Colombatti, A., Chieco-Bianchi, L., and Davis, A.J.S. 1974. T lymphocyte requirement for MSV tumour prevention or regression. Nature 249:169–70.

Collins, J.L., Patek, P.Q., and Cohn, M. 1981. Tumorigenicity and lysis by natural killers. J Exp Med 153:89–106.

Cudkowicz, G. 1981. Role of natural killer cells in natural resistance against bone marrow transplants. In: Symposium on Role of Natural Killer Cells, Macrophages and Antibody Dependent Cellular Cytotoxicity in Tumor Rejection and as Mediators of Biological Response Modifiers Activity, ed. M.A. Chirigos. Raven Press; New York. In press.

Cudkowicz, G., and Hochman, P.S. 1979. Do natural killer cells engage in regulated reactions against self to ensure homeostasis? Immunol Rev 44:13–52.

Currie, G.A. 1976. Immunological aspects of host resistance to the development and growth of cancer. Biochem Biophys Acta 458:135–62.

David, J.R., and Remold, H.G. 1979. The activation of macrophages by lymphokines. In: Biology of Lymphokines, eds. S. Cohen, E. Pick, and J.J. Oppenheim, pp. 121–40. Academic Press; New York.

Daynes, R.A., and Spellman, C.W. 1977. Evidence for the generation of suppressor cells by ultraviolet radiation. Cell Immunol 31:182–87.

Dean, J.H. 1979. Application of the micro-culture lymphocyte proliferation assay to clinical studies. In: Immunodiagnosis of Cancer, eds. R.B. Herberman and K.R. McIntire, pp. 738–69. Marcel Dekker; New York.

Dean, J.H., Connor, R., Herberman, R.B., Silva, J., McCoy, J.L., and Oldham, R.K. 1977. The relative proliferation index as a more sensitive parameter for evaluating lymphoproliferative responses of cancer patients to mitogens and alloantigens. Int J Cancer 20:359–70.

De Chatelet, L.R., Shirley, P.S., and Johnston, R.B. 1976. Effect of phorbol myristate acetate on the oxidative metabolism of human polymorphonuclear leukocytes. Blood 47:545–53.

DeLustro, F., and Argyris, B.F. 1976. Mechanism of mastocytoma-mediated suppression of lymphocyte reactivity. J Immunol 117:2073–80.

Dennert, G. 1980. Cloned lines of natural killer cells. Nature 287:47–49.

Dent, P.B., Fish, L.A., White, J.F., and Good, R.A. 1966. Chediak-Higashi syndrome. Observations on the nature of the associated malignancy. Lab Invest 15:1634–41.

Djeu, J.Y., Heinbaugh, J.A., Holden, H.T., and Herberman, R.B. 1979a. Role of macrophages in the augmentation of mouse natural killer cell activity by poly I:C and interferon. J Immunol 122:182–88.

Djeu, J.Y., Heinbaugh, J., Vieira, W.D., Holden, H.T., and Herberman, R.B. 1979b. The effect of immunopharmacological agents on mouse natural cell-mediated cytotoxicity and on its augmentation by poly I:C. Immunopharmacology 1:231–44.

Djeu, J.Y., Timonen, T., and Herberman, R.B. 1981. Augmentation of natural killer cell activity and induction of interferon by tumor cells and other biological response modifiers. In: Mediation of Cellular Immunity in Cancer by Immune Modifiers ed. M. Chirigos. M. Mitchell, M.J. Mastrangelo, and M.K. Rim Raven Press; New York. p. 161–166.

Doe, W.F., and Henson, P.M. 1979. Macrophage stimulation by bacterial lipopolysaccharides. III. Selective unresponsiveness of C3H/HeJ macrophages to the lipid A differentiation signal. J Immunol 123:2304–10.

Doll, R., and Kinlen, L. 1970. Immunosurveillance and cancer: Epidemiological evidence. Brit Med J 4:420–22.

Domzig, W., Timonen, T.T., and Stadler, B.M. 1981. Human natural killer (NK) cells produce interleukin-2 (IL-2). Proc Amer Assoc Cancer Res 22:309.

Droller, M.J., Schneider, M.V., and Perlmann, P. 1978. A possible role of prostaglandins in the inhibition of natural and antibody-dependent cell-mediated cytotoxicity against tumor cells. Cell Immunol 39:165.

Durdik, J.M., Beck, B.N., and Henney, C.S. 1980. The use of lymphoma cell variants differing in their susceptibility to NK cell mediated lysis to analyze NK cell-target cell interactions. In: Natural Cell-Mediated Immunity against Tumors, ed. R.B. Herberman, pp. 805–17. Academic Press; New York.

Easty, G.C., and Easty, D.M. 1976. Prostaglandins and cancer. Cancer Treat Rev 3:217–25.

Eccles, S.A., and Alexander, P. 1974. Macrophage content of tumors in relation to metastatic spread and host immune reaction. Nature 250:667–68.

Ehrlich, P. 1957. Über den jetzigen Stand der Karzinomforschung. The Collected Papers of Paul Ehrlich, vol. 2, ed. F. Himmelweit, pp. 550–62. Pergamon Press; London.

Ehrlich, R., Efrati, M., and Witz, I.P. 1980. Cytotoxicity and cytostasis mediated by splenocytes of mice subjected to chemical carcinogens and of mice bearing primary tumors. In: Natural Cell-Mediated Immunity against Tumors, ed. R.B. Herberman, pp. 997–1010. Academic Press; New York.

Eiras, A.S., Robins, R.A., Baldwin, R.W., and Byers, V.S. 1980. Circulating immune complexes in patients with bone tumours. Int J Cancer 25:735–39.

Eremin, O. 1980. NK cell activity in the blood, tumour-draining lymph nodes and primary tumours of women with mammary carcinoma. In: Natural Cell-Mediated Immunity against Tumors, ed. R.B. Herberman, pp. 1011–29. Academic Press; New York.

Evans, R. 1972. Macrophages in syngeneic animal tumors. Transplantation 14:468–72.

Evans, R. 1978. Macrophage requirement for growth of murine fibrosarcoma. Brit J Cancer 37:1080–88.

Evans, R. 1979. Host cells in transplanted murine tumors and their possible relevance to tumor growth. J Reticuloendothel Soc 26:427–32.

Evans, R., and Haskill, S. 1981. Activities of macrophages within and peripheral to the tumor mass. In:

The Reticuloendothelial System: A Comprehensive Treatise, vol. 8, Cancer, eds. R.B. Herberman and H. Friedman. Plenum Press; New York. In press.

Faraci, R.P., Marrone, J.C., Lesser, G.R., and Ketcham, A.S. 1975. The effect of splenectomy on tumor immunity and the metastatic spread of a murine reticulum cell sarcoma. Panminerva Med 17:59–62.

Ferrarini, M., Cadoni, A., Franzi, T., Ghigliotti, C., Leprini, A., Zicca, A., and Grossi, C.E. 1980. Ultrastructural and cytochemical markers of human lymphocytes. In: Thymus, Thymic Hormones and T Lymphocytes, ed. F.A. Iuti, pp. 39–47. Academic Press; New York.

Fidler, I.J. 1974. Inhibition of pulmonary metastases by intraveneous injection of specifically activated macrophages. Cancer Res 34:1074–79.

Fidler, I.J., Gerstein, D.M., and Hart, I.R. 1978. The biology of cancer invasion and metastasis. Adv Cancer Res 28:149–75.

Fisher, M.S., and Kripke, M.L. 1978. Further studies on the tumor-specific suppressor cells induced by ultraviolet radiation. J Immunol 121:1139–44.

Foley, E.J. 1953. Antigenic properties of methylcholanthrene-induced tumors in mice of the same strain. Cancer Res 13:835–37.

Forbes, J.T., Greco, F.A., and Oldham, R.K. 1980. Natural cell-mediated cytotoxicity in human tumor patients. In: Natural Cell-Mediated Immunity against Tumors, ed. R.B. Herberman, pp. 1031–46. Academic Press; New York.

Franceschi, C., Perocco, P., DiMarco, A.T., and Prodi, G. 1972. Lack of correlation between immunodepression and reticuloendothelial system activity in urethan or 7,12-dimethylbenz(a)-anthracene-treated rats. J Reticuloendothel Soc 12:592–98.

Fraumeni, J.F. 1969. Constitutional disorders of man predisposing to leukemia and lymphoma. Natl Cancer Inst Monogr 32:221–32.

Fujimoto, S., Greene, M.I., and Sehon, A.H. 1976a. Regulation of the immune response to tumor antigens I. Immunosuppressor cells in tumor-bearing hosts. J Immunol 116:791–99.

Fujimoto, S., Greene, M.I., and Sehon, A.H. 1976b. Regulation of the immune response to tumor antigens. II. The nature of immunosuppressor cells in tumor-bearing hosts. J Immunol 116:800–6.

Gale, R.P., Zighelboim, J., Ossorio, C., and Fahey, J. 1974. Western section immunology and connective tissue. Clin Res 22:180A.

Gallily, R., and Haran-Ghera, N. 1979. Macrophage functions in high and low cancer incidence strains of mice. A comparative study. Develop Compar Immunol 3:523–36.

Gatti, R.A., and Good, R.A. 1971. Occurrence of malignancy in immunodeficiency diseases. A literature review. Cancer 28:89–98.

Gauci, C.L., and Alexander, P. 1975. The macrophage content of some human tumors. Cancer Letters 1:20–25.

Gerson, J.M. 1980. Systemic and in situ natural killer activity in tumor-bearing mice and patients with cancer. In: Natural Cell-Mediated Immunity against Tumors, ed. R.B. Herberman, pp. 1047–62. Academic Press; New York.

Gerson, J.M., Varesio, L., and Herberman, R.B. 1981. Systemic and in situ natural killer and suppressor cell activities in mice bearing progressively growing murine sarcoma virus-induced tumors. Int J Cancer. 27:243–248.

Ghaffar, A., McBride, W.H., and Cullen, R.T. 1976. Interaction of tumor cells and activated macrophages *in vitro:* Modulation by *Corynebacterium parvum* and gold salts. J Reticuloendothel Soc 20:283–90.

Ghose, T. 1957. Effect of the blockage of reticuloendothelial system on tumor growth and metastasis. Indian J Med Sci 11:900–6.

Gillman, T., Kinns, A.M., Hallowes, R.C., and Lloyd, J.B. 1973. Malignant lymphoreticular tumors induced by trypan blue and transplanted in inbred rats. J Natl Cancer Inst 50:1179.

Glaser, M., and Herberman, R.B. 1976. Secondary cell-mediated cytotoxic response to challenge of rats with syngeneic Gross virus-induced lymphoma. J Natl Cancer Inst 56:1211–15.

Glaser, M., Lavrin, D.H., and Herberman, R.B. 1976a. *In vivo* protection against syngeneic Gross virus-induced lymphoma in rats: Comparison with *in vitro* studies of cell-mediated immunity. J Immunol 116:1507–11.

Glaser, M., Ting, C.C., and Herberman, R.B. 1976b. *In vitro* inhibition of cell-mediated cytotoxicity against syngeneic Friend virus-induced leukemia by immunoregulatory alpha globulin. J Natl Cancer Inst 55:1477–79.

Glimcher, L., Shen, F.W., and Cantor, H. 1977. Identification of a cell-surface antigen selectively expressed on the natural killer cell. J Exp Med 145:1–9.

Goldfarb, R.H., and Herberman, R.B. 1981a. Natural killer cell reactivity: Regulatory interactions among phorbol ester, interferon, cholera toxin, and retinoic acid. J Immunol 126:2129–35.

Goldfarb, R.H., and Herberman, R.B. 1982. Characteristics of natural killer cells and possible mechanisms for their cytotoxic activity. In: Advances in Inflammation Research, ed. G. Weissman. Raven Press; New York. pp. 45–72.

Goodwin, J.S., Messner, R.P., Bankhurst, A.D., Peake, G.T., Saiki, J.H., and Williams, R.C., Jr. 1977. Prostaglandin-producing suppressor cells in Hodgkin's disease. New Engl J Med 297:963–968.

Gorczynski, R.M., and Norbury, C. 1974. Immunity to murine sarcoma virus induced tumours. III.

Analysis of the cell populations involved in protection from lethal tumour progression of sublethally irradiated, MSV inoculated, mice. Brit J Cancer 30:118–28.

Gorelik, E., Fogel, M., Feldman, M., and Segal, S. 1979. Differences in resistance of metastatic tumor cells and cells from local tumor growth to cytotoxicity of natural killer cells. J Natl Cancer Inst 63:1397–1404.

Gorelik, E., and Herberman, R.B. 1981a. Assay for evaluation of *in vivo* natural cell-mediated resistance of mice to local transplantation of tumor cells. Int J Cancer. 27:207–720.

Gorelik, E., and Herberman, R.B. 1981b. Inhibition of the activity of mouse NK cells by urethane. J Natl Cancer Inst 66:543–48.

Gorelik, E., and Herberman, R.B. 1981c. Carcinogen-induced inhibition of NK activity in mice. Fed Proc 40:1093.

Grant, G., Roe, F.J.C., and Pike, M.C. 1966. Effect of neonatal thymectomy on the induction of papillomata and carcinomata by 3,4-benzopyrene in mice. Nature 210:603–4.

Greene, M.H., Young, T.I., and Clark, W.H., Jr. 1981. Malignant melanoma in renal transplant recipients. Lancet 1:1196–98.

Greene, M.I., Dorf, M.E., Pierres, M., and Benacerraf, B. 1977. Reduction of syngeneic tumor growth by an anti-I-J alloantiserum. Proc Natl Acad Sci USA 74:5118–21.

Grinwich, K.D., and Plescia, O.H. 1977. Tumor-mediated immunosuppression: Prevention by inhibitors of prostaglandin synthesis. Prostaglandins 14:1175–82.

Gross, L. 1943. Intradermal immunization of C3H mice against a sarcoma that originated in an animal of the same line. Cancer Res 3:326–33.

Gutterman, J.U., Hersh, E.M., Freireich, E.J., Rossen, R.D., Butler, W.T., McCredie, K.B., Bodey, G.P. Sr., Rodriguez, V., and Mavligit, G.M. 1973a. Cell-mediated and humoral response to acute leukemia cells and soluble leukemia antigen—relationship to immunocompetence and prognosis. Natl Cancer Inst Monogr 37:153–56.

Gutterman, J.U., Rossen, R.D., Butler, W.T., McCredie, K.B., Bodey, G.P., Freireich, E.J., and Hersh, E.M. 1973b. Immunoglobulin on tumor cells and tumor-induced lymphocyte blastogenesis in human actue leukemia. New Eng J Med 288:169–73.

Habu, S., Fukui, H., Shimamura, K., Kasai, M., Nagai, Y., Okumura, K., and Tamaoki, N. 1981. *In vivo* effects of anti-asialo GM1. I. Reduction of NK activity and enhancement of transplanted tumor growth in nude mice. J Immunol. 127:34–38.

Hafeman, D.G., and Lucas, Z.J. 1979. Polymorphonuclear leukocyte-mediated, antibody-dependent, cellular cytotoxicity against tumor cells: Dependence on oxygen and the respiratory burst. J Immunol 123:55–62.

Haller, O., Kiessling, R., Örn, A., Kärre, K., Nilsson, K., and Wigzell, H. 1977. Natural cytotoxicity to human leukemia mediated by mouse non-T cells. Int J Cancer 20:93–103.

Haller, O., Kiessling, R., Örn, A., and Wigzell, H. 1977b. Generation of natural killer cells: An autonomous function of the bone marrow. J Exp Med 145:1411–16.

Halliday, W.J. 1972. Macrophage migration inhibition with mouse tumor antigens: Properties of serum and peritoneal cells during tumor growth and after tumor loss. Cell Immunol 3:113–21.

Hanna, N., 1980. Expression of metastatic potential of tumor cells in young nude mice is correlated with low levels of natural killer cell-mediated cytotoxicity. Int J Cancer 26:675–80.

Hanna, N., and Fidler, I.J. 1980. The role of natural killer cells in the destruction of circulating tumor emboli. J Natl Cancer Inst 65:801–9.

Hanna, N., and Fidler, I.J. 1981. Expression of metastatic potential of allogeneic and xenogeneic neoplasms in young nude mice. Cancer Res 41:438–44.

Harada, M., Pearson, G., Redmon, L., Winters, E., and Kasuga, S. 1975. Antibody production and interaction with lymphoid cells in relation to tumor immunity in the Moloney sarcoma virus system. J Immunol 114:1318–22.

Haran-Ghera, N., and Lurie, M. 1971. Effect of heterologous antithymocyte serum on mouse skin tumorigenesis. J Natl Cancer Inst 46:103–12.

Haskill, J.S., and Fett, J.W. 1976. Possible evidence for antibody-dependent macrophage-mediated cytotoxicity directed against murine adenocarcinoma cells *in vivo*. J Immunol 117:1992–98.

Hellström, I. 1976. Immunological enforcement of tumor growth. In: Mechanisms of Tumor Immunity, eds. I. Green, S., Cohen, and R.T. McCluskey, pp. 276–89. J. Wiley and Sons; New York.

Herberman, R.B. 1974. Cell-mediated immunity to tumor cells. In: Advances in Cancer Research, vol. 19, eds. G Klein and S. Weinhouse, pp. 207–63. Academic Press; New York.

Herberman, R.B. 1979. Tests for tumor associated antigens and their clinical value. In: Clinical Immunology Update, ed. E.C. Franklin, pp. 23–55. Elsevier North Holland; New York.

Herberman, R.B., ed. 1980. Natural Cell-Mediated Immunology against Tumors. Academic Press; New York.

Herberman, R.B. 1981. Cells suppressing cell-mediated immune responses of cancer patients. In: Human Suppressor Cell, eds. B. Serrou and C. Rosenfeld. North Holland Publishing Co.; Amsterdam. pp. 179–211.

Herberman, R.B., Bordes, M., Lambert, P.H., Luthra, H.S., Robins, R.A., Sizaret, P., and Theofilopoulos, A. 1981a. Report on international comparative evaluation of possible value of assays for immune complexes for diagnosis of human breast cancer. Int J Cancer. 27:569–576.

Herberman, R.B., Brunda, M.J., Cannon, G.B., Djeu, J.Y., Nunn-Hargrove, M.E., Jett, J.R., Ortaldo, J.R., Reynolds, C., Riccardi, C., and Santoni, A. 1981b. Augmentation of natural killer (NK) cell activity by interferon-inducers. In: Augmenting Agents in Cancer Therapy. Current Status and Future Prospects, eds. E. Hersh, M.A. Chirigos, and M. Mastrangelo. Raven Press; New York. pp. 253–265.

Herberman, R.B:, Brunda, M.J., Djeu, J.Y., Domzig, W., Goldfarb, R.H., Holden, H.T., Ortaldo, J.R., Reynolds, C.W., Riccardi, C., Santoni, A., Stadler, B.M., and Timonen, T. 1981c. Immunoregulation and natural killer cells. In: NK Cells: Fundamental Aspects and Role in Cancer. Human Cancer Immunology, vol. 6, ed. B. Serrou. Elsevier North-Holland; Amsterdam. In press.

Herberman, R.B., Djeu, J.Y., Kay, H.D., Ortaldo, J.R., Riccardi, C., Bonnard, G.D., Holden, H.T., Fagnani, R., Santoni, A., and Puccetti, P. 1979. Natural killer cells: Characteristics and regulation of activity. Immunol Rev 44:43–70.

Herberman, R.B., and Holden, H.T. 1978. Natural cell-mediated immunity. Adv Cancer Res 27:305–77.

Herberman, R.B., Holden, H.T., Djeu, J.Y., Jerrells, T.R., Varesio, L., Tagliabue, A., White, S.L., Oehler, J.R., and Dean, J.H. 1980. Macrophages as regulators of immune responses against tumors. In: Macrophages and Lymphocytes, part B, eds. M.R. Escobar and H. Friedman, pp. 361–69. Plenum; New York.

Herberman, R.B., and McIntire, K.R., eds. 1979. Immunodiagnosis of Cancer (Part 1 and Part 2), 1258 pp. Marcel Dekker; New York.

Herberman, R.B., Nunn, M.E., and Lavrin, D.H. 1975. Natural cytotoxic reactivity of mouse lymphoid cells against syngeneic and allogeneic tumors. I. Distribution of reactivity and specificity. Int J Cancer 16:216–29.

Herberman, R.B., Ortaldo, J.R., Djeu, J.Y., Holden, H.T., Jett, J., Lang, N.P., and Pestka, S. 1980. Role of interferon in regulation of cytotoxicity by natural killer cells and macrophages. Ann NY Acad Sci 350:63–71.

Herlyn, D.M., Steplewski, Z., Herlyn, M.F., and Koprowski, H. 1980. Inhibition of growth of colorectal carcinoma in nude mice by monoclonal antibody. Cancer Res 40:717–21.

Hersey, P., Edwards, A., Honeyman, M., and McCarthy, W.H. 1979. Low natural-killer cell activity in familial melanoma patients and their relatives. Brit J Cancer 40:113–22.

Hersey, P., Edwards, A., and McCarthy, W.H. 1980. Tumour-related changes in natural killer cell activity in melanoma patients. Influence of stage of disease, tumour thickness and age of patients. Int J Cancer 25:187–94.

Hewitt, H.B., Blake, E.R., and Walder, A.S. 1976. A critique of the evidence for active host defense against cancer, based on personal studies of 27 murine tumours of spontaneous origin. Brit J Cancer 33:241–59.

Hibbs, J.B., Jr. 1974a. Discrimination between neoplastic and non-neoplastic cells *in vitro* by activated macrophages. J Natl Cancer Inst 53:1487–1493.

Hibbs, J.B., Jr. 1974b. Heterocytolysis by macrophages activated by bacillus Calmette-Guérin: Lysosome exocytosis into tumor cells. Science 184:468–71.

Hibbs, J.B. 1975. Activated macrophages as cytotoxic effector cells. I. Inhibition of specific and nonspecific tumor resistance by trypan blue. Transplantation 19:77–81.

Hibbs, J.B., Jr., Chapman, H.A., Jr., and Weinberg, J.B. 1978. The macrophage as an antineoplastic surveillance cell; Biological perspectives. J Reticuloendothel Soc 24:549–70.

Hibbs, J.B., Jr., Lambert, C.H., Jr., and Remington, J.S. 1972a. Control of carcinogenesis: A possible role for the activated macrophage. Science 177:998–1000.

Hibbs, J.B., Jr., Lambert, L.H., Jr., and Remington, J.S. 1972b. Possible role of macrophage mediated nonspecific cytotoxicity in tumor resistance. Nature New Biol 235:48–49.

Hirshaut, Y. 1977. Immune responses of patients to tumor associated antigens: Humoral immunity. In: Handbook of Clinical Immunology, eds. A. Baumgarten and F. Richards. CRC Press; Cleveland.

Hochman, P.S., Cudkowicz, G., and Dausset, J. 1978. Decline of natural killer cell activity in sublethally irradiated mice. J Natl Cancer Inst 61:265–68.

Höffken, K., Meredith, I.D., Robins, R.A., Baldwin, R.W., Davies, C.J., and Blamery, R.W. 1978. Immune complexes and prognosis of human breast cancer. Lancet 1:672–73.

Holden, H.T., Kirchner, H., and Herberman, R.B. 1975. Secondary cell-mediated cytotoxic response to syngeneic mouse tumor challenge. J Immunol 115:327–31.

Holden, H.T., Oldham, R.K., Ortaldo, J.R., and Herberman, R.B. 1976. Cryopreservation of the functional reactivity of normal and immune leukocytes and of tumor cells. In: In Vitro Methods in Cell-Mediated and Tumor Immunity, eds. B.R. Bloom and J.R. David. pp. 723–29. Academic Press; New York.

Holden, H.T., Varesio, L., Taniyama, T., and Puccetti, P. 1979. Functional heterogeneity and T cell-dependent activation of macrophages from murine sarcoma virus (MSV)-induced tumors. In: Macrophages and Lymphocytes, Part B, eds. M.R. Escobar and H. Friedman, pp. 509–20. Plenum; New York.

Houghton, A.N., Taormina, M.C., Ikeda, H., Watanabe, T., Oettgen, H.F., and Old, L.J. 1980.

Serological survey of normal humans for natural antibody to cell surface antigens of melanoma. Proc Natl Acad Sci USA 77:4260–64.

Huebner, R.J. 1963. Tumor virus study systems. Ann NY Acad Sci 108:1129–48.

Hueper, W.C. 1959. Carcinogenic studies on water-soluble and water-insoluble macromolecules. Arch Pathol 67:589–95.

Hueper, W.C. 1961. Bioassay of polyvinyl pyrrolidones with limited molecular weight range. J Natl Cancer Inst 6:229–37.

Hyman, G.A. 1969. Increased incidence of neoplasm in association with chronic lymphocytic leukemia. Scand J Haemat 6:99–104.

Ioachim, H., Keller, S., Dorsett, B., and Pearse, A. 1974. Induction of partial immunologic tolerance in rats and progressive loss of cellular antigenicity in Gross virus lymphoma. J Exp Med 139:1382–94.

Jerrells, T.R., Dean, J.H., Richardson, G., Cannon, G.B., and Herberman, R.B. 1979. Increased monocyte-mediated cytostasis of lymphoid cell lines in breast and lung cancer patients. Int J Cancer 23:768–76.

Jerrells, T.R., Dean, J.H., Richardson, G.L., McCoy, J.L., and Herberman, R.B. 1978. Role of suppressor cells in depression of *in vitro* lymphoproliferative responses of lung cancer and breast cancer patients. J Natl Cancer Inst 61:1001–9.

Jose, D.G., and Seshadri, R. 1974. Circulating immune complexes in human neuroblastoma: Direct assay and role in blocking specific cellular immunity. Int J Cancer 13:824–838.

Kaplan, H.S., Brown, M.B., and Paull, J. 1953. Influence of bone marrow injections on involution and neoplasia of mouse thymus after systemic irradiation. J Natl Cancer Inst 14:303–16.

Kaplan, J., and Callewaert, D.M. 1980. Are natural killer cells germ line V-gene encoded prothymocytes specific for self and nonself histocompatibility antigens? In: Natural Cell-Mediated Immunity against Tumors, ed. R.B. Herberman, pp. 893–907. Academic Press; New York.

Kärre, K., Klein, G.O., Kiessling, R., Klein, G., and Roder, J.C. 1980. Low natural *in vivo* resistance to syngeneic leukaemias in natural killer-deficient mice. Nature 284:624–26.

Kasai, M., Iwamori, M., Nagai, Y., Okumura, K., and Tada, T. 1980. A glycolipid on the surface of mouse natural killer cells. Eur J Immunol 10:175–80.

Kasai, M., Leclerc, J.C., McVay-Boudreau, L., Shen, F.W., and Cantor, H. 1979. Direct evidence that natural killer cells in nonimmune spleen cell populations prevent tumor growth *in vivo*. J Exp Med 149:1260–64.

Kay, H.D., and Horwitz, D.A. 1980. Evidence by reactivity with hybridoma antibodies for a possible myeloid origin of peripheral blood cells active in natural cytotoxicity and antibody-dependent cell-mediated cytotoxicity. J Clin Invest 66:847–51.

Keller, R. 1976. Promotion of tumor growth *in vivo* by anti-macrophage agents. J Natl Cancer Inst 57:1355–67.

Keller, R. 1978. Macrophage-mediated natural cytotoxicity against various target cells *in vitro*. I. Comparsion of tissue macrophages from diverse anatomic sites and from different strains of rats and mice. Brit J Cancer 37:732–41.

Keller, R. 1979. Suppression of natural antitumor defense mechanisms by phorbol esters. Nature 282:729–31.

Keller, R. 1980. Regulatory capacities of mononuclear phagocytes with particular reference to natural immunity against tumors. In: Natural Cell-Mediated Immunity against Tumors, ed. R.B. Herberman, pp. 1219–69. Academic Press; New York.

Key, M., and Haskill, J.S. 1981. Macrophage-mediated, antibody-dependent destruction of tumor cells: *in vitro* identification of an in situ mechanism. J Natl Cancer Inst. 66:103–110.

Kiessling, R., Klein, E., and Wigzell, H. 1975a. "Natural" killer cells in the mouse. I. Cytotoxic cells with specificity for mouse Moloney leukemia cells. Specificity and distribution according to genotype. Eur J Immunol 5:112–17.

Kiessling, R., Petranyi, G., Klein, G., and Wigzell, H. 1975b. Genetic variation of *in vitro* cytolytic activity and *in vivo* rejection potential of non-immunized semisyngeneic mice against a mouse lymphoma line. Int J Cancer 15:933–940.

Kiessling, R., Petranyi, G., Klein, G., and Wigzell, H. 1976. Non-T-cell resistance against a mouse Moloney lymphoma. Int J Cancer 17:275–81.

Kjaer, M. 1974. *In vitro* demonstration of cellular hypersensitivity to tumor antigens by means of the leukocyte migration technique in patients with renal carcinoma. Eur J Cancer 10:523–31.

Kjaer, M., and Christensen, N. 1977. Ability of renal carcinoma tissue extract to induce leukocyte migration inhibition in patients with nonmetastatic renal carcinoma: Correlation with clinical and histopathological findings. Cancer Immunol Immunother 2:41–48.

Klein, G. 1979. Burkitt's lymphoma and nasopharyngeal carcinoma. In: Immunodiagnosis of Cancer, eds. R.B. Herberman and K.R. McIntire. Marcel Dekker; New York, Part 2, pp. 780–800.

Klein, G., and Klein, E. 1977. Rejectability of virus induced tumors and non-rejectability of spontaneous tumors—a lesson in contrasts. Transplant Proc 9:1095–1104.

Klein, G., Klein, E., and Haughton, G. 1966. Variation of antigenic characteristics between different mouse lymphomas induced by the Moloney virus. J Natl Cancer Inst 36:607–21.

Klein, G., Sjögren, H.O., Klein, E., and Hellström,

K.E. 1960. Demonstration of resistance against methylcholanthrene-induced sarcomas in the primary autochthonous host. Cancer Res 20:1561–72.

Koo, G.C., and Hatzfeld, A. 1980. Antigenic phenotype of mouse natural killer cells. In: Natural Cell-Mediated Immunity against Tumors, ed. R.B. Herberman, pp. 105–16. Academic Press; New York.

Korec, S. 1980. The role of granulocytes in host defense against tumors. In: Natural Cell-Mediated Immunity against Tumors, ed. R.B. Herberman, pp. 1301–7. Academic Press; New York.

Kraskovsky, G., Gorelik, L., and Kagan, L. 1973. Abrogration of the immunosuppressive and carcinogenic action of urethan by transplantation of syngeneic bone marrow cells from normal mice. Proc Acad Sci BSSR 11:1052–53.

Kripke, M.L. 1974. Antigenicity of murine skin tumors induced by ultraviolet light. J Natl Cancer Inst 53:1333–36.

Kripke, M.L., and Fisher, M.S. 1976. Immunologic parameter of ultraviolet carcinogenesis. J Natl Cancer Inst 57:211–15.

Kunkel, L.A., and Welsh, R.M. 1981. Metabolic inhibitors render "resistant" target cells sensitive to natural killer cell-mediated lysis. Int J Cancer 27:73–79.

Lamon, E.W., Skurzak, H.M., Andersson, B., Whitten, H.D., and Klein, E. 1975. Antibody-dependent lymphocyte cytotoxicity in the murine sarcoma virus system: Activity of IgM and IgG with specificity for MLV determine antigen(s). J Immunol 114:1171–76.

Landazuri, M.O., Kedar, E., and Fahey, J.L. 1974. Antibody-dependent cellular cytotoxicity to a syngeneic Gross virus-induced lymphoma. J Natl Cancer Inst 52:147–52.

Landazuri, M.O., Lopez-Botet, M., Timonen, T., Ortaldo, J.R., and Herberman, R.B. 1981. Role of large granular lymphocytes in human natural cytotoxicity against monolayer target cells. J Immunol. 127:1380–1383.

Landazuri, M.O., Silva, A., Alvarez, J., and Herberman, R.B. 1979. Evidence that natural cytotoxicity and antibody dependent cellular cytotoxicity are mediated in humans by the same effector cell populations. J Immunol 123:252–258.

Langlois, A.J., Matthews, T., Roloson, G.J., Thiel, H.-J., Collins, J.J., and Bolognesi, D.P. 1981. Immunologic control of the ascites form of murine adenocarcinoma 755. V. Antibody-directed macrophages mediate tumor cell destruction. J Immunol 126:2337–41.

Lappé, M.A. 1971. Evidence for immunological surveillance during skin carcinogenesis. Inflammatory foci in immunologically competent mice. Israel J Med Sci 7:52–65.

Law, L.W. 1965. Neoplasms in thymectomized mice following room infection with polyoma virus. Nature 205:672–73.

Law, L.W. 1966. Studies of thymic functions with emphasis on the role of the thymus in oncogenesis. Cancer Res 26:551–74.

Law, L.W., and Ting, R.C. 1965. Immunologic competence and induction of neoplasms by polyoma virus. Proc Soc Exp Biol Med 119:823–30.

Levy, M.H., and Wheelock, E.F. 1974. The role of macrophages in defense against neoplastic disease. Adv Cancer Res 20:131–63.

Levy, P.C., Yhaw, G.M., and LoBuglio, A. 1979. Human monocyte, lymphocyte, and granulocyte antibody-dependent cell-mediated cytotoxicity toward tumor cells. J Immunol 123:594–99.

Lewis, M.G., Phillips, T.M., Cook, K.B., and Blake, J. 1971. Possible explanation of loss of detectable antibody in patients with disseminated malignant melanoma. Nature New Biol 232:52–54.

Liotta, L.A., Gattozzi, C., Kleinerman, J., and Saidel, G. 1977. Reduction of tumour cell entry into vessels by BCG-activated macrophages. Brit J Cancer 36:639–41.

Lipinski, M., Tursz, T., Kreis, H., Finale, Y., and Amiel, J.L. 1980. Dissociation of natural killer cell activity and antibody-dependent cell-mediated cytotoxicity in kidney allograft recipients receiving high-dose immunosuppressive therapy. Transplantation 29:214–18.

Lohmann-Matthes, M-L., and Domzig, W. 1980. Natural cytotoxicity of macrophage precursor cells and of mature macrophages. In: Natural Cell-Mediated Immunity against Tumors, ed. R.B. Herberman, pp. 117-29. Academic Press; New York.

Lotan, R. 1980. Effects of vitamin A and its analogs (retinoids) on normal and neoplastic cells. Biochim Biophys Acta 605:33–37.

Lotzová, E. 1980. C. parvum-mediated suppression of the phenomenon of natural killer and its analysis. In: Natural Cell-Mediated Immunity against Tumors, ed. R.B. Herberman, pp. 735–52. Academic Press; New York.

Lotzová, E., and Gutterman, J.U. 1979. Effect of glucan on natural killer (NK) cells: Further comparison between NK cell and bone marrow effector cell activities. J Immunol 123:607–612.

Loutit, J.F., Townsend, K.M.S., and Knowles, J.F. 1980. Tumour surveillance in beige mice. Nature 285:66.

Lupulescu, A. 1978. Enhancement of carcinogenesis by prostaglandins. Nature 272:634–36.

Lynch, N.R., Castes, M., Astoin, M., and Salomon, J.C. 1978. Mechanism of inhibition of tumour growth by aspirin and indomethacin. Brit J Cancer 38:503–12.

Lynch, N.R., and Salomon, J.C. 1979. Tumor growth inhibition and potentiation of immunotherapy by indomethacin in mice. J Natl Cancer Inst 62:117–25.

Maguire, H., Jr., Outzen, H.C., Custer, R.P., and Prehn, R.T. 1976. Invasion and metastasis of a

xenogeneic tumor in nude mice. J Natl Cancer Inst. 57:439–42.
Mahoney, K.H., Morse, S.S., and Morahan, P.S. 1980. Macrophage functions in beige (Chediak-Higashi syndrome) mice. Cancer Res 40:3934–39.
Maluish, A.E. 1979. Experiences with leukocyte adherence inhibition in human cancer. Cancer Res 39:644–48.
Mantovani, A., Allavena, P., Biondi, A., Sessa, C., and Introna, M. 1981. Natural killer activity in human ovarian carcinoma. In: NK Cells: Fundamental Aspects and Role in Cancer/ Human Cancer Immunology, vol. 6, eds. B. Serrou and R.B. Herberman. North-Holland; Amsterdam. In press.
Mantovani, A., Giavazzi, R., Polentarutti, N., Spreafico, F., and Garattini, S. 1980. Divergent effects of macrophage toxins on growth of primary tumors and lung metastasis. Int J Cancer 25:617–22.
Mantovani, A., Jerrells, T.R., Dean, J.H., and Herberman, R.B. 1979. Cytolytic and cytostatic activity on tumor cells of circulating human monocytes. Int J Cancer 23:18–27.
Marcelletti, J., and Furmanski, P. 1978. Spontaneous regression of Friend virus induced erythroleukemia. III. The role of macrophages in regression. J Immunol 120:1–9.
Martin, S.E., and Martin, W.J. 1975. Anti-tumor antibodies in normal mouse sera. Int J Cancer 15:658–664.
Mattes, M.J., Sharrow, S.O., Herberman, R.B., and Holden, H.T. 1979. Identification and separation of Thy-1 positive mouse spleen cells active in natural cytotoxicity and antibody-dependent cell-mediated cytotoxicity. J Immunol 123:2851–60.
Mavligit, G.M., Gutterman, J.U., McBride, C.M., and Hersh, E.M. 1973. Cell-mediated immunity to human solid tumors: *In vitro* detection by lymphocyte blastogenic responses to cell-associated and solubilized tumor antigens. Natl Cancer Inst Monogr 37:167–76.
McBride, W.H., Tuach, W., and Marmion, B.P. 1975. The effects of gold salts on tumor immunity and its stimulation by *Corynebacterium parvum*. Brit J Cancer 32:558–65.
McCoy, J.L. 1979. Clinical applications of assay of leukocyte migration inhibition. In: Immunodiagnosis of Cancer, Part 2, eds. R.B. Herberman and K.R. McIntire, pp. 979–98. Marcel Dekker; New York.
McCoy, J.L., Jerome, L.F., Cannon, G.B., Weese, J.L., and Herberman, R.B. 1977. Reactivity of lung cancer patients in leukocyte migration inhibition assays to 3-M potassium chloride extracts of fresh tumor and tissue-cultured cells derived from lung cancer. J Natl Cancer Inst 59:1413–18.
McCoy, J.L., Jerome, L.F., Dean, J.H., Cannon, G.B., Alford, T.C., Doering, T., and Herberman, R.B. 1974. Inhibition of leukocyte migration by tumor-associated antigens in soluble extracts of human breast carcinoma. J Natl Cancer Inst 53:11–17.
McCoy, J., Herberman, R., Perlin, E., Levine, P., and Alford, C. 1973. ^{51}Cr release cellular lymphocyte cytotoxicity as a possible measure of immunological competence of cancer patients. Proc Amer Assoc Cancer Res 14:107.
McCredie, J.A., and MacDonald, H.R. 1980. Antibody-dependent cellular cytotoxicity in cancer patients: Lack of prognostic value. Brit J Cancer 41:880–85.
Menard, S., Colnaghi, M.I., and Della Porta, G. 1977. Natural anti-tumor serum reactivity in BALB/c mice. I. Characterization and interference with tumor growth. Int J Cancer 19:267–74.
Mizel, S.B., Delarco, J.E., Todaro, G.J., Farrar, W.L., and Hilfiker, M.L. 1980. *In vitro* production of immunosuppressive factors by murine sarcoma virus-transformed mouse fibroblasts. Proc Natl Acad Sci USA 77:2205–8.
Morton, D.L., Eilber, F.R., Joseph, W.L., Wood, W.C., Trahan, E., and Ketcham, A.S. 1970. Immunological factors in human sarcomas and melanomas: A rational basis for immunotherapy. Ann Surg 172:740–49.
Morton, D.L., Malmgren, R.A., Holmes, E.C., and Ketcham, A.S. 1968. Demonstration of antibodies against human malignant melanoma by immunofluorescence. Surgery 64:233–40.
Nair, P.N.M., Fernandes, G., Onoe, K., Day, N.K. and Good, R.A. 1980. Inhibition of effector cell functions in natural killer cell activity (NK) and antibody-dependent cellular cytotoxicity (ADCC) in mice by normal and cancer sera. Int J Cancer 25:667–77.
Nairn, R.C., Nind, A.P.P., Guli, E.P.G., Davies, D.J., Little, J.H., David, N.C., and Whitehead, D. 1972. Anti-tumor immunoreactivity in patients with malignant melanoma. Med J Austr 1:397–403.
Nathan, C.F., Bruckner, L.H., Silverstein, S.C., and Cohn, Z.A. 1979. Extracellular cytolysis by activated macrophages and granulocytes. I. Pharmacologic triggering of effector cells and the release of hydrogen peroxide. J Exp Med 149:84–99.
Nepom, J.T., Hellström, I., and Hellström, K.E. 1976. Purification and partial characterization of a tumor specific blocking factor from sera of mice with growing chemically induced sarcoma. J Immunol 117:1846–54.
Norbury, K.C., and Kripke, M.L. 1979. Ultraviolet-induced carcinogenesis in mice treated with silica, trypan blue, or pyran copolymer. J Reticuloendothel Soc 26:827–32.
Nossal, G.J.V. 1980. The case history of Mr. T.I. Terminal patient or still curable? Immunology Today 1:5–9.
Nunn, M.E., and Herberman, R.B. 1979. Natural cytotoxicity of mouse, rat and human lymphocytes against heterologous target cells. J Natl Cancer Inst 62:765–71.
Nunn, M.E., Herberman, R.B., and Holden, H.T. 1977. Natural cell-mediated cytotoxicity in mice

against non-lymphoid tumor cells and some normal cells. Int J Cancer 20:381–87.

Oehler, J.R., and Herberman, R.B. 1978. Natural cell-mediated cytotoxicity in rats. III. Effects of immunopharmacologic treatments on natural reactivity and on reactivity augmented by polyinosinic-polycytidylic acid. Int J Cancer 21:221–29.

Oehler, J.R., and Herberman, R.B. 1979. Evidence for long-lasting tumor immunity in a syngeneic rat lymphoma model: Correlation of *in vitro* findings with *in vivo* observations. J Natl Cancer Inst 62:525–29.

Oehler, J.R., Herberman, R.B., and Holden, H.T. 1978. Modulation of immunity by macrophages. Pharmac Ther A 2:551–93.

Ojo, E., and Wigzell, H. 1978. Natural killer cells may be the only cells in normal mouse lymphoid populations endowed with cytolytic ability for antibody-coated tumor target cells. Scand J Immunol 7:297–306.

Old, L.J., Stockert, E., Boyse, E.A., and Kim, J.H. 1968. Antigenic modulation. Loss of TL antigen from cells exposed to TL antibody. Study of the phenomenon *in vitro*. J Exp Med 127:523–39.

Oppenheim, J.J., Northoff, H., Greenhill, A., Mathieson, B.J., Smith, K.A., and Gillis, S. 1980. Properties of human monocyte-derived lymphocyte activating factor (LAF) and lymphocyte-derived mitogenic factor (LMF). In: Biochemical Characterization of Lymphokine, ed. A. De Weck, p. 399. Academic Press; New York.

Ortaldo, J.R., and Herberman, R.B. 1981. Specificity of natural killer cells. In: NK Cells: Fundamental Aspects and Role in Cancer/Human Cancer Immunology, vol. 6, ed. B. Serrou. Elsevier North-Holland; Amsterdam. In Press.

Ortaldo, J.R., Oldham, R.K., Cannon, G.C., and Herberman, R.B. 1977. Specificity of natural cytotoxic reactivity of normal human lymphocytes against a myeloid leukemia cell line. J Natl Cancer Inst 59:77–82.

Ortaldo, J.R., Sharrow, S.O., Timonen, T., and Herberman, R.B. 1981. Analysis of surface antigens on highly purified human NK cells by flow cytometry with monoclonal antibodies. J Immunol. 127:2401–2409.

Ortaldo, J.R., and Timonen, T.T. 1981. Modification of antigen expression and surface receptors on human NK cells grown *in vitro*. In: Proceedings of the 14th International Leukocyte Culture Conference. pp 286–289.

Ortaldo, J.R., Ting, C.C., and Herberman, R.B. 1974. Modulation of fetal antigen(s) in mouse leukemia cells. Cancer Res 34:1366–71.

Ozzello, L., Sordat, B., Merenda, C., Carrell, S., Hurlimann, J., and Mach, J.P. 1974. Transplantation of a human mammary carcinoma cell line (BT 20) into nude mice. J Natl Cancer Inst 52:1669–72.

Paige, C.J., Figarella, E.F., Cuttito, M.J., Cahan, A., and Stutman, O. 1978. Natural cytotoxic cells against solid tumors in mice. II. Some characteristics of the effector cells. J Immunol 121:1827–35.

Papacharalampous, N.X. 1960. Zur frage der experimentellen induktion von tumoren am retothelialen system der ratte nach langfristigen versuchen mit intraperitonealen injektionen von trypanblau. Frankf Z Pathol 70:598–604.

Parkinson, D.R., Brightman, R.P., and Waksal, S.D. 1981. Altered natural killer cell biology in C57BL/6 mice after leukemogenic split-dose irradiation. J Immunol 126:1460–64.

Payne, L.N. 1972. Pathogenesis of Marek's disease—a review. In: Oncogenesis and Herpesviruses, eds. P.M. Briggs, G. Dethe , and L.N. Payne, pp. 21–37. International Agency for Research on Cancer; Lyon.

Penn, I., and Starzl, T.E. 1972. A summary of the status of de novo cancer in transplant recipients. Transplant Proc 4:719–32.

Perry, L.L., Kripke, M.L., Benacerraf, B., Dorf, M.E., and Greene, M.I. 1980. Regulation of the immune response to tumor antigen. VIII. The effects of host specific anti-I-J antibodies on the immune response to tumors of different origin. Cell Immunol 51:349–59.

Petrányi, G., Kiessling, R., Povey, S., Klein, G., Herzenberg, E., and Wigzell, H. 1976. The genetic control of natural killer cell activity and its association with *in vivo* resistance against a Moloney lymphoma isograft. Immunogenetics 3:15–28.

Pike, M.C., and Synderman, R. 1977. Macrophage migratory dysfunction in cancer. A mechanism for subversion of surveillance. Am J Pathol 88:727–39.

Plata, F., Cerottini, J.C., and Brunner, K.T. 1975. Primary and secondary *in vitro* generation of cytolytic T lymphocytes in the murine sarcoma virus system. Eur J Immunol 5:227–33.

Plescia, O.J., Smith, A.H., and Grinwich, K. 1975. Subversion of immune system by tumor cells and role of prostaglandins. Proc Natl Acad Sci 72:1848–51.

Pollack, S., Heppner, G., Brawn, R.J., and Nelson, K. 1972. Specific killing of tumor cells *in vitro* in the presence of normal lymphoid cells and sera from hosts immune to the tumor antigens. Int J Cancer 9:316–24.

Prather, S.O., and Lausch, R.N. 1976. Membrane-associated antigen from the SV40-induced hamster fibrosarcoma, PARA-7. I. Role in immune complex formation and effector cell blockade. Int J Cancer 18:820–28.

Prehn, R.T., and Lappé, M.A. 1971. An immunostimulation theory of tumor development. Transplant Rev 7:26–54.

Prehn, R.T., and Main, J.M. 1957. Immunity to methylcholanthrene-induced sarcomas. J Natl Cancer Inst 18:769–75.

Pross, H.F., and Baines, M.G. 1980. Natural killer cells in tumor-bearing patients. In: Natural Cell-

Mediated Immunity against Tumors, ed. R.B. Herberman, pp. 1063–72. Academic Press; New York.

Puri, H.C., and Campbell, R. 1977. Cyclophosphamide and malignancy. Lancet 1:1306.

Purtilo, D.T., De Florio D., Hutt, L.M., Bhawan, J., Yang, J.P.S., Otto, R., and Edwards, W. 1977. Variable phenotypic expression of an X-linked recessive lymphoproliferative syndrome. New Engl J Med 297:1077–81.

Rabinovitch, M., Manejias, R.E., Russo, M., and Abbey, E.E. 1977. Increased spreading of macrophages from mice treated with interferon inducers. Cell Immunol 29:86–93.

Reimer, R.R., Hoover, R., Fraumeni, J.F., Jr., and Young, R.C. 1977. Acute leukemia after alkylating-agent therapy of ovarian cancer. New Engl J Med 297:177–81.

Reinherz, E.L., Kung, P.C., Goldstein, G., Levey, R.H., and Schlossman, S.F. 1980a. Discrete stages of human intrathymic differentiation: Analysis of normal thymocytes and leukemic lymphoblasts of T-cell lineage. Proc Natl Acad Sci USA 77:1588–1592.

Reinherz, E.L., Moretta, L., Roper, M., Breard, J.M., Mingari, M.C., Cooper, M.D., and Schlossman, S.F. 1980b. Human T lymphocyte subpopulations defined by Fc receptors and monoclonal antibodies. A comparison. J Exp Med 151:969–974.

Reynolds, C.W., Sharrow, S.O., Ortaldo, J.R., and Herberman, R.B. 1981a. Natural killer activity in the rat. III. Analysis of surface antigens on LGL by flow cytometry. J Immunol. 127:2204–2208.

Reynolds, C.W., Timonen, T., and Herberman, R.B. 1981b. Natural killer (NK) cell activity in the rat. I. Isolation and characterization of the effector cell. J Immunol. 127:282–287.

Rhodes, J. 1980. Resistance of tumor cells to macrophages. Cancer Immunol Immunother 7:211–17.

Rhodes, J., Bishop, M., and Benfield, J. 1978. Tumor surveillance: How tumors may resist macrophage-mediated host defense. Science 203:179–81.

Riccardi, C., Barlozzari, T., Santoni, A., Herberman, R.B., and Cesarini, C. 1981a. Transfer to cyclophosphamide-treated mice of natural killer (NK) cells and *in vivo* natural reactivity against tumors. J Immunol 126:1284–89.

Riccardi, C., Puccetti, P., Santoni, A., and Herberman, R.B. 1979. Rapid *in vivo* assay of mouse NK cell activity. J Natl Cancer Inst 63:1041–45.

Riccardi, C., Stantoni, A., Barlozzari, T., Cesarini, C., and Herberman, R.B. 1981b. *In vivo* role of NK cells against neoplastic or non-neoplastic cells. In: NK Cells: Fundamental Aspects and Role in Cancer/Human Cancer Immunology, eds., B. Serrou and C. Rosenfeld. North Holland; Amsterdam. In press.

Riccardi, C., Santoni, A., Barlozzari, T., and Herberman, R.B. 1980a. Role of NK cells in rapid *in vivo* clearance of radiolabeled tumor cells. In: Natural Cell-Mediated Immunity against Tumors, ed. R.B. Herberman, pp. 1121–39. Academic Press; New York.

Riccardi, C., Santoni, A., Barlozzari, T., Puccetti, P., and Herberman, R.B. 1980b. *In vivo* natural reactivity of mice against tumor cells. Int J Cancer 25:475–86.

Riesenfeld, I., Orn, A., Gidlund, M., Axberg, I., Alm, G.V., and Wigzell, H. 1980. Positive correlation between *in vitro* NK activity and *in vivo* resistance towards AKR lymphoma cells. Int J Cancer 25:399–403.

Riley, V. 1975. Mouse mammary tumors: Alteration of incidence as apparent function of stress. Science 189:465–67.

Riley, V. 1981. Psychoneuroendocrine influence on immunocompetence and neoplasia. Science 212:1100–9.

Roberts, M.M., and Bell, R. 1976. Acute leukemia after immunosuppressive therapy. Lancet 2:768-70.

Roder, J., and Duwe, A. 1979. The beige mutation in the mouse selectively impairs natural killer cell function. Nature 278:451–53.

Roder, J.C., Haliotis, T., Klein, M., Korec, S., Jett, J.R., Ortaldo, J., Herberman, R.B., Katz, P., and Fauci, A.S. 1980. A new immunodeficiency disorder in humans involving NK cells. Nature 284:553–55.

Roder, J.C., Laing, L., Haliotis, T., and Kozbor, D. 1981. Genetic control of human NK function. In: NK cells: Fundamental Aspects and Role in Cancer/Human Cancer Immunology, vol. 6, eds. B. Serrou, C. Rosenfeld and R.B. Herberman. North-Holland; Amsterdam. In press.

Roder, J.C., Lohmann-Matthes, M-L, Domzig, W., and Wigzell, H. 1979. The beige mutation in the mouse. II. Selectivity of the natural killer (NK) cell defect. J Immunol 123:2174–81.

Rosenberg, E.B., Herberman, R.B., Levine, P.H., Halterman, R.H., McCoy, J.L., and Wunderlich, J.R. 1972. Lympocyte cytotoxicity reactions to leukemia-associated antigens in identical twins. Int J Cancer 9:648–58.

Rossen, R.D., Reisberg, M.A., Hersh, E.M., and Gutterman, J.U. 1977. The C1q binding test for soluble immune complexes: Clinical correlations obtained in patients with cancer. J Natl Cancer Inst 58:1205–15.

Roth, J.A., Slocum, H.K., Pellegrino, M.A., Holmes, E.C., and Reisfeld, R.A. 1976. Purification of soluble human melanoma-associated antigens. Cancer Res 36:2360–64.

Russell, S. 1981. In: Mediation of Cellular Immunity in Cancer by Immune Modifiders, ed., M.A. Chirigos, M. Mitchell, M.J. Mastrangelo and M. Krim. Raven Press; New York. pp. 49–56.

Rygaard, J., and Poulsen, C.O. 1969. Heterotransplantation of a human malignant tumor to nude mice. Acta Pathol Microbiol Scand 77:758–60.

Saksela, E., Timonen, T., Virtanen, I., and Cantell, K. 1980. Regulation of human natural killer activity by interferon. In: Natural Cell-Mediated Immunity against Tumors, ed. R.B. Herberman, pp. 645–53. Academic Press; New York.

Santoni, A., Riccardi, C., Barlozzari, T., and Herberman, R.B. 1980a. Suppression of activity of mouse natural killer (NK) cells by activated macrophages from mice treated with pyran copolymer. Int J Cancer 26:837–43.

Santoni, A., Riccardi, C., Barlozzari, T., and Herberman, R.B. 1980b. Inhibition as well as augmentation of mouse NK activity by pyran copolymer and adriamycin. In: Natural Cell-Mediated Immunity against Tumors, ed. R.B. Herberman, pp. 753–63. Academic Press; New York.

Sbarra, A.J., and Strauss, P.R., ed. 1980. The Reticuloendothelial System: A Comprehensive Treatise, vol. 2. Plenum Press; New York.

Schmidt, M., and Good, R.A. 1976. Cancer xenografts in nude mice. Lancet 1:39.

Schultz, R.M., Stoychkov, J.N., Pavlidis, N., Chirigos, M.A., and Olkowski, Z.L. 1979. J Reticuloendothel Soc 26:93–102.

Sendo, F., Aoki, T., Boyse, E.A., and Buafo, C.K. 1975. Natural occurrence of lymphocytes showing cytotoxic activity to BALB/c radiation-induced leukemia RLo1 cells. J Natl Cancer Inst 55:603–9.

Serrate, S., and Herberman, R.B. 1981. Natural cell-mediated cytotoxicity against primary mammary tumors. Fed Proc. 40:1007.

Sethi, J., and Hirshaut, Y. 1976. Complement-fixing antigen of human sarcomas. J Natl Cancer Inst 57:489–93.

Sharkey, F.E., and Fogh, J. 1979. Metastasis of human tumors in athymic nude mice. Int J Cancer 24:733–38.

Shin, H.S., Economou, J.S., Pasternack, G.R., Johnson, R.J., and Hayden, M. 1976. Antibody mediated suppression of grafted lymphoma. IV. Influence of time of tumor residency *in vivo* and tumor size upon the effectiveness of suppression by syngeneic antibody. J Exp Med 144:1274–83.

Shin, H.S., Hayden, M.L., Langley, S., Kaliss, N., and Smith, M.R. 1975. Antibody-mediated suppression of grafted lymphoma. III. Evaluation of the role of thymic function, non-thumus-derived lymphocytes, macrophages, platelets and polymorphonuclear leukocytes in syngeneic and allogeneic hosts. J Immunol 114:1255.

Shin, H.S., Johnson, R.J., Pasternack, G.R., and Economou, J.S. 1978. Mechanisms of tumor immunity: The role of antibody and nonimmune effectors. Prog Allergy 25:163–210.

Shope, T.C., and Kaplan, J. 1979. Inhibition of the *in vitro* outgrowth of Epstein-Barr virus-infected lymphocytes by T_G lymphocytes. J Immunol 123:2150–55.

Sjögren, H.O. 1974. Blocking and unblocking of cell-mediated tumor immunity. Methods Cancer Res 10:19–32.

Sones, P.D.E., and Castro, J.E. 1977. Immunological mechanisms in metastatic spread and the antimetastatic effect of *C. parvum*. Brit J Cancer 35:519–26.

Stern, K. 1981. Control of tumors by the RES. In: The Reticuloendothelial System: A Comprehensive Treatise, vol. 8, Cancer, eds. R.B. Herberman and H. Friedman. Plenum Press; New York. In press.

Stjernswärd, J., and Vánky, F. 1972. Stimulation of lymphocytes by autochthonous cancer. Natl Cancer Inst Monogr 35:237–42.

Strausser, H.R., and Humes, J.L. 1975. Prostaglandin synthesis inhibition: Effect on bone changes and sarcoma tumor induction in BALB/c mice. Int J Cancer 15:724–30.

Stutman, O. 1975a. Tumor development after polyoma infection in athymic nude mice. J Immunol 114:1213–17.

Stutman, O. 1975b. Immunodepression and malignancy. In: Advances in Cancer Research, vol. 22, eds. G. Klein, S. Weinhouse, and A. Haddow, pp. 261–422. Academic Press; New York.

Stutman, O. 1979. Chemical carcinogenesis in nude mice: Comparison between nude mice from homozygous matings and heterozygous matings and effect of age and carcinogen dose. J Natl Cancer Inst 62:353–58.

Stutman, O., Dien, P., Wisun, R., Pecoraro, G., and Lattime, E.C. 1980a. Natural cytotoxic (NC) cells against solid tumors in mice: Some target cell characteristics and blocking of cytoxicity by D-mannose. In: Natural Cell-Mediated Immunity against Tumors, ed. R.B. Herberman, pp. 949–61. Academic Press; New York.

Stutman, O., Figarella, E.F., Paige, C.J., and Lattime, E.C. 1980b. Natural cytotoxic (NC) cells against solid tumors in mice: General characteristics and comparison to natural killer (NK) cells. In: Natural Cell-Mediated Immunity against Tumors, ed. R.B. Herberman, pp. 187–229. Academic Press; New York.

Stutman, O., Figarella, E.F., and Wisun, R. 1980c. Natural cytotoxic (NC) cells in tumor-bearing mice. In: Natural Cell-Mediated Immunity against Tumors, ed. R.B. Herberman, pp. 1073–79. Academic Press; New York.

Sullivan, J.L., Byron, K.S., Brewster, F.E., and Purtilo, D.T. 1980. Deficient natural killer cell activity in X-linked lymphoproliferative syndrome. Science 210:543–45.

Tagliabue, A., Mantovani, A., Kilgallen, M., Herberman, R.B., and McCoy, J.L. 1979. Natural cytotoxicity of mouse monocytes and macrophages. J Immunol 122:2363–70.

Tai, A., and Warner, N.L. 1980. Biophysical and serological characterization of murine NK cells. In: Natural Cell-Mediated Immunity against Tumors, ed. R.B. Herberman, pp. 241–55. Academic Press; New York.

Takasugi, M., Ramseyer, A., and Takasugi, J. 1977. Decline of natural nonselective cell-mediated cytotoxicity in patients with tumor progression. Cancer Res 37:413–18.

Takei, F., Levy, J.G., and Kilburn, D.G. 1976. *In vitro* induction of cytotoxicity against syngeneic mastocytoma and its suppression by spleen and thymus cells from tumor-bearing mice. J Immunol 116:288–93.

Talmadge, J.E., Meyers, K.M., Prieur, D.J., and Starkey, J.R. 1980. Role of NK cells in tumor growth and metastasis in beige mice. Nature 284:622–24.

Tam, M.R., Emmons, S.L., and Pollack, S.B. 1980. FACS analysis and enrichment of NK effector cells. In: Natural Cell-Mediated Immunity against Tumors, ed. R.B. Herberman, pp. 265–76. Academic Press; New York.

Tchernia, G., Mielot, F., and Subtil, E. 1976. Acute myeloblastic leukemia after immunodepressive therapy for primary nonmalignant disease. Blood Cells 2:67–80.

Terman, D.S. 1981. Tumoricidal responses in spontaneous canine neoplasms after extracorporeal perfusion over immobilized protein A. Fed Proc 40:45–49.

Teshima, H., Wanebo, H., Prinsky, C., and Day, N.K. 1977. Circulating immune complexes detected by I-125-C1q deviation test in sera of cancer patients. J Clin Invest 59:1134–1142.

Tewari, R.P., Balint, J.P., and Brown, K.A. 1979. Suppressive effect of 3-methylcholanthrene on phagocytic activity of mouse peritoneal macrophages for Torulopsis glabrata. J Natl Cancer Inst 62:983–90.

Theofilopoulos, A.N., and Dixon, F.J. 1979. Immune complexes associated with neoplasia. In: Immunodiagnosis of Cancer, Part 2, eds. R.B. Herberman and K.R. McIntire, pp. 896–937. Marcel Dekker; New York.

Thomas, L. 1959. Discussion. In: Cellular and Humoral Aspects of the Hypersensitive State, ed. H.S. Lawrence, pp. 529–30. Harper; New York.

Thomson, D.M.P. 1975. Soluble tumor-specific antigen and its relationship to tumor growth. Int J Cancer 15:1016–29.

Thomson, D.M.P., Tataryn, D.N., Lopez, M., Schwartz, R., and MacFarlane. 1979. Human tumor-specific immunity assayed by a computerized tube leukocyte adherence inhibition. Cancer Res 39:638–43.

Thor, D.E., Reichert, D.F., and Flippen, J.H. 1977. The interaction of chemical carcinogens and the immune response. J Reticuloendothel Soc 22:243–52.

Timonen, T., Ortaldo, J.R., Bonnard, G.D., and Herberman, R.B. 1981a. Cultures of human natural killer cells in the presence of T cell growth factor (TCGF) containing medium (CM). In: Proceedings of the 14th International Leukocyte Culture Conference. pp 286–289.

Timonen, T., Ortaldo, J.R., and Herberman, R.B. 1981b. Characteristics of human large granular lymphocytes and relationship to natural killer and K cells. J Exp Med 153:569–82.

Timonen, T., and Saksela, E. 1980. Isolation of human natural killer cells by discontinuous gradient centrifugation. J Immunol Methods 36:285–91.

Ting, A., and Terasaki, P.I. 1974. Depressed lymphocyte mediated killing of sensitized targets in cancer patients. Cancer Res 34:2694–98.

Ting, C.C., and Bonnard, G.D. 1976. Cell-mediated immunity to Friend virus-induced leukemia. IV. *In vitro* generation of primary and secondary cell-mediated cytotoxic responses. J Immunol 116:1419–25.

Ting, C.C., and Herberman, R.B. 1976. Humoral host defense mechanisms against tumors. In: International Review of Experimental Pathology, vol. 15, eds. G.W. Richter and M.A. Epstein, pp. 93–152. Academic Press; New York.

Ting. C.C., Lavrin, D.H., Takemoto, K.K., Ting, R.C., and Herberman, R.B. 1972. Expression of various tumor-specific antigens in polyoma virus-induced tumors. Cancer Res 32:1–6.

Trinchieri, G., and Santoli, D. 1978. Anti-viral activity induced by culturing lymphocytes with tumor-derived or virus-transformed cells. Enhancement of human natural killer cell activity by interferon and antagonistic inhibition of susceptibility of target cells to lysis. J Exp Med 147:1314–33.

Tursz, T., Dokhelar, M.-C., Lipinski, M., and Amiel, J.-L. 1981. Low natural killer (NK) cell activity in patients with malignant lymphoma or with a high risk of lymphoid tumors. In: NK Cells: Fundamental Aspects and Role in Cancer/Human Cancer Immunology, vol. 6, eds. B. Serrou and R.B. Herberman. Elsevier North-Holland; Amsterdam.

Vánky, F.T., Argov, S.A., Einhorn, S.A., and Klein, E. 1980. Role of alloantigens in natural killing. Allogeneic but not autologous tumor biopsy cells are sensitive for interferon-induced cytotoxicity of human blood lymphocytes. J Exp Med 151:1151–1165.

Vánky, F.T., and Stjernswa¨rd, J. 1979. Lymphocyte stimulation (by autologous tumor biopsy cells). In: Immunodiagnosis of Cancer, Part 2, eds. R.B. Herberman and K.R. McIntire, pp. 998–1032. Marcel Dekker; New York.

Varesio, L., Herberman, R.B., Gerson, J.M., and Holden, H.T. 1979. Suppression of lymphokine production by macrophages infiltrating murine virus-induced tumors. Int J Cancer 24:97–102.

Varesio, L., Holden, H.T., and Taramelli, D. 1980.

Mechanism of lymphocyte activation. II. Requirements for macromolecular synthesis in the production of lymphokines. J Immunol 125:2810–17.

Vose, B.M. 1980. Natural killers in human cancer: Activity of tumor-infiltrating and draining node lymphocytes. In: Natural Cell-Mediated Immunity against Tumors, ed. R.B. Herberman, pp. 1081–97. Academic Press; New York.

Vose, B.M., and Moore, M. 1979. Suppressor cell activity of lymphocytes infiltrating human lung and breast tumors. Int J Cancer 24:579–85.

Walpole, A.L. 1962. Observations upon the induction of subcutaneous sarcomas in rats. In: The Morphological Precursors of Cancer, ed. L. Severi, pp. 83–88. University of Perugia Division of Cancer Research; Perugia.

Weese, J.L., Herberman, R.B., Hollinshead, A.C., Cannon, G.B., Keels, M., Kibrite, A., Morales, A., Char, D.H., and Oldham, R.K. 1978. Specificity of delayed cutaneous hypersensitivity reactions to extracts of human tumor cells. J Natl Cancer Inst 60:255–63.

Welsh, R.M., Jr., and Kiessling, R.W. 1980. Natural killer cell response to lymphocytic choriomeningitis virus in beige mice. Scand J Immunol 11:363–367.

West, W.H., Cannon, G.B., Kay, H.D., Bonnard, G.D., and Herberman, R.B. 1977. Natural cytotoxic reactivity of human lymphocytes against a myeloid cell line: Characterization of effector cells. J Immunol 118:355–61.

Wood, G.W., and Gillespie, G.Y. 1973. Studies on the role of macrophages in regulation of growth and metastases of murine chemically induced fibrosarcomas. Int J Cancer 16:1022–29.

Wright, P.W., Hellström, K.E., and Hellström, I. 1976. Serotherapy of malignant disease. Med Clin N Amer 60:607–30.

Young, W.W., Jr., Hakomori, S.-I., Durdik, J.M., and Henney, C.S. 1980. Identification of ganglio-N-tetrasylceramide as a new cell surface marker for murine natural killer (NK) cells. J Immunol 124:199–201.

Yunis, E.J., Martinez, C., Smith, J., Stutman, O., and Good, R.A. 1969. Spontaneous mammary adenocarcinoma in mice: Influence of thymectomy and reconstitution with thymus grafts or spleen cells. Cancer Res 29:174–78.

Zarling, J.M., Eskra, L., Borden, E.C., Horoszewicz, J., and Carter, W.A. 1979. Activation of human natural killer cells cytotoxic for human leukemia cells by purified interferon. J Immunol 123:63–70.

Zarling, J.M., and Kung, P.C. 1980. Monoclonal antibodies which distinguish between human NK cells and cytotoxic T lymphocytes. Nature 288:394–96.

Zwilling, B.S., Filippi, J.A., and Chorpenning, F.W. 1978. Chemical carcinogenesis and immunity: Immunologic studies of rats treated with methylnitrosourea. J Natl Cancer Inst 61:731–38.

Index